Reactive Sulfur Species in Biology and Medicine

Reactive Sulfur Species in Biology and Medicine

Editors

John P. Toscano
Vinayak S. Khodade

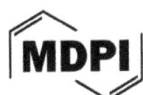

Basel • Beijing • Wuhan • Barcelona • Belgrade • Novi Sad • Cluj • Manchester

Editors
John P. Toscano
Department of Chemistry
Johns Hopkins University
Baltimore, USA

Vinayak S. Khodade
Department of Chemistry
Johns Hopkins University
Baltimore, USA

Editorial Office
MDPI
St. Alban-Anlage 66
4052 Basel, Switzerland

This is a reprint of articles from the Special Issue published online in the open access journal *Antioxidants* (ISSN 2076-3921) (available at: https://www.mdpi.com/journal/antioxidants/special_issues/reactive_sulfur_species_medicine).

For citation purposes, cite each article independently as indicated on the article page online and as indicated below:

Lastname, A.A.; Lastname, B.B. Article Title. *Journal Name* **Year**, *Volume Number*, Page Range.

ISBN 978-3-0365-9120-9 (Hbk)
ISBN 978-3-0365-9121-6 (PDF)
doi.org/10.3390/books978-3-0365-9121-6

© 2023 by the authors. Articles in this book are Open Access and distributed under the Creative Commons Attribution (CC BY) license. The book as a whole is distributed by MDPI under the terms and conditions of the Creative Commons Attribution-NonCommercial-NoDerivs (CC BY-NC-ND) license.

Contents

About the Editors . . . . **vii**

Vinayak S. Khodade and John P. Toscano
Reactive Sulfur Species in Biology and Medicine
Reprinted from: *Antioxidants* 2023, 12, 1759, doi:10.3390/antiox12091759 1

You-Lin Tain, Chih-Yao Hou, Guo-Ping Chang-Chien, Sufan Lin and Chien-Ning Hsu
Protection by Means of Perinatal Oral Sodium Thiosulfate Administration against Offspring Hypertension in a Rat Model of Maternal Chronic Kidney Disease
Reprinted from: *Antioxidants* 2023, 12, 1344, doi:10.3390/antiox12071344 7

Eleni A. Kisty, Emma C. Saart and Eranthie Weerapana
Identifying Redox-Sensitive Cysteine Residues in Mitochondria
Reprinted from: *Antioxidants* 2023, 12, 992, doi:10.3390/antiox12050992 21

Qamarul Hafiz Zainol Abidin, Tomoaki Ida, Masanobu Morita, Tetsuro Matsunaga, Akira Nishimura, Minkyung Jung, et al.
Synthesis of Sulfides and Persulfides Is Not Impeded by Disruption of Three Canonical Enzymes in Sulfur Metabolism
Reprinted from: *Antioxidants* 2023, 12, 868, doi:10.3390/antiox12040868 37

Daniela Claudia Maresca, Lia Conte, Benedetta Romano, Angela Ianaro and Giuseppe Ercolano
Antiproliferative and Proapoptotic Effects of Erucin, a Diet-Derived H_2S Donor, on Human Melanoma Cells
Reprinted from: *Antioxidants* 2023, 12, 41, doi:10.3390/antiox12010041 51

Mariko Ezaka, Eizo Marutani, Yusuke Miyazaki, Eiki Kanemaru, Martin K. Selig, Sophie L. Boerboom, et al.
Oral Administration of Glutathione Trisulfide Increases Reactive Sulfur Levels in Dorsal Root Ganglion and Ameliorates Paclitaxel-Induced Peripheral Neuropathy in Mice
Reprinted from: *Antioxidants* 2022, 11, 2122, doi:10.3390/antiox11112122 67

Brenna J. C. Walsh, Sofia Soares Costa, Katherine A. Edmonds, Jonathan C. Trinidad, Federico M. Issoglio, José A. Brito and David P. Giedroc
Metabolic and Structural Insights into Hydrogen Sulfide Mis-Regulation in *Enterococcus faecalis*
Reprinted from: *Antioxidants* 2022, 11, 1607, doi:10.3390/antiox11081607 87

Bindu D. Paul and Andrew A. Pieper
Protective Roles of Hydrogen Sulfide in Alzheimer's Disease and Traumatic Brain Injury
Reprinted from: *Antioxidants* 2023, 12, 1095, doi:10.3390/antiox12051095 111

Qiwei Hu and John C. Lukesh III
H_2S Donors with Cytoprotective Effects in Models of MI/R Injury and Chemotherapy-Induced Cardiotoxicity
Reprinted from: *Antioxidants* 2023, 12, 650, doi:10.3390/antiox12030650 131

Biswajit Roy, Meg Shieh, Geat Ramush and Ming Xian
Organelle-Targeted Fluorescent Probes for Sulfane Sulfur Species
Reprinted from: *Antioxidants* 2023, 12, 590, doi:10.3390/antiox12030590 157

Jianyun Liu, Fikir M. Mesfin, Chelsea E. Hunter, Kenneth R. Olson, W. Christopher Shelley, John P. Brokaw, et al.
Recent Development of the Molecular and Cellular Mechanisms of Hydrogen Sulfide Gasotransmitter
Reprinted from: *Antioxidants* **2022**, *11*, 1788, doi:10.3390/antiox11091788 . . . . **173**

Miriam M. Cortese-Krott
The Reactive Species Interactome in Red Blood Cells: Oxidants, Antioxidants, and Molecular Targets
Reprinted from: *Antioxidants* **2023**, *12*, 1736, doi:10.3390/antiox12091736 . . . . **191**

About the Editors

John P. Toscano

Dr. John P. Toscano received his bachelor's degree in chemistry from Princeton University and completed his doctoral studies in organic chemistry at Yale University. Following a National Institutes of Health postdoctoral fellowship at Ohio State University, he started his independent research career in the Department of Chemistry at Johns Hopkins University in 1995 and was promoted to full Professor in 2003. During his time at Hopkins, he has taken on several leadership roles, including as department chair, vice dean for natural sciences, and interim dean of the school of arts and sciences. His research has focused on the fundamental chemistry and biology of small-molecule bioactive signaling agents, with a particular focus on reactive nitrogen and reactive sulfur species, including, most recently, nitroxyl (HNO), hydrogen sulfide (H_2S), and related hydropersulfides (RSSH), especially with respect to exploring their cardioprotective properties.

Vinayak S. Khodade

Vinayak S. Khodade earned his Bachelor of Science degree in 2008, followed by a Master of Science degree in 2010, both from Savitribai Phule University, Pune. In 2016, he successfully completed his doctoral studies at the Indian Institute of Science Education and Research (IISER), Pune. While conducting his doctoral research, he specialized in the development of small molecules capable of generating redox signaling molecules and employed them for studying and targeting antibiotic resistance. Currently, he holds the position of Assistant Research Scientist at Johns Hopkins University, where he works with Professor John P. Toscano. His research is primarily centered on designing innovative precursors to hydropersulfides (RSSH) with a focus on uncovering their fundamental chemical properties and exploring their therapeutic potential in addressing various pathological conditions.

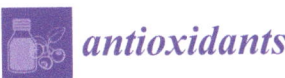

Editorial
Reactive Sulfur Species in Biology and Medicine

Vinayak S. Khodade * and John P. Toscano *

Department of Chemistry, Johns Hopkins University, Baltimore, MD 21218, USA
* Correspondence: vkhodad1@jhu.edu (V.S.K.); jtoscano@jhu.edu (J.P.T.)

Hydrogen sulfide (H_2S) has emerged as a third small-molecule bioactive signaling agent, along with nitric oxide (NO) and carbon monoxide (CO). It regulates diverse physiological processes such as cell differentiation, development, and immune responses. H_2S is produced mainly by cystathionine-β-synthase (CBS), cystathionine-γ-lyase (CSE), and 3-mercapto-sulfurtransferase (3-MST) in mammals. Despite being highly toxic at elevated concentrations, emerging evidence highlights a distinct cytoprotective role of endogenously produced H_2S, and intensive studies have focused on its potential as a therapeutic agent for cardiovascular, inflammatory, infectious, and neuropathological diseases. Furthermore, emerging evidence shows that many biological effects initially ascribed to H_2S may instead be due to other reactive sulfur species (RSS), including hydropersulfides (RSSH) and other higher-order polysulfur species (RSS_nH, RSS_nR, HS_nH, n > 1). Importantly, these RSS are highly prevalent in biological systems. RSS have intriguing biochemical properties, such as the ability to modify protein cysteine residues and efficiently scavenge reactive oxygen species and electrophiles. Moreover, RSS donors have begun to demonstrate therapeutic potential in treating a range of maladies, including cancer, neurological disorders, and cardiovascular disease. Nonetheless, the chemistry of RSS is complicated due to their reactive nature, and their accurate measurement in biological systems remains a challenge. This Special Issue focuses on studies that highlight recent advances in H_2S/RSS chemical biology, including six original research articles and five reviews aimed at exploring the therapeutic applications of H_2S/RSS donors, understanding the molecular mechanisms and physiological roles of RSS, and methods that measure the concentration and distribution of RSS in biological systems.

Paul and Pieper summarize the latest discoveries regarding the neuroprotective function of H_2S in Alzheimer's disease (AD) and traumatic brain injury (TBI) [1]. Initially, they delve into H_2S biosynthesis in the brain, followed by an exploration of its role in these major neuropsychiatric conditions characterized by cognitive impairment. The authors review the existing literature that underscores the significance of adequate H_2S signaling in modulating neuronal health and reveal how deficiencies in this signaling molecule contribute to the pathology of AD and TBI. They also highlight the mechanism of the underlying physiological effects of H_2S through the persulfidation of cysteine residues on target proteins. The authors underscore the potential of H_2S donors as therapeutic agents in alleviating symptoms associated with AD, TBI, and analogous neurodegenerative disorders characterized by compromised H_2S signaling pathways.

H_2S also plays a pivotal role in the cardiovascular system, exerting profound influence over vasodilation and blood pressure regulation. Lukesh and Hu present a comprehensive review that delves into H_2S donors with promising cardioprotective effects against myocardial ischemia-reperfusion (MI/R) injury and chemotherapy-induced cardiotoxicity, a frequent and often lethal complication of chemotherapy [2]. They provide a systematic categorization of donors based on mechanisms triggering H_2S release, encompassing hydrolysis, pH, thiol, enzyme, and ROS. A detailed explanation of the H_2S-releasing mechanism for each donor is provided, along with an overview of their therapeutic effects across various models of MI/R injury. The potential benefits of H_2S and H_2S-conjugated codrugs in mitigating anthracycline-induced cardiotoxicity are also discussed.

Citation: Khodade, V.S.; Toscano, J.P. Reactive Sulfur Species in Biology and Medicine. *Antioxidants* **2023**, *12*, 1759. https://doi.org/10.3390/antiox12091759

Received: 11 September 2023
Accepted: 11 September 2023
Published: 13 September 2023

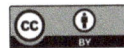

Copyright: © 2023 by the authors. Licensee MDPI, Basel, Switzerland. This article is an open access article distributed under the terms and conditions of the Creative Commons Attribution (CC BY) license (https://creativecommons.org/licenses/by/4.0/).

Recent research has indicated the potential benefits of H_2S in alleviating hypertension. In this context, Hsu and colleagues present their study that investigates the protective effects of sodium thiosulfate (STS) in a rat model of hypertension induced by maternal chronic kidney disease (CKD) [3]. Thiosulfate, a member of the sulfane sulfur family, is known to undergo enzymatic reduction to generate H_2S. The researchers induced CKD in rats by exposing them to a diet enriched with 0.5% adenine for three weeks prior to mating. Subsequently, pregnant rats received sodium thiosulfate (2 g/kg/day) during both gestation and lactation. The study demonstrated that administering STS effectively counteracted the development of hypertension in the offspring. Employing HPLC–mass spectrometry, the investigators observed significant increases in the plasma H_2S concentrations and renal tissue levels of the 3MST protein in the CKD offspring. The authors suggest that the positive effects of STS treatment can be attributed, at least in part, to enhancements in the signaling pathways of H_2S and NO. Furthermore, the researchers delved into the impact of STS on the composition of gut microbiota. A particularly intriguing finding was that maternal CKD led to a reduction in the population of the *Enterococcus* genus, coupled with an elevation in the abundance of *Erysipelatoclostridium* and *Dorea* genera. Conversely, administering maternal rats with STS resulted in higher proportions of the *Dorea*, *Streptococcus*, and *Anaerotruncus* genera. Importantly, the favorable impact of STS on offspring hypertension correlated with an increase in beneficial microbial species. Thus, this study underscores the potential efficacy of early-life STS intervention in mitigating hypertension among offspring born to mothers with CKD.

H_2S-releasing compounds have also emerged as potential therapeutics for various types of cancers. Ianaro, Ercolano, and co-workers examine the effects of erucin (ERU), a compound derived from the dietary source, on human melanoma cell lines [4]. ERU was found to exert a significant inhibitory effect on human melanoma cell lines. Notably, ERU was shown to induce apoptosis in A375 melanoma cells. Expanding on ERU's proapoptotic attributes, the researchers delved into its effect on cadherins and transcription factors central to the epithelial-to-mesenchymal transition (EMT) process, a critical event in cancer progression. They demonstrated that ERU significantly enhances the expression of the epithelial protein E-CAD while reducing the expression of the mesenchymal protein N-CAD. Beyond its effects on apoptosis and cell cycle regulation, ERU exhibited remarkable inhibition of A375 melanoma cell migration, invasiveness, and clonogenic potential. Intriguingly, ERU also demonstrated the ability to diminish melanin levels and downregulate genes associated with melanogenesis, hinting at its potential to interfere with melanoma-specific pathways. An intriguing facet of ERU's mechanism was its capacity to attenuate the generation of intracellular ROS in A375 cells.

Beyond its presence in mammals, H_2S is also produced by bacteria. Recent studies have demonstrated its pivotal role in bacterial physiology, particularly in bacterial responses toward host-induced stressors like ROS and antibiotics during infections. Recent studies, however, suggest that the physiological benefits of H_2S are likely attributed to its downstream sulfur derivatives, i.e., RSS. Brito, Giedroc, and co-workers present their investigation of H_2S/RSS homeostasis in the microbial pathogen *Enterococcus faecalis*, probing the pathophysiological response of elevated H_2S levels [5]. Employing proteomic analysis, they demonstrated a notable increase in the cellular abundance of enzymes reliant on coenzyme A (CoA) and acyl-CoA. They also examined protein persulfidation, revealing that approximately 13% of the proteome undergoes persulfidation and is significantly augmented by exogenous sulfide introduction. Prominent among the proteins persulfidated were CstR, a sensor for RSS, and CoAPR, an enzyme intricately associated with the reduction of coenzyme A persulfide (CoASSH). Furthermore, they demonstrated the impact of exogenous sulfide on the speciation of fatty acid composition and cellular acetyl-CoA concentrations. Collectively, these insights augment our understanding of the intricate interplay encompassing H_2S/RSS signaling, protein persulfidation, and the metabolic pathways governed by coenzyme A and acyl-CoA in *Enterococcus faecalis*.

The molecular mechanisms underlying the physiological effects of H_2S are complex and remain an active area of research. Markel and colleagues present a review that delves into the molecular and cellular mechanisms of H_2S within mammalian systems [6]. In their exploration of potential direct targets, the authors focus on H_2S interactions with reactive oxygen/nitrogen species, which is critical in redox signaling. Furthermore, H_2S interaction with hemeproteins and its role in modulating metal ions containing complexes are highlighted. The post-translational modification of cysteine residue in proteins via oxidized derivative of H_2S, i.e., persulfidation, is emphasized. The H_2S-mediated significant impact on cell structure and many cellular functions, such as tight junctions, autophagy, apoptosis, vesicle trafficking, cell signaling, epigenetics, and inflammasomes is discussed. Importantly, the authors also indicate that several biological effects initially ascribed to H_2S might instead be attributed to other RSS. In recent years, RSS has remained an active area of research with a focus on their biosynthetic pathways and physiological functions.

Recently, Akaike and colleagues have revealed that cysteinyl-tRNA synthetase (CARS) functions as a cysteine hydropersulfide synthase (CPERS), which is primarily responsible for generating RSSH in biological systems. However, some researchers have proposed that H_2S-producing enzymes 3-MST, CBS, and CSE also contribute to RSSH production. To determine hydropersulfide biosynthesis, Tsutsui, Akaike, and co-workers conducted research to elucidate the relative contributions of these enzymes to cysteine hydropersulfide biosynthesis [7]. They initiated their investigation by creating 3-MST knockout mice, which surprisingly exhibited no statistically significant differences in RSSH production when compared to wild-type mice. Then, they generated triple-knockout mice lacking the CBS, CSE, and 3-MST genes by crossbreeding them with single-knockout mice of each of these enzymes. Using LC–MS/MS analysis, they quantified levels of CysSSH and GSSH in various tissues and plasma from both the triple-knockout and control mice. Remarkably, the absence of CBS, CSE, and 3-MST genes did not appear to hinder RSSH synthesis. The researchers also turned their attention to CARS2-deficient heterozygous mice ($Cars2^{+/-}$) mice and found significantly reduced levels of CysSSH, GSSH, and related compounds in liver and lung tissues of these mice compared to their wild-type counterparts, pointing to the reliance on CARS2 for the synthesis of RSSH and sulfide derivatives in mouse tissues. Western blot assays conducted on tissues from $Cars2^{+/-}$ mice indicated unchanged protein expression levels of 3-MST, CBS, and CSE between wild-type and CARS2-deficient mice, suggesting the absence of compensatory upregulation in the expression of these canonical enzymes. Thus, this study highlights the critical role of CARS as the primary enzyme responsible for biosynthesizing RSSH. The findings provide substantial evidence regarding the relative involvement of various enzymes in RSSH production, clarifying the complex landscape of sulfur metabolism in biological systems.

In the last decade, RSS donors have been tested for their therapeutic potential across a spectrum of disorders, including cancer, neurological disorders, and cardiovascular disease. Ichinose and co-workers present a study examining the potential neuroprotective effects of glutathione trisulfide (GSSSG) within a murine model of paclitaxel-induced peripheral neuropathy (PIPN) [8]. These researchers showed that oral administration of GSSSG at 50 mg/kg/day over 28 days effectively mitigates the mechanical allodynia induced by PIPN. Through liquid chromatography coupled with tandem mass spectrometry analysis, the study demonstrated the presence of ^{34}S-labeled GSSSG within the lumbar dorsal root ganglia (DRG) and lumbar spinal cord for two hours following oral administration. Additionally, the researchers showcased several pivotal outcomes in paclitaxel-treated mice following GSSSG administration. These included the upregulation of antioxidant gene expression in the lumbar DRG, the preservation of unmyelinated axons, and the attenuation of sciatic nerve mitochondria degeneration. Moreover, GSSSG effectively counteracted paclitaxel-induced superoxide generation, mitigated the loss of axonal mitochondria, and attenuated axonal degeneration in primary neurons derived from both the cortex and DRG. These collective findings strongly suggest that the oral administration of GSSSG effectively counters PIPN by safeguarding peripheral sensory nerve axons and maintaining the structural integrity of mitochondria.

Within the domain of redox biology, biological sulfane sulfur (S^0) species, including RSSH, RSS$_n$SR, H$_2$S$_n$, $n \geq 2$, and protein-bound elemental sulfur (S_8), have emerged as pivotal RSS. Despite their important roles in redox signaling, the exploration of sulfane sulfur species remains difficult, given their inherent instability and low concentrations in biological systems. Xian and co-workers present a review article that delves into organelle-targeted fluorescent probes for sulfane sulfur species [9]. The scope of the review encompasses a variety of probes designed for distinct organelles, including mitochondria, endoplasmic reticulum, and lysosomes. The strategies employed to direct these probes to specific cellular locales are thoroughly examined. An overview of organelle-targeted sulfane sulfur probes is presented, encompassing their underlying mechanisms, capacity for colocalization, sensitivities, and efficacy in detecting endogenous and exogenous sulfane sulfur under physiological circumstances. The authors highlight a predominant focus on mitochondria among the organelle-targeted probes, with relatively limited attention directed toward lysosomes and the endoplasmic reticulum. The authors further identify a significant gap in the availability of sulfane sulfur probes for additional organelles, such as the Golgi apparatus and nucleus, thereby proposing directions for future research.

Beyond the modification of cysteine residues on proteins through interactions with sulfane sulfur species, ROS also mediate the oxidative post-translational modifications of cysteines that are pivotal in cell signaling. Notably, ROS-mediated cell signaling is particularly prominent within mitochondria, given that ROS constitute natural byproducts of cellular respiration. While various sites of cysteine oxidation on mitochondrial proteins have been identified, a notable interest in identifying uncharacterized redox-sensitive cysteines persists. In a contribution by Weerapana and colleagues, an approach combining mitochondrial enrichment with redox proteomic methodologies was employed to identify the cysteines sensitive to redox alterations by ROS [10]. They utilized an isotopic tandem orthogonal proteolysis-activity-based protein profiling (isoTOP-ABPP) platform for the indirect identification of oxidation sites by tracking the loss of cysteine reactivity. Additionally, the oxidative isotopically coded affinity tag (OxICAT) platform was employed to monitor reversible cysteine oxidation through differential labeling. Within the isoTOP-ABPP framework, mitochondrial cysteines were systematically evaluated for their responsiveness to hydrogen peroxide exposure. The outcomes revealed a set of approximately 700 mitochondrial cysteines exhibiting varying degrees of susceptibility to peroxide-triggered oxidation. These cysteines were effectively classified into categories of low, moderate, and high sensitivity, revealing distinct patterns of reactivity. Furthermore, the study explored the spatial distribution of redox-sensitive cysteines within crucial mitochondrial pathways. Particularly, the tricarboxylic acid (TCA) cycle and proteins involved in mitochondrial transcription and translation were noted for harboring noteworthy concentrations of highly redox sensitive cysteines.

Emerging evidence suggests that reactive species generated from the metabolism of oxygen, NO, and H$_2$S have the potential to interact with each other. This interaction, in turn, has the capacity to influence shared biological targets. These complex interplays are termed the "reactive species interactome". Cortese-Krott presents a review article that examines the reactive species interactome, specifically focusing on its relevance to the intricate landscape of redox biology in red blood cells (RBCs) [11]. The review investigates multiple facets, including the generation and detoxification of reactive species, their interactions, and their ultimate molecular targets. It is also noted that future research endeavors should be directed towards unraveling how modulation of the reactive species interactome intricately regulates the biology, physiology, and systemic repercussions of RBCs.

In summary, this Special Issue compiles original research articles as well as review articles that collectively illuminate the rich significance of H$_2$S and RSS within biological systems. These reports serve not only as a testament to the current state of research, but also as a catalyst for the further exploration of important, unanswered questions.

Author Contributions: Writing, review, and editing—V.S.K. and J.P.T. All authors have read and agreed to the published version of the manuscript.

Acknowledgments: We would like to thank all contributors for their submissions to this Special Issue, and the reviewers for their valuable input in improving the articles. We also thank the Editorial Office for their helpful support during the compilation of this Special Issue.

Conflicts of Interest: The authors declare no conflict of interest.

References

1. Paul, B.D.; Pieper, A.A. Protective Roles of Hydrogen Sulfide in Alzheimer's Disease and Traumatic Brain Injury. *Antioxidants* **2023**, *12*, 1095. [CrossRef] [PubMed]
2. Hu, Q.; Lukesh, J.C. H_2S Donors with Cytoprotective Effects in Models of MI/R Injury and Chemotherapy-Induced Cardiotoxicity. *Antioxidants* **2023**, *12*, 650. [CrossRef]
3. Tain, Y.-L.; Hou, C.-Y.; Chang-Chien, G.-P.; Lin, S.; Hsu, C.-N. Protection by Means of Perinatal Oral Sodium Thiosulfate Administration against Offspring Hypertension in a Rat Model of Maternal Chronic Kidney Disease. *Antioxidants* **2023**, *12*, 1344. [CrossRef] [PubMed]
4. Maresca, D.C.; Conte, L.; Romano, B.; Ianaro, A.; Ercolano, G. Antiproliferative and Proapoptotic Effects of Erucin, a Diet-Derived H2S Donor, on Human Melanoma Cells. *Antioxidants* **2023**, *12*, 41. [CrossRef] [PubMed]
5. Walsh, B.J.C.; Costa, S.S.; Edmonds, K.A.; Trinidad, J.C.; Issoglio, F.M.; Brito, J.A.; Giedroc, D.P. Metabolic and Structural Insights into Hydrogen Sulfide Mis-Regulation in Enterococcus faecalis. *Antioxidants* **2022**, *11*, 1607. [CrossRef] [PubMed]
6. Liu, J.; Mesfin, F.M.; Hunter, C.E.; Olson, K.R.; Shelley, W.C.; Brokaw, J.P.; Manohar, K.; Markel, T.A. Recent Development of the Molecular and Cellular Mechanisms of Hydrogen Sulfide Gasotransmitter. *Antioxidants* **2022**, *11*, 1788. [CrossRef] [PubMed]
7. Zainol Abidin, Q.H.; Ida, T.; Morita, M.; Matsunaga, T.; Nishimura, A.; Jung, M.; Hassan, N.; Takata, T.; Ishii, I.; Kruger, W.; et al. Synthesis of Sulfides and Persulfides Is Not Impeded by Disruption of Three Canonical Enzymes in Sulfur Metabolism. *Antioxidants* **2023**, *12*, 868. [CrossRef] [PubMed]
8. Ezaka, M.; Marutani, E.; Miyazaki, Y.; Kanemaru, E.; Selig, M.K.; Boerboom, S.L.; Ostrom, K.F.; Stemmer-Rachamimov, A.; Bloch, D.B.; Brenner, G.J.; et al. Oral Administration of Glutathione Trisulfide Increases Reactive Sulfur Levels in Dorsal Root Ganglion and Ameliorates Paclitaxel-Induced Peripheral Neuropathy in Mice. *Antioxidants* **2022**, *11*, 2122. [CrossRef] [PubMed]
9. Roy, B.; Shieh, M.; Ramush, G.; Xian, M. Organelle-Targeted Fluorescent Probes for Sulfane Sulfur Species. *Antioxidants* **2023**, *12*, 590. [CrossRef] [PubMed]
10. Kisty, E.A.; Saart, E.C.; Weerapana, E. Identifying Redox-Sensitive Cysteine Residues in Mitochondria. *Antioxidants* **2023**, *12*, 992. [CrossRef] [PubMed]
11. Cortese-Krott, M.M. The Reactive Species Interactome in Red Blood Cells: Oxidants, Antioxidants, and Molecular Targets. *Antioxidants* **2023**, *12*, 1736. [CrossRef]

Disclaimer/Publisher's Note: The statements, opinions and data contained in all publications are solely those of the individual author(s) and contributor(s) and not of MDPI and/or the editor(s). MDPI and/or the editor(s) disclaim responsibility for any injury to people or property resulting from any ideas, methods, instructions or products referred to in the content.

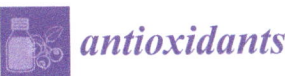

Article

Protection by Means of Perinatal Oral Sodium Thiosulfate Administration against Offspring Hypertension in a Rat Model of Maternal Chronic Kidney Disease

You-Lin Tain [1,2,3], Chih-Yao Hou [4], Guo-Ping Chang-Chien [5,6,7], Sufan Lin [5,6,7] and Chien-Ning Hsu [8,9,*]

1. Department of Pediatrics, Kaohsiung Chang Gung Memorial Hospital, Kaohsiung 833, Taiwan; tainyl@cgmh.org.tw
2. Institute for Translational Research in Biomedicine, Kaohsiung Chang Gung Memorial Hospital, Kaohsiung 833, Taiwan
3. College of Medicine, Chang Gung University, Taoyuan 330, Taiwan
4. Department of Seafood Science, National Kaohsiung University of Science and Technology, Kaohsiung 811, Taiwan; chihyaohou@webmail.nkmu.edu.tw
5. Center for Environmental Toxin and Emerging-Contaminant Research, Cheng Shiu University, Kaohsiung 833, Taiwan; guoping@csu.edu.tw (G.-P.C.-C.)
6. Institute of Environmental Toxin and Emerging-Contaminant, Cheng Shiu University, Kaohsiung 833, Taiwan
7. Super Micro Mass Research and Technology Center, Cheng Shiu University, Kaohsiung 833, Taiwan
8. Department of Pharmacy, Kaohsiung Chang Gung Memorial Hospital, Kaohsiung 833, Taiwan
9. School of Pharmacy, Kaohsiung Medical University, Kaohsiung 807, Taiwan
* Correspondence: cnhsu@cgmh.org.tw; Tel.: +886-975-368-975

Abstract: Hydrogen sulfide (H_2S) and related reactive sulfur species are implicated in chronic kidney disease (CKD) and hypertension. Offspring born to CKD-afflicted mothers could develop hypertension coinciding with disrupted H_2S and nitric oxide (NO) signaling pathways as well as gut microbiota. Thiosulfate, a precursor of H_2S and an antioxidant, has shown anti-hypertensive effects. This study aimed to investigate the protective effects of sodium thiosulfate (STS) in a rat model of maternal CKD-induced hypertension. Before mating, CKD was induced through feeding 0.5% adenine chow for 3 weeks. Mother rats were given a vehicle or STS at a dosage of 2 g/kg/day in drinking water throughout gestation and lactation. Perinatal STS treatment protected 12-week-old offspring from maternal CKD-primed hypertension. The beneficial effects of STS could partially be explained by the enhancement of both H_2S and NO signaling pathways and alterations in gut microbiota. Not only increasing beneficial microbes but maternal STS treatment also mediates several hypertension-associated intestinal bacteria. In conclusion, perinatal treatment with STS improves maternal CKD-primed offspring hypertension, suggesting that early-life RSS-targeting interventions have potential preventive and therapeutic benefits, awaiting future translational research.

Keywords: thiosulfate; hydrogen sulfide; asymmetric dimethylarginine; gut microbiota; hypertension; chronic kidney disease; developmental origins of health and disease (DOHaD)

1. Introduction

Reactive sulfur species (RSS) have emerged as important molecules in redox regulation and have significant roles in health and disease [1,2]. Various biochemical forms of RSS are closely linked biochemically, including hydrogen sulfide (H_2S), iron–sulfur clusters, sulfane sulfur, etc. [3].

The production of H_2S can occur via three pathways—enzymatic, non-enzymatic, and bacterial origins. H_2S is synthesized from L-cysteine via three enzymes, which are cystathionine γ-lyase (CSE), cystathionine β-synthase (CBS), and 3-mercaptopyruvate sulfurtransferase (3MST) [4]. H_2S can also be produced in the gastrointestinal tract by sulfate- reducing bacteria (SRB), which use reduced compounds as a source of energy, reducing sulfate to H_2S [5]. Additionally, non-enzymatic H_2S production occurs through sulfane sulfur.

Thiosulfate, belonging to the sulfane sulfur family, is a major oxidation product of H_2S. On the other hand, thiosulfate can be reduced to recreate H_2S. Thiosulfate has been clinically used in the form of sodium thiosulfate (STS). Its indications include calciphylaxis, carbon monoxide toxicity, acute cyanide poisoning, and cisplatin toxicities [4]. In addition to being an H_2S donor, STS has antioxidant and anti-inflammatory properties. Accordingly, STS has become a potential treatment candidate for several diseases [6].

An estimated 10% of people have chronic kidney disease (CKD) [7]. As CKD can originate in early life through so-called renal programming [8], a superior strategy to improve kidney health worldwide is to avert, not just treat, kidney disease. CKD is reported to influence up to 3–4% of women of reproductive age [9]. Maternal CKD is intimately tied to adverse outcomes of pregnancy and the health of the offspring [10]. Previously, we observed that adult rats born from dams with CKD develop hypertension, which perinatal L-cysteine supplementation prevented [11]. The beneficial actions of cysteine are accompanied by a restoration of H_2S signaling, a reduction of oxidative stress, and the alteration of gut microbiota composition [11].

As an H_2S donor as well as an antioxidant, STS treatment has revealed benefits against kidney disease and hypertension in several animal models [12–14]. Given this background, we hypothesize that STS treatment during gestation and lactation can prevent offspring hypertension induced by maternal CKD. The protective mechanisms of maternal STS treatment were also evaluated.

2. Materials and Methods

2.1. Animal Experiments

All animal experiments were conducted with approval from the Institutional Animal Ethics Committee at our hospital (Permit #2020110202); the procedures were consistent with the recommendations of the Care and Use of Laboratory Animals of the National Institutes of Health and following Animal Research: Reporting of In Vivo Experiments (ARRIVE) guidelines. Timed-pregnant Sprague Dawley (SD) rats were obtained from BioLASCO Taiwan Co. Ltd. (Taipei, Taiwan) for breeding. Upon arrival at our AAALAC-accredited animal facility, rats were housed individually in cages provided with standard laboratory chow and tap water ad libitum.

We used an established model of maternal CKD consisting of feeding with chow containing 0.5% adenine protein to the dam for three weeks before gestation as previously described [15]. At 11 weeks old, female rats were mated. The day of copulatory plug detection was designated as gestational day 0. We randomly divided the dams into one of four treatments (n = 3 per group): a normal diet (ND), a diet containing 0.5% adenine (CKD), a normal diet with STS (NDST), and a diet containing 0.5% adenine with STS (CKDST). STS was orally administered in drinking water at a dosage of 2 g/kg/day during gestation and lactation. The dosage and route chosen rely on previous studies in rats [13,14]. Following parturition, litters from each dam were culled to eight pups to maintain consistency in pup growth. As males are more likely to be hypertensive than females [16], only male offspring were included in the experiment.

BP was determined using the CODA rat tail-cuff system (Kent Scientific Corporation, Torrington, CT, USA) in offspring over time at ages ranging from 3 to 12 weeks. To ensure accuracy and reproducibility, the rats were acclimated to restraint and tail-cuff inflation for one week before the measurement. For each rat, five measurements were recorded at each time point. Three stable consecutive measures were taken and averaged [14]. A total of 32 rats (n = 8 per group) were sacrificed at 12 weeks of age. Before sacrifice, fresh fecal samples were collected in the morning and stored at $-80\ °C$. Rats were anesthetized using an intraperitoneal injection of xylazine (10 mg/kg) and ketamine (50 mg/kg), then euthanized with an intraperitoneal overdose of pentobarbital. Kidneys were removed, and the cortex and inner medulla were then dissected and snap-frozen in liquid nitrogen. Kidney samples were stored at −80 °C. Blood samples were collected using heparin tubes.

2.2. NO Parameters

Several biochemical parameters of the NO pathway were determined via Agilent 1100 HPLC (Santa Clara, CA, USA) with the OPA-3MPA derivatization reagent [14]. Plasma concentrations of L-arginine and symmetric and asymmetric dimethylarginine (SDMA and ADMA, inhibitors of NO synthase) were analyzed in duplicate. The L-arginine-to-ADMA ratio was calculated to denote NO bioavailability [17].

2.3. Plasma H_2S and Thiosulfate

We used a validated method using HPLC–Mass Spectrometry to measure H_2S and thiosulfate, as described previously [11]. The HPLC system (Agilent Technologies 1290) was coupled to an Agilent 6470 Triple Quadrupole LC/MS and an electrospray ionization source. The solvent system consisted of water and acetonitrile with 0.1% formic acid and an eluent flow rate of 300 µL/min was used. We measured thiosulfate derivative pentafluorobenzyl (PFB)-S_2O_3H and H_2S derivative sulfide dibimane (SDB). Phenyl 4-hydroxybenzoate (PHB) was utilized as an internal standard. Selected reaction monitoring mode was utilized to detect target compounds with a targeted m/z 212.99 → 93, m/z 415 → 223, and m/z 292.99 → 81, for PHB, SDB, and PFB-S_2O_3H, respectively. The intra-assay variability for H_2S and thiosulfate was 4% and 6%, respectively.

2.4. H_2S-Producing Enzymes

Western blotting was performed according to our earlier report [18]. Renal cortex tissues were homogenized, and equal amounts of protein were loaded into each well (200 µg per gel well). After transferring from gel to membrane, Ponceau S staining (PonS, Sigma-Aldrich, Darmstadt, Germany) was applied as a total protein normalization method to detect all sample proteins. Antibodies used to detect H_2S-producing enzymes are listed in Table 1. Quantitative integrated optical density (IOD) analysis of the Western blot densitometry band was performed through Quantity One Analysis software version 4.6.3 (Bio-Rad, Hercules, CA, USA). The relative protein abundance was presented as the IOD/PonS to correct protein loading variations.

Table 1. List of antibodies used for Western blot.

Antigen	Clonality	Source	Dilution
CSE	Polyclonal rabbit	Proteintech Group	1:1000
CBS	Monoclonal mouse	Abnova Corporation	1:1000
3MST	Monoclonal rabbit	Novus Biologicals	1:500

CSE = cystathionine γ-lyase; CBS = cystathionine β-synthase; 3MST = 3-mercaptopyruvate sulfurtransferase.

2.5. 16S rRNA Gene Sequencing and Analysis

As we described previously, metagenomic DNA was isolated from frozen fecal samples. V1–V9 full-length 16S gene sequencing and analysis were performed at the Biotools Co., Ltd. (New Taipei City, Taiwan) [18]. PCR amplification was performed with barcoded 16S gene-specific primers for multiplexed SMRTbell library (PacBio, Menlo Park, CA, USA) preparation and sequencing procedure. The QIIME2 was applied to analyze data from high-throughput 16S rRNA sequencing [19]. From the amplicon sequence variant (ASV) sequences, a phylogenetic tree was formed via FastTree (QIIME2).

Sequencing analysis included alpha and beta diversity analysis and different taxa analysis. As alpha diversity indices, Faith's phylogenetic diversity (PD) index and Shannon index were utilized to determine the microbiota richness and evenness. Beta diversity analysis was conducted based on principal coordinate analysis (PCoA) with unweighted UniFrac distance and Analysis of Similarities (ANOSIM) for comparison of the differences in bacterial composition between groups. Linear discriminant analysis effect size (LEfSe) difference analysis was applied to find differentially abundant taxa [20].

2.6. Statistics

Quantitative data are presented as means ± the standard error of the mean (SEM). Statistical analyses were conducted with one-way ANOVA. A *p*-value less than 0.05 was considered statistically significant, and Tukey's post hoc test was applied if the *p*-value was less than 0.05. QIIME2 was performed to generate phylogenetic beta diversity, and further to perform PCoA using the R program based on unweighted Unifrac distance. LEfSe used the two-tailed nonparametric Kruskal–Wallis test to evaluate the significance of differences in ASVs in 2 groups. A set of pairwise tests among 2 groups was performed using the unpaired Wilcoxon test. Finally, linear discriminant analysis (LDA) was performed to estimate the effect size of each differentially abundant taxa. For stringency, the gut microbiotas were considered significantly different if their differences had a *p*-value < 0.05 and an LDA score (log10) > 4. Statistical analysis was carried out using SPSS (SPSS Inc., Chicago, IL, USA).

3. Results

3.1. Offspring Outcomes

We observed no difference in offspring in terms of mortality, sex ratio, or litter size between the four treatments. The offspring born to dams treated with the adenine diet or STS weighed significantly less than their control counterparts (Figure 1A). A similar pattern was observed for kidney weight (Figure 1B). However, the kidney weight to body weight ratio was lowest in the ND group compared to others (Figure 1C). The plasma concentration of creatinine was comparable between the four groups (Figure 1D). Systolic blood pressure (SBP) in offspring, measured via the tail-cuff method at different ages, is presented in Figure 1E. Maternal CKD elicited a rise in SBP during 8–12 weeks of age, which maternal STS treatment prevented. Collectively, these findings indicated that maternal CKD induced hypertension, renal hypertrophy, and low body weights in adult progeny. Maternal STS administration similarly caused renal hypertrophy and low body weights in normal control offspring but prevented maternal CKD-induced offspring hypertension.

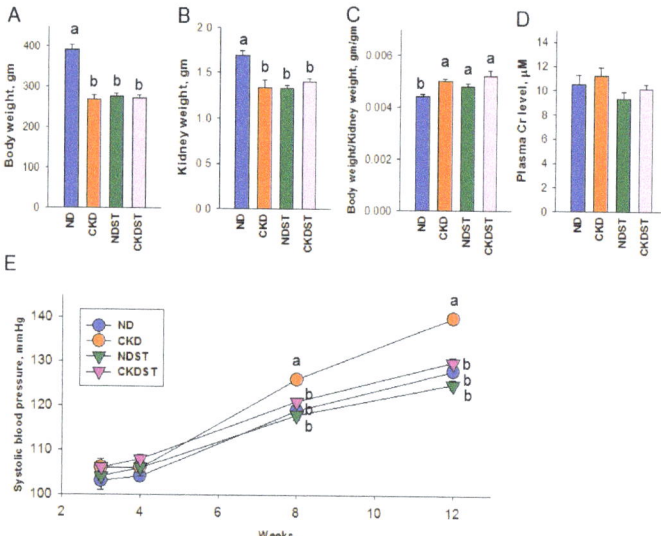

Figure 1. Offspring (**A**) body weight, (**B**) kidney weight, (**C**) body-weight-to-kidney-weight ratio, (**D**) plasma creatinine (Cr) level, and (**E**) systolic blood pressure. N = 8/group. Different letters above the column show significant differences between groups.

3.2. H$_2$S Pathway

To determine the influence of maternal CKD and STS administration on the H$_2$S pathway, we determined plasma concentrations of H$_2$S and thiosulfate and protein abundance of H$_2$S-producing enzymes in the offspring's kidneys (Figure 2).

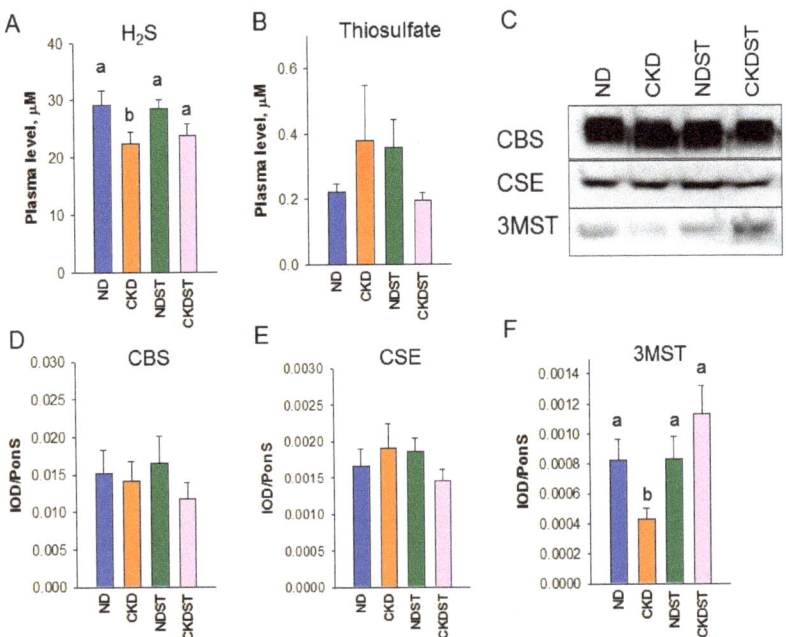

Figure 2. Plasma concentrations of (**A**) H$_2$S and (**B**) thiosulfate, and renal protein abundance of H$_2$S-producing enzymes. (**C**) Representative Western blot protein bands demonstrate immunoreactivity to CBS (61 kDa), CSE (45 kDa), and 3MST (52 kDa). Renal cortical protein abundance of (**D**) CBS, (**E**) CSE, and (**F**) 3MST was calculated. N = 8/group. Different letters above the column show significant differences between groups. CBS = cystathionine β-synthase; CSE = cystathionine γ-lyase; 3MST = 3-mercaptopyruvate sulfurtransferase.

Male offspring in the CKD group exhibited plasma H$_2$S concentration lower than controls at 12 weeks of age (Figure 2A), while plasma thiosulfate concentration was comparable among the four groups (Figure 2B). No differences were observed for renal protein levels of H$_2$S-producing enzymes CBS and CSE among the four groups (Figure 2C). Nevertheless, exposure to maternal CKD diminished renal 3MST protein abundance, which was averted via maternal STS treatment (Figure 2F). Altogether, these observations reveal that the protective actions of STS treatment are relevant to increases in plasma H$_2$S concentrations and the 3MST protein amount in the kidneys.

3.3. NO Pathway

As summarized in Figure 3, no differences in NO-related parameters were observed in terms of L-arginine and SDMA. Maternal CKD programming substantially increased plasma ADMA concentrations in adult offspring (Figure 3B). Additionally, maternal CKD reduced the L-arginine-to-ADMA ratio (AAR) in the CKD group (Figure 3D), which was prevented by means of maternal STS treatment. This observation, together with the fact that AAR represents NO bioavailability [17], suggests that STS protects adult offspring from hypertension and is possibly related to the restoration of NO.

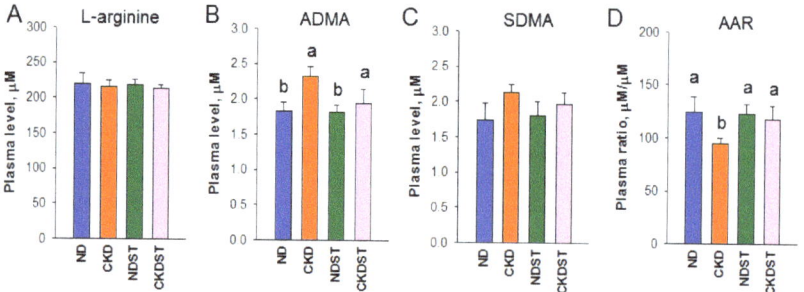

Figure 3. Plasma concentrations of nitric oxide (NO) parameters include (**A**) L-arginine, (**B**) asymmetric dimethylarginine (ADMA), (**C**) symmetric dimethylarginine (SDMA), and (**D**) L-arginine-to-ADMA ratio (AAR). N = 8/group. Different letters above the column show significant differences between groups.

3.4. Gut Microbiota Composition

Alpha diversity analysis was performed utilizing Faith's PD index (Figure 4A) and the Shannon index (Figure 4B) to determine the species richness and evenness. Alpha diversity revealed that maternal CKD and STS have a negligible effect on each group. Beta diversity analysis (Figure 4C) was carried out utilizing PCoA plots to illustrate the phylogenetic distance of the bacterial communities of the fecal samples. The beta diversity analysis revealed that four groups had distinct clustering. However, the ND group samples were further apart. Additionally, ANOSIM revealed that the four groups differ greatly from each other (All $p < 0.01$).

Consistent with prior animal studies [11,18], the major phyla are *Firmicutes* and *Bacteroidetes*, with subsequent *Deferribacteres* and *Actinobacteria*. The *Firmicutes/Bacteroidetes* (F/B) ratio was considered a microbial marker for hypertension [21]. Our data revealed the F/B ratio did not differ among the four groups (Figure 4D). At the genus level, the top ten dominant genera were comparable among the four groups (Figure 4E).

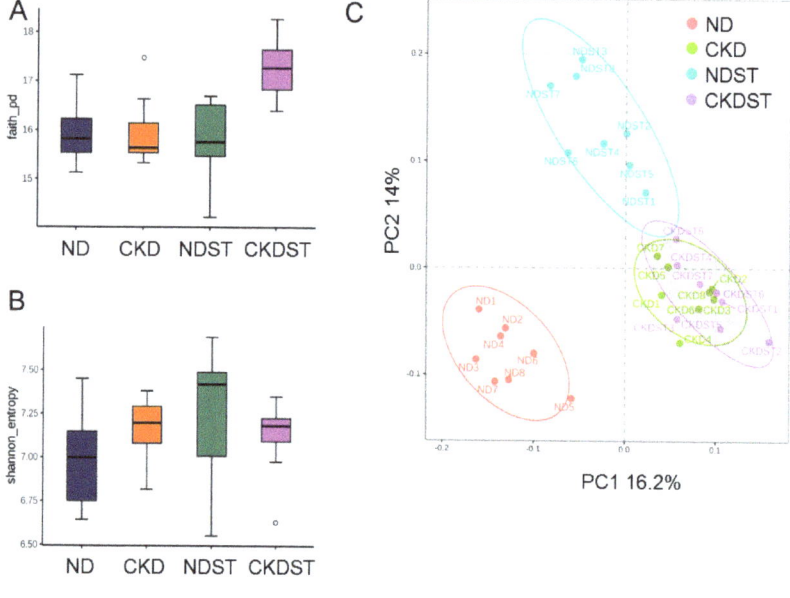

Figure 4. *Cont.*

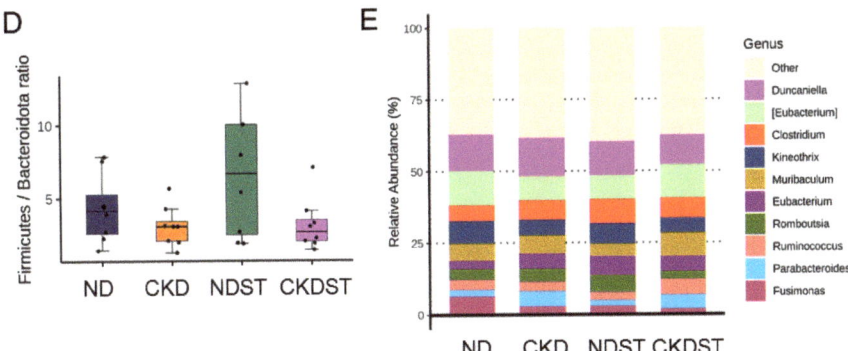

Figure 4. Box plots of (**A**) Faith's phylogenetic diversity (PD) index and (**B**) Shannon index show alpha diversity in the gut microbiota of the four groups. (**C**) Principal coordinate analysis (PCoA) plots of beta diversity. Each data point represents one sample, and each color represents each group. (**D**) Variability in the *Firmicutes/Bacteroidetes* ratio in the gut microbiota. Each circle represents the data of a single sample. (**E**) 16s rRNA gene sequencing analysis of gut microbiota composition at the genus level.

Maternal CKD caused a decrease in genus *Enterococcus* and increases in genera of *Erysipelatoclostridium* and *Dorea* vs. the ND group (Figure 5A–C). Conversely, maternal CKD-induced reduction in genus *Dorea* was restored after STS treatment (Figure 5D). Compared with the CKD group, the abundance of genera *Streptococcus* and *Anaerotruncus* was higher in the CKDST group (Figure 5E,F).

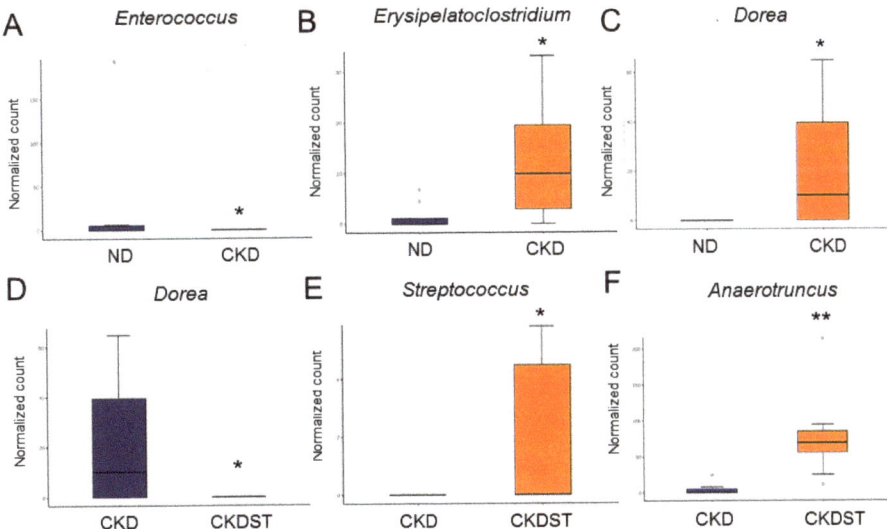

Figure 5. Composition of gut microbiota demonstrating different communities at the genus level. Relative abundance of (**A**) *Enterococcus*, (**B**) *Erysipelatoclostridium*, (**C**) *Dorea*, (**D**) *Dorea*, (**E**) *Streptococcus*, and (**F**) *Anaerotruncus*. * $p < 0.05$. ** $p < 0.01$.

To analyze the reasons for the protective effects of STS treatment and explore in more detail the gut microbiota component, we next illustrate the significant changes between the CKD and CKDST groups at the species level. We found that compared with the CKD group, *Akkermansia muciniphila* (Figure 6A), *Blautia schinkii* (Figure 6B), and *Ruminococcus champanellensis* (Figure 6C) were significantly increased in the CKDST group.

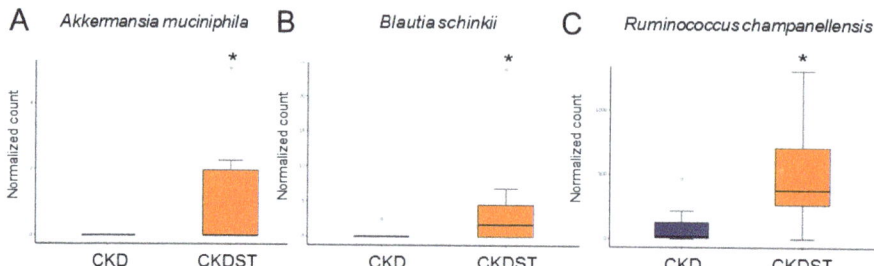

Figure 6. Composition of gut microbiota revealing different communities at the species level. Relative abundance of (**A**) *Akkermansia muciniphila*, (**B**) *Blautia schinkii*, and (**C**) *Ruminococcus champanellensis*. * $p < 0.05$.

LEfSe analysis was undertaken to further discover the differentially abundant taxa between groups (Figure 7). The CKD group exhibited a significant rise in the proportion of the genus *Parabacteroides*. STS treatment caused an increase in the genera *Eubacterium*, *Oscillibacter*, *Lactobacillus*, and *Turicibacter*. Additionally, LEfSe analysis identified the proportion of the genus *Alistipes* was augmented in the CKDST group.

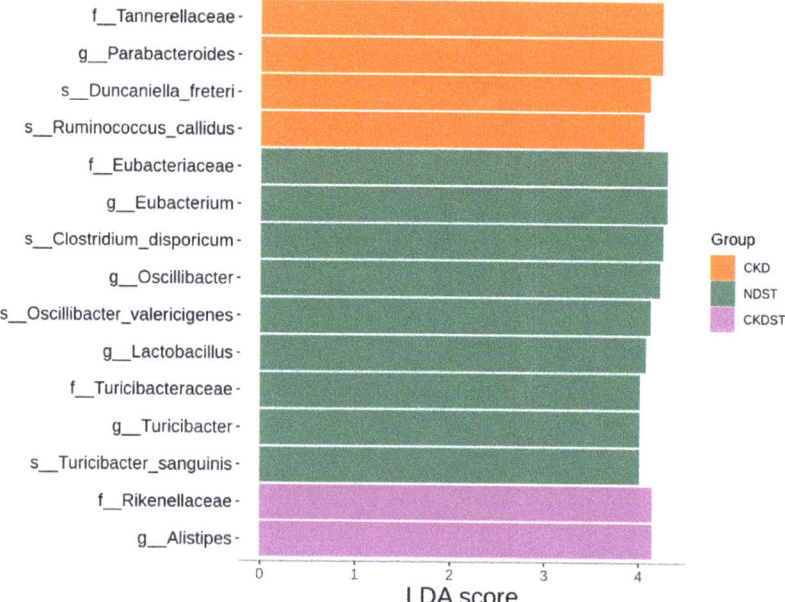

Figure 7. Linear discriminant analysis effect size (LEfSe) to identify the differentially abundant taxa between groups. It mainly shows the significantly different taxa with the linear discriminant analysis (LDA) score > 4. The color of the horizontal bar denotes the respective group.

4. Discussion

Our findings demonstrate that (i) maternal STS treatment prevented adult offspring from exhibiting hypertension induced by maternal CKD; (ii) treatment with STS during pregnancy and lactation restores maternal CKD-induced reduction of renal 3MST protein levels and plasma H₂S concentration; (iii) the benefits of STS for offspring hypertension are connected to increased NO bioavailability; (iv) maternal treatment with STS alters microbiota beta diversity and composition in adult progeny; (v) maternal CKD reduced genus *Enterococcus* and increased genera of *Erysipelatoclostridium* and *Dorea*, while maternal STS treatment increased genus *Dorea*, *Streptococcus*, and *Anaerotruncus*; and (vi) the beneficial effect of STS against offspring hypertension coincided with increases of beneficial microbes such as *Akkermansia muciniphila*, *Blautia schinkii*, and *Ruminococcus champanellensis*. The protective effects and putative mechanisms are presented in Figure 8.

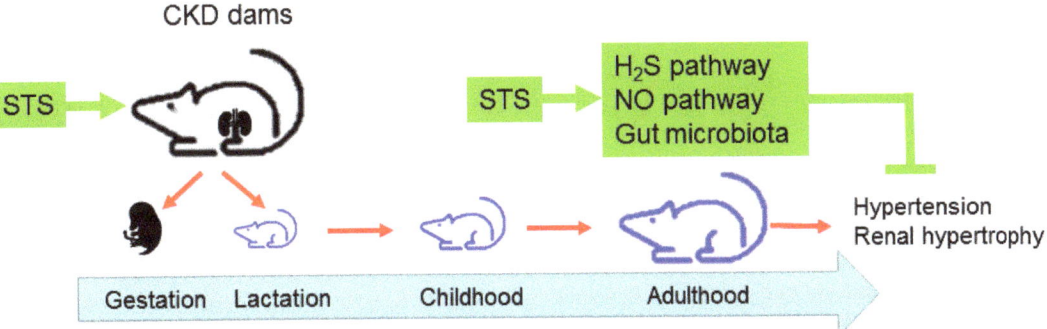

Figure 8. Schematic illustration of protective effects of sodium thiosulfate (STS) treatment and putative mechanisms underlying maternal chronic kidney disease (CKD)-induced offspring hypertension.

In support of prior research indicating that maternal illness results in long-term adverse offspring outcomes [8–10], we found that adult progeny born from CKD mothers developed hypertension, renal hypertrophy, and low body weight. That treatment with STS throughout gestation and lactation was able to improve offspring hypertension in a maternal CKD model is a novel finding. There was, however, no differential impact on body weight and the kidney-weight-to-body-weight ratio between the CKD and CKDST groups.

Though the anti-hypertensive effect of STS has been reported in CKD [13], our report goes beyond prior research and reveals maternal treatment with STS enables the prevention of offspring hypertension induced by maternal CKD. In most former studies, STS has been delivered via i.p. or i.v. administration. The novel observation that oral administration of STS exerts anti-hypertensive actions in the maternal CKD model offers opportunities for translation into clinical practice.

Considering STS is a precursor of H₂S [6], our observations are in line with prior work that supports the role played by H₂S in the development of hypertension [22]. Importantly, H₂S-related interventions, such as H₂S donors and precursors of H₂S, have shown preventive and therapeutic potential for adult diseases of developmental origins [23]. In the present study, the use of STS was ceased after weaning. Therefore, its actions are only due to reprogramming instead of direct effects.

The beneficial actions of STS against maternal CKD-primed offspring hypertension might be associated with plasma H₂S concentrations and increased renal 3MST protein abundance. Although oral administration of STS can directly increase urinary excretion of thiosulfate and sulfate [13], our results go beyond prior research showing that the use of STS in early life can have long-term effects on offspring's H₂S-generating system to increase H₂S bioavailability later in life.

The BP-lowering effect of maternal STS treatment on adult offspring was achieved in the face of an increase in NO bioavailability. H₂S is a physiological vasorelaxant through an enhancement of NO signaling [22]. This notion is supported by our data presenting that the beneficial action of STS was accompanied by decreased ADMA levels and increased AAR, a NO bioavailability index. Given that H₂S has been proposed to exert an anti-oxidative effect against oxidative stress [1], and that impaired ADMA/NO pathway mediates oxidative stress implicating in hypertension [24], how the crosstalk between H_2S and NO in the control of offspring's BP is reprogrammed through STS treatment deserves further clarification.

Another advantageous action of STS could be changes in gut microbiota composition. According to the available human and animal studies [25–28], genera *Streptococcus*, *Enterococcus*, *Anaerotruncus*, *Alistipes*, and *Eubacterium* were depleted, while genera *Parabacteroides*, *Dorea*, and *Erysipelatoclostridium* were enriched in hypertension.

Consistent with previous reports, maternal CKD-induced offspring hypertension coincides with a high abundance of the genera *Parabacteroides*, *Dorea*, and *Erysipelatoclostridium*, and a low abundance of *Enterococcus*. Conversely, maternal STS treatment enriched several genera that are reported as negatively associated with BP, including *Streptococcus*, *Anaerotruncus*, and *Alistipes*. Importantly, maternal STS treatment increased the abundance of several beneficial microbes with potential probiotic properties, including *Akkermansia muciniphia* [29], *Blautia schinkii* [30], and *Ruminococcus champanellensis* [31]. Of note is that several studies have highlighted the positive role of *Akkermansia muciniphila* in improving hypertension [29]. To further understand the impact of STS on programmed hypertension, further research should be investigated to truly explore its actions on beneficial microbes and their interactions with BP regulation.

Moreover, we determined microbial taxa involved in sulfur metabolism. Our data indicated that all SRBs (e.g., *Desulfovibrio* or *Desulfobacter*) were not noticeable in both STS-treated groups. In the gut, several species with sulfite reductase can also participate in H_2S production, including *E coli*, *Klebsiella*, *Bacillus*, *Corynebacterium*, *Salmonella*, *Rhodococcus*, etc. [32]. We observed that STS has a neglectable effect on the abundance of sulfite-reducing microbes. Therefore, it is not known whether the protective role of STS is connected to intestinal microbe-derived H_2S and alterations of sulfite- or sulfate-reducing microorganisms.

In addition to gut microbiota dysbiosis, oxidative stress and inflammation also contribute to the pathogenesis of CKD and have been identified as molecular mechanisms for H_2S effects [4,33]. Using the maternal CKD model, our previous study showed perinatal resveratrol therapy prevented offspring hypertension and is connected to the reduction of oxidative stress and an altered gut microbiome and microbe-derived metabolites [34]. Resveratrol, a natural polyphenol, exhibits antioxidant and anti-inflammatory properties. Considering the beneficial effect of STS in the present study, whether the application of nutraceuticals with anti-inflammatory or antioxidant properties could provide renoprotection and thereby avert maternal CKD-induced hypertension deserves to be investigated further.

Short-chain fatty acids (SCFAs) are the main microbiota-derived metabolites [35]. As we mentioned earlier, the beneficial effects of perinatal resveratrol therapy also contributed to the mediation of SCFA and their receptors [34]. Another study indicated that maternal CKD-induced offspring hypertension can be averted through the perinatal use of propionate, one of the predominant SCFAs [36]. Accordingly, targeting microbial metabolite SCFAs might also be an interesting mechanism to explore. Future studies should assess microbial metabolites and evaluate their connections with the protective actions of STS against maternal CKD-induced hypertension.

Our study has a few limitations. Firstly, we did not assess the impact of STS treatment on sex differences, since only male progeny was used in the present study. Another limitation is that the microbiome data do not provide information on whether or not oral administration of STS during pregnancy and lactation could alter gut microbiota in mothers or neonate offspring. Whether STS treatment could regulate gut microbiota-derived fecal H_2S connected to offspring hypertension awaits further clarification. Thirdly, we analyzed renal outcomes and gut microbiota in adult offspring at the time hypertension appeared, but not in dams. Our previous research indicated that adenine-fed mother rats displayed renal dysfunction, glomerular and tubulointerstitial damage, hypertension, and placental abnormalities [15]. Considering STS treatment has shown benefits against kidney disease and hypertension [12–14], additional research is needed to clarify whether STS treatment could also improve renal outcomes for mother rats. Whether STS treatment during pregnancy and lactation might alter the gut microbiota in both dams and offspring, and whether maternal alterations in renal outcomes and gut microbiota are connected with offspring outcomes, both require further evaluation. As several inflammatory mediators, such as NF-κB, NLRP3, and mitogen-activated protein kinase (MAPK) signaling pathways, were all activated in CKD and could represent a potential target for STS [37,38], studying these mechanisms might also be an interesting alternative target to explore. Lastly, the findings presented in our study are valuable for revealing that STS has beneficial effects on offspring programmed by maternal CKD but are limited to testing in this model. Further studies are needed in other animal models of CKD and humans before STS can be translated into clinical practice. Considering the significant progress that has been made over the last decade in RSS-related drugs [39–41], the reprogramming effects of other RSS-based interventions on maternal CKD-primed hypertension also deserve further attention.

5. Conclusions

To conclude, our results suggest that oral administration of STS during gestation and lactation improved offspring hypertension induced by maternal CKD via augmentation of both the H_2S and NO pathways and changes in gut microbiota composition. As such, early-life intervention strategies specifically targeting the H_2S signaling pathway could be considered for preventing hypertension in progeny born from mothers with CKD.

Author Contributions: Y.-L.T. and C.-N.H. designed the whole study. C.-Y.H., G.-P.C.-C. and S.L. contributed to the methodology and data analysis. Y.-L.T., C.-Y.H., S.L., G.-P.C.-C. and C.-N.H. contributed to the drafting of the manuscript, comments, and revision of the manuscript. All authors have read and agreed to the published version of the manuscript.

Funding: This work was supported by grant MOST 110-2314-B-182-020-MY3 (Y.-L.T.) from the Ministry of Science and Technology, Taiwan.

Institutional Review Board Statement: Animal experiments were approved by the Institutional Animal Ethics Committee of Kaohsiung Chang Gung Memorial Hospital (Permit #2020110202).

Informed Consent Statement: Not applicable.

Data Availability Statement: The data that support the findings of this study are contained within the article.

Acknowledgments: We would like to thank the Institute of Environmental Toxin and Emerging-Contaminant, the Super Micro Mass Research and Technology Center, and the Center for Environmental Toxin and Emerging Contaminant Research, Cheng Shiu University, Kaohsiung, for technical support. We also sincerely appropriate the support provided by the Center for Laboratory Animals, Kaohsiung Chang Gung Memorial Hospital.

Conflicts of Interest: The authors declare no conflict of interest.

References

1. Olson, K.R. Hydrogen sulfide, reactive sulfur species and coping with reactive oxygen species. *Free Radic. Biol. Med.* **2019**, *140*, 74–83. [CrossRef] [PubMed]
2. Giles, G.I.; Nasim, M.J.; Ali, W.; Jacob, C. The Reactive Sulfur Species Concept: 15 Years On. *Antioxidants* **2017**, *6*, 38. [CrossRef]
3. Iciek, M.; Bilska-Wilkosz, A.; Górny, M. Sulfane sulfur—New findings on an old topic. *Acta Biochim. Pol.* **2019**, *66*, 533–544. [CrossRef] [PubMed]
4. Kimura, H. Signaling molecules: Hydrogen sulfide and polysulfide. *Antioxid. Redox Signal.* **2015**, *22*, 362–376. [CrossRef] [PubMed]
5. Linden, D.R. Hydrogen Sulfide Signaling in the Gastrointestinal Tract. *Antioxid. Redox Signal.* **2014**, *20*, 818–830. [CrossRef]
6. Zhang, M.Y.; Dugbartey, G.J.; Juriasingani, S.; Sener, A. Hydrogen Sulfide Metabolite, Sodium Thiosulfate: Clinical Applications and Underlying Molecular Mechanisms. *Int. J. Mol. Sci.* **2021**, *22*, 6452. [CrossRef]
7. Luyckx, V.A.; Tonelli, M.; Stanifer, J.W. The global burden of kidney disease and the sustainable development goals. *Bull. World Health Organ.* **2018**, *96*, 414D–422D. [CrossRef]

8. Tain, Y.L.; Hsu, C.N. Developmental origins of chronic kidney disease: Should we focus on early life? *Int. J. Mol. Sci.* **2017**, *18*, 381. [CrossRef]
9. Munkhaugen, J.; Lydersen, S.; Romundstad, P.R.; Widerøe, T.-E.; Vikse, B.E.; Hallan, S. Kidney function and future risk for adverse pregnancy outcomes: A population-based study from HUNT II, Norway. *Nephrol. Dial. Transplant.* **2009**, *24*, 3744–3750. [CrossRef]
10. Piccoli, G.B.; Alrukhaimi, M.; Liu, Z.H.; Zakharova, E.; Levin, A.; World Kidney Day Steering Committee. What we do and do not know about women and kidney diseases; Questions unanswered and answers unquestioned: Reflection on World Kidney Day and International Woman's Day. *Physiol. Int.* **2018**, *105*, 199–209. [CrossRef]
11. Hsu, C.N.; Hou, C.Y.; Chang-Chien, G.P.; Lin, S.; Tain, Y.L. Dietary Supplementation with Cysteine during Pregnancy Rescues Maternal Chronic Kidney Disease-Induced Hypertension in Male Rat Offspring: The Impact of Hydrogen Sulfide and Microbiota Derived Tryptophan Metabolites. *Antioxidants* **2022**, *11*, 483. [CrossRef]
12. Snijder, P.M.; Frenay, A.-R.S.; Koning, A.M.; Bachtler, M.; Pasch, A.; Kwakernaak, A.J.; Berg, E.V.D.; Bos, E.M.; Hillebrands, J.-L.; Navis, G.; et al. Sodium thiosulfate attenuates angiotensin II-induced hypertension, proteinuria and renal damage. *Nitric Oxide* **2014**, *42*, 87–98. [CrossRef]
13. Nguyen, I.T.; Klooster, A.; Minnion, M.; Feelisch, M.; Verhaar, M.C.; van Goor, H.; Joles, J.A. Sodium thiosulfate improves renal function and oxygenation in L-NNA–induced hypertension in rats. *Kidney Int.* **2020**, *98*, 366–377. [CrossRef]
14. Hsu, C.N.; Hou, C.Y.; Chang-Chien, G.P.; Lin, S.; Yang, H.W.; Tain, Y.L. Sodium Thiosulfate Improves Hypertension in Rats with Adenine-Induced Chronic Kidney Disease. *Antioxidants* **2022**, *11*, 147. [CrossRef]
15. Hsu, C.N.; Yang, H.W.; Hou, C.Y.; Chang-Chien, G.P.; Lin, S.; Tain, Y.L. Maternal Adenine-Induced Chronic Kidney Disease Programs Hypertension in Adult Male Rat Offspring: Implications of Nitric Oxide and Gut Microbiome Derived Metabolites. *Int. J. Mol. Sci.* **2020**, *21*, 7319. [CrossRef]
16. Reckelhoff, J.F. Gender differences in the regulation of blood pressure. *Hypertension* **2001**, *37*, 1199–1208. [CrossRef]
17. Bode-Böger, S.M.; Scalera, F.; Ignarro, L.J. The L-arginine paradox: Importance of the L-arginine/asymmetrical dimethylarginine ratio. *Pharmacol. Ther.* **2007**, *114*, 295–306. [CrossRef] [PubMed]
18. Tain, Y.L.; Hou, C.Y.; Chang-Chien, G.P.; Lin, S.; Hsu, C.N. Perinatal Garlic Oil Supplementation Averts Rat Offspring Hypertension Programmed by Maternal Chronic Kidney Disease. *Nutrients* **2022**, *14*, 4624. [CrossRef] [PubMed]
19. Bolyen, E.; Rideout, J.R.; Dillon, M.R.; Bokulich, N.A.; Abnet, C.C.; Al-Ghalith, G.A.; Alexander, H.; Alm, E.J.; Arumugam, M.; Asnicar, F.; et al. Reproducible, interactive, scalable and extensible microbiome data science using QIIME 2. *Nat. Biotechnol.* **2019**, *37*, 852–857. [CrossRef]
20. Segata, N.; Izard, J.; Waldron, L.; Gevers, D.; Miropolsky, L.; Garrett, W.S.; Huttenhower, C. Metagenomic biomarker discovery and explanation. *Genome Biol.* **2011**, *12*, R60. [CrossRef] [PubMed]
21. Yang, T.; Richards, E.M.; Pepine, C.J.; Raizada, M.K. The gut microbiota and the brain-gut-kidney axis in hypertension and chronic kidney disease. *Nat. Rev. Nephrol.* **2018**, *14*, 442–456. [CrossRef] [PubMed]
22. Wang, R. Roles of Hydrogen Sulfide in Hypertension Development and Its Complications: What, So What, Now What. *Hypertension* **2023**, *80*, 936–944. [CrossRef]
23. Hsu, C.N.; Tain, Y.L. Preventing Developmental Origins of Cardiovascular Disease: Hydrogen Sulfide as a Potential Target? *Antioxidants* **2021**, *10*, 247. [CrossRef] [PubMed]
24. Tain, Y.L.; Hsu, C.N. Targeting on Asymmetric Dimethylarginine-Related Nitric Oxide-Reactive Oxygen Species Imbalance to Reprogram the Development of Hypertension. *Int. J. Mol. Sci.* **2016**, *17*, 2020. [CrossRef]
25. Palmu, J.; Salosensaari, A.; Havulinna, A.S.; Cheng, S.; Inouye, M.; Jain, M.; Salido, R.A.; Sanders, K.; Brennan, C.; Humphrey, G.C.; et al. Association Between the Gut Microbiota and Blood Pressure in a Population Cohort of 6953 Individuals. *J. Am. Heart Assoc.* **2020**, *9*, e016641. [CrossRef]
26. Guo, Y.; Li, X.; Wang, Z.; Yu, B. Gut Microbiota Dysbiosis in Human Hypertension: A Systematic Review of Observational Studies. *Front. Cardiovasc. Med.* **2021**, *8*, 650227. [CrossRef]
27. Naik, S.S.; Ramphall, S.; Rijal, S.; Prakash, V.; Ekladios, H.; Mulayamkuzhiyil Saju, J.; Mandal, N.; Kham, N.I.; Shahid, R.; Venugopal, S. Association of Gut Microbial Dysbiosis and Hypertension: A Systematic Review. *Cureus* **2022**, *14*, e29927. [CrossRef]
28. Muralitharan, R.R.; Jama, H.A.; Xie, L.; Peh, A.; Snelson, M.; Marques, F.Z. Microbial Peer Pressure: The Role of the Gut Microbiota in Hypertension and Its Complications. *Hypertension* **2020**, *76*, 1674–1687. [CrossRef] [PubMed]
29. Lakshmanan, A.P.; Murugesan, S.; Al Khodor, S.; Terranegra, A. The potential impact of a probiotic: Akkermansia muciniphila in the regulation of blood pressure-the current facts and evidence. *J. Transl. Med.* **2022**, *20*, 430. [CrossRef] [PubMed]
30. Liu, X.; Mao, B.; Gu, J.; Wu, J.; Cui, S.; Wang, G.; Zhao, J.; Zhang, H.; Chen, W. Blautia-a new functional genus with potential probiotic properties? *Gut Microbes* **2021**, *13*, 1875796. [CrossRef]
31. Moraïs, S.; Cockburn, D.W.; Ben-David, Y.; Koropatkin, N.M.; Martens, E.C.; Duncan, S.H.; Flint, H.J.; Mizrahi, I.; Bayer, E.A. Lysozyme activity of the Ruminococcus champanellensis cellulosome. *Environ. Microbiol.* **2016**, *18*, 5112–5122. [CrossRef]
32. Tomasova, L.; Konopelski, P.; Ufnal, M. Gut Bacteria and Hydrogen Sulfide: The New Old Players in Circulatory System Homeostasis. *Molecules* **2016**, *21*, 1558. [CrossRef]

33. Calabrese, V.; Scuto, M.; Salinaro, A.T.; Dionisio, G.; Modafferi, S.; Ontario, M.L.; Greco, V.; Sciuto, S.; Schmitt, C.P.; Calabrese, E.J.; et al. Hydrogen Sulfide and Carnosine: Modulation of Oxidative Stress and Inflammation in Kidney and Brain Axis. *Antioxidants* **2020**, *9*, 1303. [CrossRef]
34. Hsu, C.N.; Hou, C.Y.; Chang-Chien, G.P.; Lin, S.; Yang, H.W.; Tain, Y.L. Perinatal Resveratrol Therapy Prevents Hypertension Programmed by Maternal Chronic Kidney Disease in Adult Male Offspring: Implications of the Gut Microbiome and Their Metabolites. *Biomedicines* **2020**, *8*, 567. [CrossRef]
35. Pluznick, J.L. Microbial short-chain fatty acids and blood pressure regulation. *Curr. Hypertens. Rep.* **2017**, *19*, 25. [CrossRef] [PubMed]
36. Tain, Y.L.; Hou, C.Y.; Chang-Chien, G.P.; Lin, S.F.; Hsu, C.N. Perinatal Propionate Supplementation Protects Adult Male Offspring from Maternal Chronic Kidney Disease-Induced Hypertension. *Nutrients* **2022**, *14*, 3435. [CrossRef] [PubMed]
37. Castelblanco, M.; Lugrin, J.; Ehirchiou, D.; Nasi, S.; Ishii, I.; So, A.; Martinon, F.; Busso, N. Hydrogen sulfide inhibits NLRP3 inflammasome activation and reduces cytokine production both in vitro and in a mouse model of inflammation. *J. Biol. Chem.* **2018**, *293*, 2546–2557. [CrossRef] [PubMed]
38. Fan, H.N.; Wang, H.J.; Ren, L.; Ren, B.; Dan, C.R.; Li, Y.F.; Hou, L.Z.; Deng, Y. Decreased expression of p38 MAPK mediates protective effects of hydrogen sulfide on hepatic fibrosis. *Eur. Rev. Med. Pharmacol. Sci.* **2013**, *17*, 644–652.
39. Li, Z.; Polhemus, D.J.; Lefer, D.J. Evolution of Hydrogen Sulfide Therapeutics to Treat Cardiovascular Disease. *Circ. Res.* **2018**, *123*, 590–600. [CrossRef]
40. Zaorska, E.; Tomasova, L.; Koszelewski, D.; Ostaszewski, R.; Ufnal, M. Hydrogen Sulfide in Pharmacotherapy, Beyond the Hydrogen Sulfide-Donors. *Biomolecules* **2020**, *10*, 323. [CrossRef]
41. Khodade, V.S.; Aggarwal, S.C.; Eremiev, A.; Bao, E.; Porche, S.; Toscano, J.P. Development of Hydropersulfide Donors to Study Their Chemical Biology. *Antioxid. Redox Signal.* **2022**, *36*, 309–326. [CrossRef] [PubMed]

Disclaimer/Publisher's Note: The statements, opinions and data contained in all publications are solely those of the individual author(s) and contributor(s) and not of MDPI and/or the editor(s). MDPI and/or the editor(s) disclaim responsibility for any injury to people or property resulting from any ideas, methods, instructions or products referred to in the content.

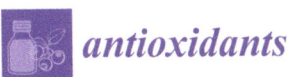

Article

Identifying Redox-Sensitive Cysteine Residues in Mitochondria

Eleni A. Kisty, Emma C. Saart and Eranthie Weerapana *

Department of Chemistry, Boston College, Chestnut Hill, MA 02467, USA
* Correspondence: eranthie@bc.edu

Abstract: The mitochondrion is the primary energy generator of a cell and is a central player in cellular redox regulation. Mitochondrial reactive oxygen species (mtROS) are the natural byproducts of cellular respiration that are critical for the redox signaling events that regulate a cell's metabolism. These redox signaling pathways primarily rely on the reversible oxidation of the cysteine residues on mitochondrial proteins. Several key sites of this cysteine oxidation on mitochondrial proteins have been identified and shown to modulate downstream signaling pathways. To further our understanding of mitochondrial cysteine oxidation and to identify uncharacterized redox-sensitive cysteines, we coupled mitochondrial enrichment with redox proteomics. Briefly, differential centrifugation methods were used to enrich for mitochondria. These purified mitochondria were subjected to both exogenous and endogenous ROS treatments and analyzed by two redox proteomics methods. A competitive cysteine-reactive profiling strategy, termed isoTOP-ABPP, enabled the ranking of the cysteines by their redox sensitivity, due to a loss of reactivity induced by cysteine oxidation. A modified OxICAT method enabled a quantification of the percentage of reversible cysteine oxidation. Initially, we assessed the cysteine oxidation upon treatment with a range of exogenous hydrogen peroxide concentrations, which allowed us to differentiate the mitochondrial cysteines by their susceptibility to oxidation. We then analyzed the cysteine oxidation upon inducing reactive oxygen species generation via the inhibition of the electron transport chain. Together, these methods identified the mitochondrial cysteines that were sensitive to endogenous and exogenous ROS, including several previously known redox-regulated cysteines and uncharacterized cysteines on diverse mitochondrial proteins.

Keywords: mitochondria; cysteine; ROS; oxidation; mass spectrometry; isoTOP-ABPP; OxICAT

Citation: Kisty, E.A.; Saart, E.C.; Weerapana, E. Identifying Redox-Sensitive Cysteine Residues in Mitochondria. *Antioxidants* **2023**, *12*, 992. https://doi.org/10.3390/antiox12050992

Academic Editors: John Toscano, Vinayak Khodade and Naphtali Savion

Received: 2 March 2023
Revised: 18 April 2023
Accepted: 20 April 2023
Published: 25 April 2023

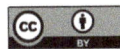

Copyright: © 2023 by the authors. Licensee MDPI, Basel, Switzerland. This article is an open access article distributed under the terms and conditions of the Creative Commons Attribution (CC BY) license (https://creativecommons.org/licenses/by/4.0/).

1. Introduction

Mitochondria are the sites of essential cellular metabolic pathways, including the tricarboxylic acid (TCA) cycle and the electron transport chain (ETC). Mitochondria comprise distinct membranes, where the outer (OMM) and inner (IMM) mitochondrial membranes envelop the intermembrane space (IMS) [1]. The IMS is critical for the import and folding of mitochondrial proteins, as well as for apoptotic signaling [2–5]. The innermost compartment, the matrix, hosts the bioenergetic machinery essential for ATP production [6].

In addition to the central role of mitochondria in cellular metabolism, mitochondria are well-characterized hubs of redox signaling. As one of the primary sites of reactive oxygen species (ROS) production in the cell [7], mitochondria balance the ROS production and metabolism to maintain cellular redox homeostasis. ROS production in the mitochondria results from incomplete electron transfer during aerobic respiration, forming superoxide, and ultimately, a variety of different ROS, including hydrogen peroxide [8]. These ROS can regulate the diverse metabolic and signaling pathways in the mitochondria through cysteine oxidation events. In the presence of ROS, cysteines undergo reversible and irreversible oxidative post-translational modifications (oxPTMs) [9] that transiently affect the protein structure, catalytic activity, complex formation, localization, and degradation [10–14]. There are several characterized sites of cysteine oxidation that affect the mitochondrial protein function [15], including C385 on aconitase (ACO2), which regulates the TCA cycle [16,17], C39 on ND3 subunit of complex I (MT-ND3), which tunes the ETC electron flux [18,19], and C253 on uncoupling protein 1 (UCP1), which disrupts the IMM proton gradient [20,21]. These oxidation events underscore the importance of cysteine oxidation in regulating the metabolic flux as a feedback mechanism for maintaining cell homeostasis.

High levels of mtROS are associated with a variety of pathologies, including cancer [22], diabetes [23,24], neurodegeneration [25], and cardiac disease [26]. Therefore, identifying redox-sensitive cysteines within the mitochondria can provide insight into the redox-regulated metabolic and signaling pathways implicated in disease pathogenesis. Redox proteomics approaches facilitate the identification of redox-sensitive cysteines within a complex proteome. One challenge in performing redox proteomic studies on mitochondrial proteins is the low abundance of these proteins relative to the highly abundant cytosolic and nuclear proteins. Mitochondrial proteins account for only 6% of the human proteome [27,28]; therefore, proteomic analyses of whole-cell lysates result in poor coverage of the mitochondrial proteome. The enrichment of mitochondrial proteins through organelle fractionation [29], targeted probes [30–35], proximity labeling (BioID [36,37], APEX [38–40], and small molecules [41]) significantly improves this mitochondrial protein coverage.

Coupling these mitochondrial enrichment methods with redox proteomic workflows can facilitate the identification of redox-sensitive cysteines within the mitochondria. Several redox proteomic strategies exist that either directly or indirectly monitor cysteine oxidation. Reactive cysteine profiling, using the isotopic tandem orthogonal proteolysis-activity-based protein profiling (isoTOP-ABPP) platform, indirectly identifies redox-sensitive cysteines by monitoring the oxidation-induced losses in cysteine reactivity. Briefly, isoTOP-ABPP applies a thiol-reactive iodoacetamide-alkyne (IA) probe to monitor the decreases in the cysteine reactivity resulting from oxPTMs. In previous work, isoTOP-ABPP has been used to map the sites of cysteine nitrosation within mitochondrial proteins upon mitochondrial enrichment via differential centrifugation [42]. An alternative redox proteomic approach is the use of oxidative isotopically coded affinity tags (OxICAT [43]), which applies the differential isotopic tagging of reduced and oxidized cysteines to determine the percentage of oxidation. Variations of the OxICAT method have been applied to monitor the cysteine oxidation in the mammalian endoplasmic reticulum [44], yeast [45], bacteria [43], and drosophila [46]. Lastly, mitochondria-targeted probes for sulfinic and sulfenic acids have identified these specific oxidation events within mitochondrial proteins [30–35].

Here, we combine differential centrifugation to isolate the mitochondria with the isoTOP-ABPP and OxICAT redox proteomic strategies, in order to study the oxidation of mitochondrial cysteines. Specifically, we rank mitochondrial cysteines by their susceptibility to oxidation with hydrogen peroxide and identify the oxidation events that occur upon the inhibition of the ETC using antimycin A (AMA). The redox-sensitive cysteines we identify comprise well-characterized sites of mitochondrial redox regulation, as well as proteins and pathways that have yet to be fully evaluated for their redox sensitivity.

2. Materials and Methods

2.1. Biological and Chemical Materials

All the reagents were purchased from Sigma-Aldrich (St. Louis, MO, USA) and Fisher Scientific (Waltham, MA, USA), unless otherwise indicated. All the antibodies (Anti-GAPDH (14C10), Anti-ATPIF1 (D6P1Q), Anti-Histone-H3 (D1H2), Anti-CALR (D3E6), and Anti-DYKDDDK (FLAG)) were purchased from Cell Signaling Technology (Danvers, MA, USA). IA-light (IA-L) and IA-heavy (IA-H) were synthesized in-house according to Abo, M. et al. [47].

2.2. Mammalian Cell Culture

HEK293T cells were maintained at 37 °C under an atmosphere of 5% CO_2 in a DMEM medium (Corning, Corning, NY, USA) supplemented with 10% FBS (Biotechne, Minneapolis, MN, USA) and 1% Anti-Anti (Gibco, Waltham, MA, USA).

2.3. Isolation of Mitochondria

HEK293T pellets were washed 3 times with a mitochondrial isolation buffer (10 mM Tris-MOPS, 1 mM EDTA/Tris, 200 mM Sucrose, pH 7.4, IBC). Crude and pure mitochondria (Mito-C and Mito-P) were obtained following the general protocol of differential centrifugation and isopycnic separation by Frezza, C. et al. [29] and Bak, D. et al. [42].

2.4. Western Blot Analysis of GAPDH, CALR, Histone H3 and ATPIF1

A Western blot analysis was performed on 25 μg of whole cell (WC), cytosolic (Cyto), crude mitochondrial (Mito-C) and pure mitochondrial (Mito-P) lysates using rabbit anti-GAPDH (1:1000, TBST and 5% bovine serum albumin (BSA)), rabbit anti-Histone H3 (1:1000, TBST and 5% milk)), rabbit anti-CALR (1:1000, TBST and 5% milk)), or rabbit anti-ATPIF1 (1:1000, TBST and 5% bovine serum albumin (BSA)) primary antibodies, followed by an anti-rabbit IgG HRP conjugate (1:2000).

2.5. Treatment of HEK293T Cells with Antimycin A

Confluent HEK293T cells were incubated with either 100 μM of Antimycin A in DMSO or an equivalent volume of DMSO for a total of 1 h at 37 °C.

2.6. Mass Spectrometry Sample Preparation

2.6.1. isoTOP-ABPP Analysis

The analysis using isoTOP-ABPP was performed according to Weerapana, E. et al. [48], Bak, D. et al. [42], and Abo, M. et al. [47]. For the hydrogen peroxide treatments, 0.5 mg of isolated Mito-P lysates in 500 μL were pretreated in the dark with 1 μL of 100× stocks of hydrogen peroxide or water on ice, for 20 min prior to the IA labeling. For the Antimycin A studies, the IA labeling was performed on 0.5 mg of intact Mito-P fractions prior to lysis.

2.6.2. OxICAT Studies and Cysteine Oxidation Analysis

The OxICAT studies were performed with 4 mg of isolated Mito-P using the protocol described in Bechtel, T. et al. [44].

2.7. Tandem MS Analysis

An MS analysis was performed on a Thermo Fisher LTQ Orbitrap Discovery mass spectrometer coupled with an Agilent 1200 series HPLC, as previously described [48].

2.8. LC/LC-MS/MS Data Processing

The MS/MS data were analyzed using the SEQUEST algorithm, filtered using DTASelect 2.0 [49,50], and the light:heavy ratios were obtained using CIMAGE [48], as previously described [48]. A dynamic modification of the cysteine for the IA-L (306.14806 m/z) and IA-H (312.16819 m/z) adducts was included.

2.8.1. MS Data Analysis: isoTOP-ABPP for Peroxide Treatment

Two replicates of each peroxide concentration (1, 2.5, 5, and 10 mM of H_2O_2) were analyzed. The average ratios were calculated for the peptides with ratios present in both replicates, and values exhibiting > 2-fold changes and coefficients of variation of >50% were removed. The data were filtered via mitochondrial localization through a comparison with the Uniprot [51] and MitoCarta3.0 [52] databases.

2.8.2. MS Data Analysis: isoTOP-ABPP for AMA Treatment

Three replicates were analyzed. L:H Ratios were required to be in 2 out of 3 of the replicates. The average ratios of a >2-fold change were filtered by a coefficient of variation cut-off of 50%. Only peptides from the mitochondria-annotated proteins were included.

2.8.3. MS Data Analysis: OxICAT

Three replicates were analyzed to obtain the L:H and H:L ratios. The data were filtered to include only the mitochondrial proteins and peptides that appeared in two out of the three replicates. The L:H and H:L ratios were converted to % oxidation values by using the equations: $1 - (L:H/(L:H + 1))$ or $H:L/(H:L + 1)$. The average % oxidation values were determined for each peptide and those with a standard deviation of mean of >30% were removed.

2.9. Statistical Analysis of Overrepresented GO Biological Processes Using Panther

Protein ID lists from the whole cell cysteine reactivity data from Weerapana, E. et al. [48] and the Mito-P cysteine reactivity data from the 1 mM peroxide studies were analyzed using Panther 16.0 overrepresentation tests (http://pantherdb.org (accessed on 21 May 2021)) [53].

3. Results

3.1. Differential Centrifugation to Increase Coverage of Mitochondrial Cysteines

To enrich the intact mitochondria, we adapted the established methods of differential centrifugation [29,42] to fractionate the HEK293T cell lysates to generate a crude mitochondrial sample (Mito-C) (Figure S1A). The Mito-C fraction was further purified with an isopycnic percoll gradient to produce a pure mitochondrial sample (Mito-P), with minimal cytosolic and nuclear contamination (Figure S1B). An analysis by Western blot using antibodies against the nuclear (histone H3), ER (calreticulin), cytosolic (GAPDH), and mitochondrial (ATPIF1) proteins demonstrated the successful enrichment of the mitochondrial proteins and a loss of the nuclear and cytosolic proteins in the Mito-C and Mito-P fractions. The ER marker, calreticulin, was still present in the Mito-P sample, likely due to the inability of differential centrifugation to disrupt ER–mitochondrial contact sites.

The enrichment of the mitochondrial proteins in the Mito-P fraction was further confirmed by enriching and identifying the reactive cysteines using mass spectrometry (MS) [50]. Briefly, the Mito-P lysates were treated with an iodoacetamide-alkyne (IA) probe to covalently modify their reactive cysteines. The IA-modified proteins were conjugated to a chemically cleavable biotin linker (Figure S2B) using a copper (I)-catalyzed azide-alkyne cycloaddition (CuAAC). Biotinylated proteins were enriched on streptavidin beads, subjected to on-bead trypsin digestion, and there was a subsequent release of the IA-modified peptides using a sodium dithionite treatment. The resulting IA-modified peptides were analyzed with tandem liquid chromatography–mass spectrometry (LC/LC-MS/MS). The mitochondrial cysteine coverage in the Mito-P sample was determined to be similar to that in previous fractionation reports [42], with a total of 1563 cysteines identified from the 481 proteins that were identified to localize to the mitochondria by Uniprot [51] and MitoCarta2.0 [54] (Table S1). Previously reported reactive cysteine profiling studies on unfractionated whole-cell lysates [48] have identified 278 cysteines from 172 mitochondrial proteins. Therefore, mitochondrial isolation resulted in a ~three-fold increase in the mitochondrial proteins and ~five-fold increase in the mitochondrial peptides identified (Figure S1D). Additionally, 57% of the spectral counts in the Mito-P sample originated from the mitochondrial proteins, compared to 11% in the whole-cell sample (Figure S1C). A gene ontology (GO) analysis of the Mito-P sample revealed a robust enrichment for common mitochondrial processes such as mitochondrial protein translation, mitochondrial gene expression, and the TCA cycle, none of which were enriched in the whole-cell sample (Tables S2 and S3, Figure S1E). Together, our data confirm differential centrifugation to be a valuable method for mitochondrial proteome enrichment.

3.2. Monitoring the Redox Sensitivity of Mitochondrial Cysteines

Upon confirming this mitochondrial enrichment, we applied the isoTOP-ABPP platform to rank the mitochondrial cysteines by their sensitivity to hydrogen peroxide (Figure 1A) [47,48]. IsoTOP-ABPP compared the cysteine reactivity across two biological samples through the application of isotopically labeled IA probes, IA-L (light), and IA-H (heavy) (Figure S2A). The Mito-P fractions were treated with 1, 2.5, 5, and 10 mM of hydrogen peroxide for 20 min. These peroxide-treated samples were then labeled with IA-H, and a corresponding untreated control sample was labeled with IA-L. The peroxide-treated and untreated samples were mixed together prior to the streptavidin enrichment, trypsin digestion, and sodium dithionite elution. The resulting peptide mixtures were analyzed using LC/LC-MS/MS. For every cysteine-containing peptide that was identified, the relative IA-labeling in the untreated controls versus the peroxide-treated experimental samples could be determined by the light:heavy (L:H) ratios. An L:H ratio of >1 corresponded to a decrease in the cysteine reactivity upon the peroxide treatment, and was indicative of cysteine oxidation. An L:H ratio equivalent to 1 indicated an unchanged cysteine reactivity upon the peroxide treatment. Importantly, the use of this isoTOP-ABPP analysis allowed for a determination of the extent of oxidation, whereby the higher the L:H ratio value, the greater the stoichiometry of the oxidation. The peroxide concentrations used were supraphysiological, but were selected such that minimal oxidation was observed at the lowest concentration (1 mM) and a high-stoichiometry oxidation for a subset of cysteines was present at the highest peroxide concentration (10 mM). Importantly, we ensured that, at the highest (10 mM) concentration of peroxide, we did not see the complete oxidation of all the cysteines, indicating that we were not completely overwhelming the oxidation capacity of the system.

The isoTOP-ABPP analysis identified ~700 mitochondrial cysteines (Tables S4–S7) with robust L:H ratios in each of the peroxide treatments. As expected, increasing median L:H ratios were observed with increasing peroxide concentrations (Figure 1B), indicating proteome-wide decreases in cysteine reactivity. For example, a 1 mM peroxide treatment led to very minor changes in cysteine reactivity (a median L:H ratio of 1.1). In contrast, the 10 mM peroxide treatments displayed pronounced decreases in cysteine reactivity (a median L:H ratio of 2.3). The treatments of 2.5 mM and 5 mM peroxide gave median L:H ratios of 1.3 and 1.7, respectively.

Importantly, the effect of the peroxide was not uniform across the identified cysteines, allowing us to group the cysteines within groupings of a low, moderate, and high sensitivity to the peroxide treatments. A subset of cysteines displayed no change in their cysteine reactivity (L:H ratios ~1), regardless of the peroxide concentration, indicating a resistance to oxidation with hydrogen peroxide. These cysteines included C536 on succinate dehydrogenase A (SDHA) (Figure 1C). The cysteines that were oxidation-sensitive displayed variations in their concentration dependence, underscoring the unique redox susceptibilities of each individual cysteine. Some cysteines, such as C348 on Mitofusin 2 (MFN2), displayed steep linear decreases in their reactivity, indicating a high susceptibility to oxidation. MFN2 is an OMM protein central to mitochondrial network remodeling and inter-organelle contact (Figure 1C). MFN2 dysfunction has been implicated in mitophagy, unfolded protein responses, and the metabolic dysregulation characteristics of neurodegeneration, cardiomyopathy, and cancer [55]. C348 has not been previously identified to be redox-sensitive, but C684 is known to form an intermolecular disulfide with a cysteine on MFN1 to promote mitochondrial fusion [56]. Notably, C348 on MFN2 is located prior to an HR1 (heptad-repeating coiled-coil) domain analogous to the positioning of C684 and the HR2 domain, thereby supporting a potential redox function for C348, similar to C684 [57]. The cysteines that displayed a moderate peroxide sensitivity included C126 on the matrix-residing GrpE protein homolog 2 (GRPEL2) and C590 on mitochondrial aspartate tRNA ligase (DARS2) (Figure 1C). The trends in the cysteine redox sensitivity were further visualized with extracted ion chromatograms for each IA-L- and IA-H-labeled peptide (Figure 1D). Together, these concentration-dependent analyses enabled the ranking of the mitochondrial cysteines by their sensitivity to peroxide-mediated oxidation.

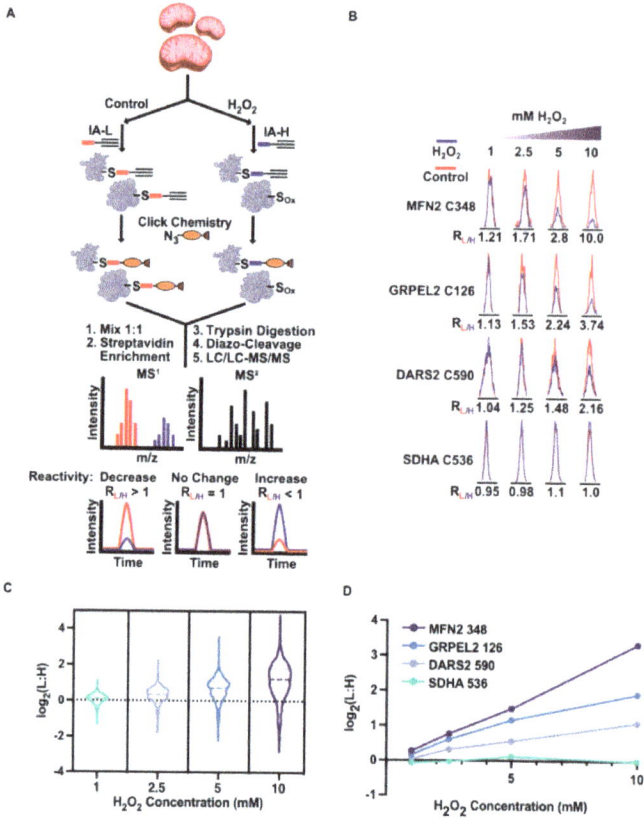

Figure 1. Analysis of mitochondrial cysteine reactivity in the presence of peroxide. (**A**) Workflow for evaluating peroxide-dependent changes in cysteine reactivity in isolated mitochondrial lysates using isoTOP-ABPP. Cysteines from control or peroxide-treated Mito-P lysates are labeled with IA-L or IA-H, respectively. Cleavable biotin-azide tags are then appended followed by enrichment of labeled cysteine-containing proteins on streptavidin resin, trypsin digestion, and isolation of labeled cysteine-containing peptides for quantitative MS analysis to identify and quantify cysteine reactivity changes due to oxidation by peroxide. (**B**) Violin plot displaying median L:H ratios for all identified cysteines with increasing concentrations of peroxide (1 mM, 2.5 mM, 5 mM, and 10 mM H_2O_2). (**C**) Plotted average L:H ratios ($\log_2$ L:H) of mitochondrial cysteines with increasing peroxide treatments. (**D**) Representative extracted ion chromatograms of cysteines from (**C**) alkylated by IA-L (red) or IA-H (blue) in the control and peroxide-treated samples, respectively.

3.3. Cysteine-Reactivity Changes of Known Redox-Sensitive Proteins

We focused on the dataset for the Mito-P lysates that were exposed to 10 mM of the peroxide (Figure 2A, Table S7), where the largest extent of cysteine oxidation was observed. Of the 785 cysteines that generated robust L:H ratios, 454 (58%) revealed at least a two-fold decrease in their reactivity, including 65 (8%) cysteines that displayed a higher than five-fold decrease. Within these highly peroxide-sensitive cysteines were well-characterized sites of oxidation, including C385 on aconitase 2 (ACO2) (an L:H ratio of 13.3) and C395 on 2-oxoglutarate dehydrogenase (OGDH) (an L:H ratio of 17.3) (Figure 2B). The oxidation of ACO2 and OGDH is known to inhibit protein function and attenuate the TCA cycle [17,58]. Interestingly, OGDH catalyzes the rate-limiting step of the TCA cycle and is the highest generator of mtROS outside of the ETC. OGDH is also known to be self-regulated through cysteine modifications such as glutathionylation [59,60]. The precise site(s) of cysteine oxidation that result in OGDH inhibition remain uncharacterized, however, C395 on OGDH has been previously shown to undergo S-nitrosation in a biotin-switch study on cardiac mitochondria [60].

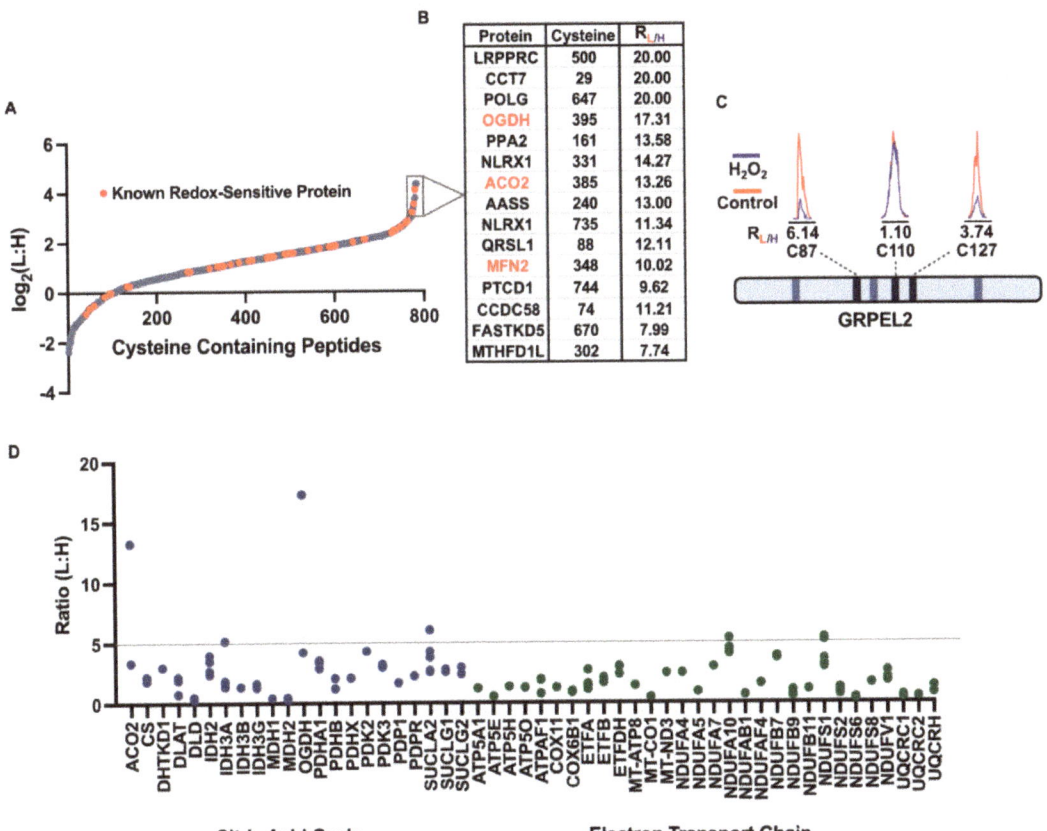

Figure 2. Evaluation of cysteine reactivity changes under 10 mM peroxide treatment using IsoTOP-ABPP. (**A**) L:H ratio plot (log$_2$L:H) of mitochondrial cysteines identified by isoTOP-ABPP upon 10 mM peroxide treatment. Previously characterized redox-sensitive proteins are annotated in red. (**B**) Inset highlights cysteine-containing peptides with the highest L:H ratios and previously characterized redox-sensitive proteins are in red. (**C**) Representative extracted ion chromatograms for cysteines identified from GRPEL2. Blue traces are from the untreated control and red traces are from the peroxide-treated sample. (**D**) Average L:H ratios for cysteines identified on proteins belonging to mitochondrial bioenergetic pathways including the citric acid cycle (blue), urea cycle (red), and electron transport chain (green) in the 10 mM peroxide isoTOP-ABPP dataset. High peroxide sensitivity (L:H ratio of 5) is denoted by a gray line.

Our data confirm that cysteines within a single protein can display widely divergent redox sensitivities. For instance, we identified three cysteines on GRPEL2 with varying redox sensitivities (Figure 2C). In the presence of the peroxide, the reactivity of C110 was preserved (an L:H ratio of 1.1), while C87 and C127 displayed L:H ratios of 6.1 and 3.7, respectively. The most redox-sensitive cysteine, C87, is known to facilitate a GRPEL2 dimer formation that protects against proteolysis during oxidative stress [61]. The identification of well-characterized sites of cysteine oxidation serves to validate the ability of our platform to accurately report on the redox sensitivities of mitochondrial cysteines.

3.4. Levels of Cysteine Oxidation within Key Mitochondrial Pathways

The most well-characterized redox-sensitive cysteines are known to reside within known ROS-regulated pathways [15]. Therefore, we sought to explore if the highly redox-sensitive cysteines that we identified were concentrated within specific mitochondrial processes or pathways. The cysteines identified from the 10 mM peroxide dataset were binned into 12 well-established biochemical classifications: the TCA cycle, innate immunity, transport, the urea cycle, fatty acid oxidation, redox regulation, Fe-S biogenesis, apoptosis, tRNA-ligases, mitochondrial (mt) ribosomal subunits, ETC, and mitochondrial transcription and translation (Figures 2D and S4). We observed that the redox-sensitive cysteines were distributed across these pathways and processes, but that some pathways had an increased number of highly redox-sensitive cysteines (>five-fold decrease in reactivity). Within the known redox-regulated metabolic pathways, the TCA cycle contained four proteins with highly redox-sensitive cysteines. These included the characterized redox-sensitive C385 on ACO2 and C395 on OGDH, which were mentioned previously, as well as poorly characterized cysteines on isocitrate dehydrogenase, IDH3A, and succinyl-CoA ligase, SUCLA2. Several subunits of the ETC (NDUFA10 and NDUFS1) also contained cysteines with a high redox sensitivity. Interestingly, the proteins involved in mitochondrial transcription and translation contained a high abundance of these redox-sensitive cysteines, including subunits of the mitochondrial ribosome, mRNA-processing enzymes, and DNA polymerase subunits. In support of this observation, the recent literature indicates that mtROS can regulate mitochondrial ribosome and aminoacyl tRNA complex formation [45,62]. Together, our data identify the highly redox-sensitive cysteines within the pathways that are known to be redox-regulated.

3.5. Inhibition of the Electron Transport Chain Induces ROS Generation and Cysteine Oxidation

The hydrogen peroxide treatments were geared toward enabling the ranking of the mitochondrial cysteines by their relative susceptibility to oxidation. The concentrations of peroxide that were used were supraphysiological, so as to push the levels of oxidation to a high stoichiometry that would differentiate the cysteines with high, medium, and low sensitivities to oxidation. The highly redox-sensitive cysteines that we identified correlated with the cysteines that were previously shown to be oxidized within (patho)physiological systems, suggesting that a high redox susceptibility in vitro can be predictive of in vivo sensitivity. To further evaluate this cysteine oxidation under physiological ROS conditions, we applied isoTOP-ABPP to assess the changes in cysteine reactivity and oxidation upon the inhibition of complex III with Antimycin A (AMA) (Figure 3A) [63], in order to release mtROS into the matrix and IMS.

To investigate the cysteine oxidation upon ETC inhibition, the cells were incubated with either AMA or DMSO (control) for 1 h prior to the fractionation and Mito-P isolation. The intact Mito-P fractions from the AMA-treated cells were labeled with IA-H, while the Mito-P from the control cells was labeled with IA-L. After lysis, the isoTOP-ABPP workflow was followed as previously described (Figure S3). The AMA-induced oxidation of a cysteine resulted in an increased L:H ratio. The resulting MS analysis provided robust L:H ratios for 828 cysteines on 432 mitochondrial proteins (Table S8). The proteome-wide impact of AMA on the cysteine reactivity was much less severe than that with an exogenous 10 mM peroxide treatment, generating a median L:H ratio of 1.4 compared to 2.3 for the peroxide.

The majority of the cysteines displayed L:H ratios of ~1 and were not affected by AMA. However, a small subset of 31 cysteines displayed >two-fold decreases in their reactivity, signifying increased oxidation upon the AMA treatment. Interestingly, C146 on Mitochondrial Ribosomal Protein L39 (MRPL39) exhibited the highest L:H value of 19.1 in the AMA-treated dataset. Based on the available structural data, C146 on MRPL39 is located proximal to C275 and could potentially form a disulfide bond under oxidative stress. Although MRPL39 has not been shown to be redox-regulated, proximal cysteines on adjacent MRPs have been identified to form disulfide bonds [64]. Furthermore, in yeast OxICAT studies [45], numerous proteins involved in mitochondrial translation have demonstrated high oxidation in the presence of peroxide, including MRPL32, indicating the potential for the MRP family, in general, to be regulated by mtROS [45,65].

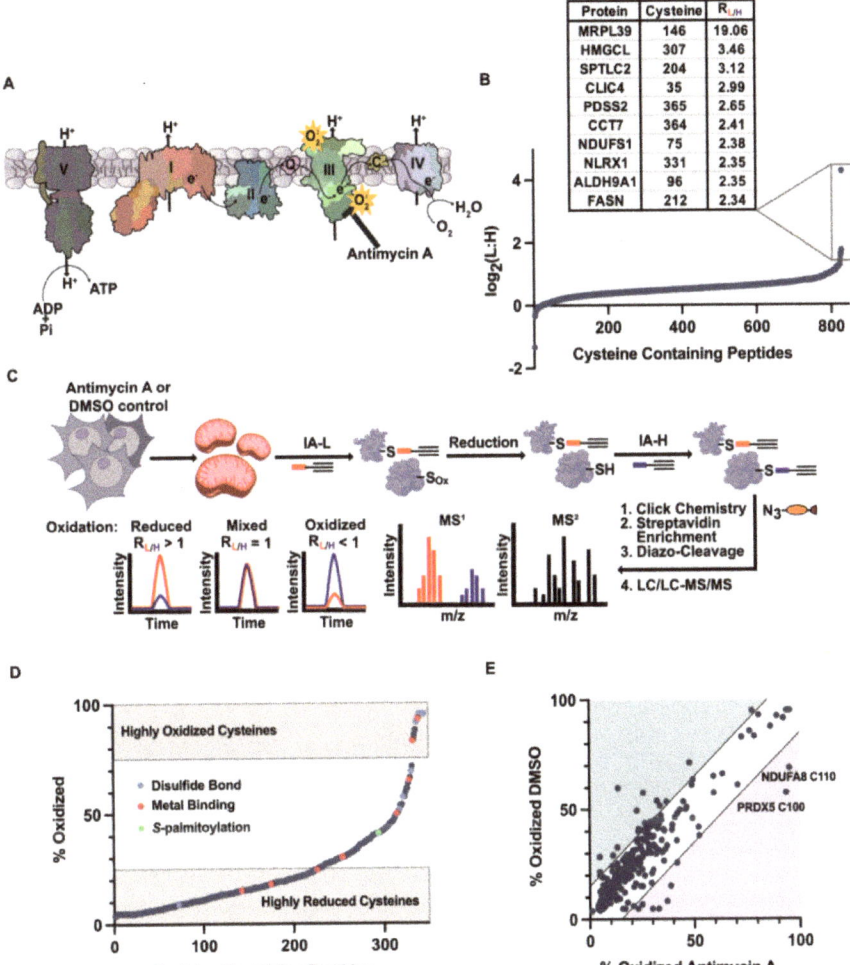

Figure 3. Cysteine reactivity and oxidation profiling under ETC inhibition. (A) Depiction of ETC inhibition of complex III by Antimycin A (AMA). Electron leakage and superoxide production occurs in both the mitochondrial matrix and IMS. (B) L:H ratio plot ($\log_2$L:H) of mitochondrial cysteine-containing peptides identified in isoTOP-ABPP analysis of Mito-P from AMA-treated cells. (C) OxICAT workflow in isolated mitochondria from DMSO-treated cells (control) or AMA-treated cells. Workflow includes differential alkylation of reduced and oxidized cysteine thiols with IA-L or IA-H followed by incorporation of cleavable biotin-azide tag for labeled cysteine-containing protein enrichment, trypsin digestion, and labeled cysteine-containing peptide isolation. L:H ratios directly correspond to percent oxidation values of cysteines. (D) Percent oxidation values for DMSO-treated mitochondria (control). UniProt annotation of cysteine residues that are disulfide linked (blue), metal binding (red) and s-palmitoylation (green). Percent oxidation is directly calculated from L:H and H:L ratios. (E) Percent oxidation values for DMSO- and AMA-treated mitochondria.

The correlation of the peroxide and AMA datasets identified cysteines that displayed decreases in their reactivity under both conditions. For instance, C331 on NLR Family Member X1 (NLRX1) displayed an average L:H ratio of 14.3 with 10 mM peroxide and 2.4 with AMA. NLRX1 is involved in antiviral signaling and injury prevention via the potentiation of ROS-driven immune activation [66]. NLRX1 is also known to negatively regulate the mitochondrial anti-viral signaling protein (MAVS), which is a redox-regulated protein that undergoes ROS-dependent oligomerization. Despite the implication of NLRX1 in ROS-dependent pathways, there has been no report of NLRX1 cysteines being the target of oxidation. Our studies identify C331 as a potential site of oxidation on NLRX1.

3.6. Monitoring Mitochondrial Cysteine Oxidation with OxICAT

Cysteine reactivity changes, as measured by isoTOP-ABPP, provide an indirect measure of cysteine oxidation through the observed decreases in the cysteine reactivity. A more direct method for analyzing this cysteine oxidation is through OxICAT [39], which uses the differential isotopic tagging of reduced and oxidized cysteines to directly monitor the cysteine oxidation within a single sample. Briefly, the proteins were denatured and the free thiols were alkylated with IA-L, followed by a reduction in the reversibly oxidized thiols and a subsequent labeling with IA-H (Figure 3C). Upon MS analysis, the resulting L:H ratios could be converted into % oxidation values to report on the stoichiometry of the oxidation for each identified cysteine. The Mito-P isolated from the AMA- or DMSO (control)-treated whole cells were subjected to OxICAT analyses.

In the control cells (Figure 3D, Table S9), a small subset of cysteines (8%) were found to be over 50% oxidized and included several annotated disulfide-linked and metal-binding cysteines. The disulfide-linked cysteines included C50 on mitochondrial import inner membrane translocase subunit TIMM13, which was 95% oxidized. This cysteine lies within a Cx3C motif and is predicted to participate in an intramolecular disulfide bond with C65. Additionally, the active site C80 on dihydrolipoamide dehydrogenase (DLD) was found to be highly oxidized (95%). This cysteine is known to form a redox-active disulfide bond with C85. Lastly, several disulfide-linked cysteines, C30, C54, and C65, on cytochrome C oxidase subunit 6B1 (COX6B1), were identified, and each were 95% oxidized.

AMA treatment results in an observable increase in the oxidation for several cysteines (Figure 3E, Table S9). The cysteines that displayed increased oxidation upon AMA treatment included the peroxidatic cysteine, C100, on peroxiredoxin 5, PRDX5, with a 58% oxidation in the control sample compared to a 94% oxidation in the AMA-treated sample. PRDX5 is an antioxidant enzyme critical in the regulation of peroxide levels and protection of the cell from irreversible oxidative damage under high levels of oxidative stress [67]. C100 is known to become sulfenylated and form a redox-active disulfide bond with C204 [68,69]. Interestingly, the resolving cysteine of PRDX5, C204, was identified to have a 92% oxidation in both the control and AMA-treated samples. Lastly, C110 on NADH dehydrogenase 1 alpha subcomplex subunit (NDUFA8), a complex I subunit, displayed increased oxidation upon the AMA treatment (95% oxidized) compared to the control treatment (70% oxidized). This cysteine is a part of the four CX_9C motifs on NDUFA8 that undergo a disulfide exchange, which is dependent on the redox conditions of the IMS [70,71]. The identification of the known sites of cysteine oxidation supports the use of mitochondrial fractionation and OxICAT to directly monitor these sites upon the induction of endogenous oxidative stress.

4. Discussion

Mitochondria are intricate organelles central to a variety of cellular functions, including aerobic respiration. Many mitochondrial processes can be regulated by an ROS-mediated oxidation of the key mitochondrial cysteines. Although several sites of cysteine oxidation on mitochondrial proteins and the functional consequences of this oxidation have been identified, there is a continued interest in globally assessing the redox sensitivity of these mitochondrial cysteines. Identifying new sites of cysteine oxidation in mitochondria can unearth uncharacterized redox-regulated proteins and pathways.

Here, we describe the use of mitochondrial enrichment by differential centrifugation coupled with redox proteomic platforms, such as isoTOP-ABPP and OxICAT, to identify redox-sensitive cysteines under exogenous and endogenous ROS treatments. The differential centrifugation afforded Mito-P fractions that were analyzed using mass spectrometry and confirmed to be highly enriched in mitochondrial proteins, relative to the whole-cell samples. These Mito-P fractions were then subjected to exogenous hydrogen peroxide treatments and analyzed using isoTOP-ABPP. The hydrogen peroxide concentrations used were supraphysiological, but were chosen to differentiate the cysteines with a high sensitivity to oxidation (highly oxidized at the lowest peroxide concentration used) from those with moderate and low sensitivities to oxidation. Our data enabled the rank ordering of the mitochondrial cysteines by their sensitivity to oxidation and identified the mitochondrial pathways that were enriched in highly redox-sensitive cysteines. Importantly, many of the cysteines identified within the high redox sensitivity category had been previously reported to be oxidized under physiologically relevant levels of oxidative stress.

We then treated cells with the ETC inhibitor Antimycin and applied isoTOP-ABPP and OxICAT to identify the cysteines that were oxidized upon the induction of endogenous reactive oxygen species. The isoTOP-ABPP platform is an indirect method that identifies sites of oxidation through a loss of cysteine reactivity, whereas OxICAT more directly monitors reversible cysteine oxidation events through differential cysteine labeling. These two methods are complementary to each other and differ in their cysteine coverage and the types of oxPTMs that are detectable. Their key differences include the fact that OxICAT will only identify reversible oxidation events (i.e., sulfenic acids and disulfides), whereas isoTOP-ABPP can identify both reversible and irreversible sites of oxidation. Additionally, fully oxidized cysteines, such as those engaged in stable disulfide linkages, can only be identified via an OxICAT analysis, as cysteines that are 100% oxidized are not captured by an isoTOP-ABPP analysis. Lastly, isoTOP-ABPP applies low (100 uM) concentrations of a cysteine-reactive probe to fully folded proteins, resulting in the labeling of only highly reactive cysteines. In contrast, OxICAT applies high (10 mM) concentrations of a cysteine-alkylating agent to fully denatured proteomes, resulting in the labeling of all cysteines, regardless of their reactivity. For these reasons, the cysteines identified by these two methods do not show a complete overlap (Figure S5) and provide access to different subsets of cysteines. The use of both platforms provides a broader snapshot of the cysteine oxidation events that occur in the mitochondria upon the induction of reactive oxygen species. As with the exogenous peroxide treatment, many of the cysteines that were identified to be oxidized in the isoTOP-ABPP and OxICAT analyses of the antimycin-treated mitochondria were previously reported as sites of cysteine oxidation.

5. Conclusions

In summary, we combine isoTOP-ABPP and oxICAT redox proteomic methods, together with mitochondrial isolation, to provide a snapshot of the cysteine oxidation events that accompany both exogenous and endogenous ROS exposure. Our combined datasets identify many previously characterized sites of oxidation, but also unearth unannotated sites of oxidation on proteins that could potentially regulate diverse mitochondrial processes under oxidative stress. This work sets the foundation for a more extensive exploration of mitochondrial cysteine oxidation. The use of more stringent mitochondrial fractionation methods, as well as an improved MS sensitivity, will likely serve to improve mitochondrial cysteine coverage.

Supplementary Materials: The following supporting information can be downloaded at: https://www.mdpi.com/article/10.3390/antiox12050992/s1, Figure S1: Evaluation of mitochondrial isolation by differential centrifugation; Figure S2: Probe structures used for MS experiments; Figure S3: Workflow for quantifying redox-dependent changes in cysteine reactivity in isolated mitochondria using IsoTOP-ABPP; Figure S4: L:H ratios plotted from isoTOP-ABPP analysis of 10 mM peroxide treated Mito-P samples; Figure S5: Overlap between isoTOP-ABPP analysis and OxICAT analysis for all identified cysteines; Table S1: Annotated list of mitochondrial peptides identified in the Mito-P sample; Table S2: Gene ontology (GO) analysis for enrichment of biological processes for proteins identified in whole cell sample; Table S3: Gene ontology (GO) analysis for enrichment of biological processes for proteins identified in whole cell sample; Table S4: Filtered list of L:H ratio values obtained for isoTOP-ABPP analysis of all mitochondrial cysteines identified in Mito-P lysates treated with 1 mM H_2O_2; Table S5: Filtered list of L:H ratio values obtained for isoTOP-ABPP analysis of all mitochondrial cysteines identified in Mito-P lysates treated with 2.5 mM H_2O_2; Table S6: Filtered list of L:H ratio values obtained for isoTOP-ABPP analysis of all mitochondrial cysteines identified in Mito-P lysates treated with 5 mM H_2O_2; Table S7: Filtered list of L:H ratio values obtained for isoTOP-ABPP analysis of all mitochondrial cysteines identified in Mito-P lysates treated with 10 mM H_2O_2; Table S8: Filtered list of L:H ratio values obtained from IsoTOP-ABPP analysis of all mitochondrial cysteines identified in Mito-P isolated from whole cells treated with Antimycin A (AMA) or DMSO for 1 h; Table S9: Filtered list of L:H ratios and % oxidation values calculated for mitochondrial cysteines identified in OxICAT analysis of Mito-P isolated from whole cells treated with Antimycin A (AMA) or DMSO for 1 h.

Author Contributions: Conceptualization, E.A.K. and E.W.; Methodology, E.A.K. and E.W.; Software, E.A.K.; Validation, E.A.K. and E.W.; Formal Analysis, E.A.K. and E.C.S.; Investigation E.A.K.; Resources, E.W.; Data Curation, E.A.K.; Writing—Original Draft Preparation, E.A.K. and E.W.; Writing—Review and Editing, E.A.K. and E.W.; Visualization, E.A.K.; Supervision, E.W.; Project Administration, E.A.K. and E.W.; Funding Acquisition, E.W. All authors have read and agreed to the published version of the manuscript.

Funding: This research was funded by NIH grant number R35GM134964.

Institutional Review Board Statement: Not applicable.

Informed Consent Statement: Not applicable.

Data Availability Statement: All data in the manuscript are available from the corresponding author.

Acknowledgments: This work was supported by NIH R35GM134964 to E.W. We thank members of the Weerapana Lab for helpful discussions and critical reading of the manuscript.

Conflicts of Interest: E.W. is a paid consultant for Odyssey Therapeutics. E.A.K and E.C.S. have no competing interests to declare.

References

1. FFriedman, J.R.; Nunnari, J. Mitochondrial form and function. *Nature* **2014**, *505*, 335–343. [CrossRef] [PubMed]
2. Riemer, J.; Bulleid, N.; Herrmann, J.M. Disulfide Formation in the ER and Mitochondria: Two Solutions to a Common Process. *Science* **2009**, *324*, 1284–1287. [CrossRef] [PubMed]
3. Hell, K. The Erv1–Mia40 disulfide relay system in the intermembrane space of mitochondria. *Biochim. Biophys. Acta (BBA)—Mol. Cell Res.* **2008**, *1783*, 601–609. [CrossRef]
4. Redza-Dutordoir, M.; Averill-Bates, D.A. Activation of apoptosis signalling pathways by reactive oxygen species. *Biochim. Biophys. Acta (BBA)—Mol. Cell Res.* **2016**, *1863*, 2977–2992. [CrossRef]
5. Wang, C.; Youle, R.J. The Role of Mitochondria in Apoptosis. *Annu. Rev. Genet.* **2009**, *43*, 95–118. [CrossRef]
6. Spinelli, J.B.; Haigis, M.C. The multifaceted contributions of mitochondria to cellular metabolism. *Nature* **2018**, *20*, 745–754. [CrossRef] [PubMed]
7. Lane, N.; Martin, W. The energetics of genome complexity. *Nature* **2010**, *467*, 929–934. [CrossRef]
8. Ott, M.; Gogvadze, V.; Orrenius, S.; Zhivotovsky, B. Mitochondria, oxidative stress and cell death. *Apoptosis* **2007**, *12*, 913–922. [CrossRef]
9. Paulsen, C.E.; Carroll, K.S. Cysteine-Mediated Redox Signaling: Chemistry, Biology, and Tools for Discovery. *Chem. Rev.* **2013**, *113*, 4633–4679. [CrossRef]
10. Bechtel, T.J.; Weerapana, E. From structure to redox: The diverse functional roles of disulfides and implications in disease. *Proteomics* **2017**, *17*, 1600391. [CrossRef]
11. Morgan, M.J.; Liu, Z.-G. Crosstalk of reactive oxygen species and NF-kappaκB signaling. *Cell Res.* **2011**, *21*, 103–115. [CrossRef] [PubMed]
12. Canet-Avilés, R.M.; Wilson, M.A.; Miller, D.W.; Ahmad, R.; McLendon, C.; Bandyopadhyay, S.; Baptista, M.J.; Ringe, D.; Petsko, G.A.; Cookson, M.R. The Parkinson's disease protein DJ-1 is neuroprotective due to cysteine-sulfinic acid-driven mitochondrial localization. *Proc. Natl. Acad. Sci. USA* **2004**, *101*, 9103–9108. [CrossRef]
13. Aiken, C.T.; Kaake, R.M.; Wang, X.; Huang, L. Oxidative Stress-Mediated Regulation of Proteasome Complexes. *Mol. Cell. Proteom.* **2011**, *10*, R110.006924. [CrossRef] [PubMed]

14. Sena, L.A.; Chandel, N.S. Physiological roles of mitochondrial reactive oxygen species. *Mol. Cell* **2012**, *48*, 158–167. [CrossRef] [PubMed]
15. Groitl, B.; Jakob, U. Thiol-based redox switches. *Biochim. Biophys. Acta (BBA)—Proteins Proteom.* **2014**, *1844*, 1335–1343. [CrossRef] [PubMed]
16. Cantu, D.; Schaack, J.; Patel, M. Oxidative Inactivation of Mitochondrial Aconitase Results in Iron and H_2O_2-Mediated Neurotoxicity in Rat Primary Mesencephalic Cultures. *PLoS ONE* **2009**, *4*, e7095. [CrossRef]
17. Lushchak, O.V.; Piroddi, M.; Galli, F.; Lushchak, V.I. Aconitase post-translational modification as a key in linkage between Krebs cycle, iron homeostasis, redox signaling, and metabolism of reactive oxygen species. *Redox Rep.* **2014**, *19*, 8–15. [CrossRef]
18. Chouchani, E.T.; Methner, C.; Nadtochiy, S.M.; Logan, A.; Pell, V.R.; Ding, S.; James, A.M.; Cochemé, H.M.; Reinhold, J.; Lilley, K.S.; et al. Cardioprotection by S-nitrosation of a cysteine switch on mitochondrial complex I. *Nat. Med.* **2013**, *19*, 753–759. [CrossRef]
19. Burger, N.; James, A.M.; Mulvey, J.F.; Hoogewijs, K.; Ding, S.; Fearnley, I.M.; Loureiro-López, M.; Norman, A.A.; Arndt, S.; Mottahedin, A.; et al. ND3 Cys39 in complex I is exposed during mitochondrial respiration. *Cell Chem. Biol.* **2021**, *29*, 636–649.e14. [CrossRef]
20. Chouchani, E.T.; Kazak, L.; Jedrychowski, M.P.; Lu, G.Z.; Erickson, B.K.; Szpyt, J.; Pierce, K.A.; Laznik-Bogoslavski, D.; Vetrivelan, R.; Clish, C.B.; et al. Mitochondrial ROS regulate thermogenic energy expenditure and sulfenylation of UCP1. *Nature* **2016**, *532*, 112–116. [CrossRef]
21. Ježek, P.; Jabůrek, M.; Porter, R.K. Uncoupling mechanism and redox regulation of mitochondrial uncoupling protein 1 (UCP1). *Biochim. Biophys. Acta (BBA)—Bioenerg.* **2019**, *1860*, 259–269. [CrossRef] [PubMed]
22. Sullivan, L.B.; Chandel, N.S. Mitochondrial reactive oxygen species and cancer. *Cancer Metab.* **2014**, *2*, 17. [CrossRef] [PubMed]
23. Chen, J.; Stimpson, S.; Fernandez-Bueno, G.A.; Mathews, C.E. Mitochondrial Reactive Oxygen Species and Type 1 Diabetes. *Antioxid. Redox Signal.* **2018**, *29*, 1361–1372. [CrossRef] [PubMed]
24. Kaludercic, N.; Di Lisa, F. Mitochondrial ROS Formation in the Pathogenesis of Diabetic Cardiomyopathy. *Front. Cardiovasc. Med.* **2020**, *7*, 12. [CrossRef]
25. Lin, M.T.; Beal, M.F. Mitochondrial dysfunction and oxidative stress in neurodegenerative diseases. *Nature* **2006**, *443*, 787–795. [CrossRef] [PubMed]
26. Moris, D.; Spartalis, M.; Spartalis, E.; Karachaliou, G.-S.; Karaolanis, G.I.; Tsourouflis, G.; Tsilimigras, D.I.; Tzatzaki, E.; Theocharis, S. The role of reactive oxygen species in the pathophysiology of cardiovascular diseases and the clinical significance of myocardial redox. *Ann. Transl. Med.* **2017**, *5*, 326. [CrossRef]
27. Thul, P.J.; Åkesson, L.; Wiking, M.; Mahdessian, D.; Geladaki, A.; Ait Blal, H.; Alm, T.; Asplund, A.; Björk, L.; Breckels, L.M.; et al. A subcellular map of the human proteome. *Science* **2017**, *356*, eaal3321. [CrossRef]
28. Uhlén, M.; Fagerberg, L.; Hallström, B.M.; Lindskog, C.; Oksvold, P.; Mardinoglu, A.; Sivertsson, Å.; Kampf, C.; Sjöstedt, E.; Asplund, A.; et al. Tissue-based map of the human proteome. *Science* **2015**, *347*, 1260419. [CrossRef]
29. Frezza, C.; Cipolat, S.; Scorrano, L. Organelle isolation: Functional mitochondria from mouse liver, muscle and cultured filroblasts. *Nat. Protoc.* **2007**, *2*, 287–295. [CrossRef]
30. Shi, Y.; Fu, L.; Yang, J.; Carroll, K.S. Wittig reagents for chemoselective sulfenic acid ligation enables global site stoichiometry analysis and redox-controlled mitochondrial targeting. *Nat. Chem.* **2021**, *13*, 1140–1150. [CrossRef]
31. Yasueda, Y.; Tamura, T.; Fujisawa, A.; Kuwata, K.; Tsukiji, S.; Kiyonaka, S.; Hamachi, I. A Set of Organelle-Localizable Reactive Molecules for Mitochondrial Chemical Proteomics in Living Cells and Brain Tissues. *J. Am. Chem. Soc.* **2016**, *138*, 7592–7602. [CrossRef]
32. Alcock, L.J.; Oliveira, B.L.; Deery, M.J.; Pukala, T.L.; Perkins, M.V.; Bernardes, G.J.L.; Chalker, J.M. Norbornene Probes for the Detection of Cysteine Sulfenic Acid in Cells. *ACS Chem. Biol.* **2019**, *14*, 594–598. [CrossRef] [PubMed]
33. Akter, S.; Fu, L.; Jung, Y.; Conte, M.L.; Lawson, J.R.; Lowther, W.T.; Sun, R.; Liu, K.; Yang, J.; Carroll, K.S. Chemical proteomics reveals new targets of cysteine sulfinic acid reductase. *Nat. Chem. Biol.* **2018**, *14*, 995–1004. [CrossRef] [PubMed]
34. Meng, J.; Fu, L.; Liu, K.; Tian, C.; Wu, Z.; Jung, Y.; Ferreira, R.B.; Carroll, K.S.; Blackwell, T.K.; Yang, J. Global profiling of distinct cysteine redox forms reveals wide-ranging redox regulation in C. elegans. *Nat. Commun.* **2021**, *12*, 1415. [CrossRef] [PubMed]
35. Paulsen, C.E.; Carroll, K.S. Chemical Dissection of an Essential Redox Switch in Yeast. *Chem. Biol.* **2009**, *16*, 217–225. [CrossRef] [PubMed]
36. Roux, K.J.; Kim, D.I.; Raida, M.; Burke, B. A promiscuous biotin ligase fusion protein identifies proximal and interacting proteins in mammalian cells. *J. Cell Biol.* **2012**, *196*, 801–810. [CrossRef]
37. Branon, T.C.; Bosch, J.A.; Sanchez, A.D.; Udeshi, N.D.; Svinkina, T.; Carr, S.A.; Feldman, J.L.; Perrimon, N.; Ting, A.Y. Efficient proximity labeling in living cells and organisms with TurboID. *Nat. Biotechnol.* **2018**, *36*, 880–887. [CrossRef]
38. Hung, V.; Udeshi, N.D.; Lam, S.S.-M.; Loh, K.H.; Cox, K.J.; Pedram, K.; Carr, S.A.; Ting, Y. Spatially resolved proteomic mapping in living cells with the engineered peroxidase APEX2. *Nat. Protoc.* **2016**, *11*, 456–475. [CrossRef]
39. Hung, V.; Zou, P.; Rhee, H.-W.; Udeshi, N.D.; Cracan, V.; Svinkina, T.; Carr, S.A.; Mootha, V.K.; Ting, A.Y. Proteomic Mapping of the Human Mitochondrial Intermembrane Space in Live Cells via Ratiometric APEX Tagging. *Mol. Cell* **2014**, *55*, 332–341. [CrossRef]
40. Rhee, H.-W.; Zou, P.; Udeshi, N.D.; Martell, J.D.; Mootha, V.K.; Carr, S.A.; Ting, A.Y. Proteomic Mapping of Mitochondria in Living Cells via Spatially Restricted Enzymatic Tagging. *Science* **2013**, *339*, 1328–1331. [CrossRef]

41. Wang, H.; Zhang, Y.; Zeng, K.; Qiang, J.; Cao, Y.; Li, Y.; Fang, Y.; Zhang, Y.; Chen, Y. Selective Mitochondrial Protein Labeling Enabled by Biocompatible Photocatalytic Reactions inside Live Cells. *JACS Au* **2021**, *1*, 1066–1075. [CrossRef] [PubMed]
42. Bak, D.W.; Pizzagalli, M.D.; Weerapana, E. Identifying Functional Cysteine Residues in the Mitochondria. *ACS Chem. Biol.* **2017**, *12*, 947–957. [CrossRef] [PubMed]
43. Leichert, L.I.; Gehrke, F.; Gudiseva, H.V.; Blackwell, T.; Ilbert, M.; Walker, A.K.; Strahler, J.R.; Andrews, P.C.; Jakob, U. Quantifying changes in the thiol redox proteome upon oxidative stress in vivo. *Proc. Natl. Acad. Sci. USA* **2008**, *105*, 8197–8202. [CrossRef] [PubMed]
44. Bechtel, T.J.; Li, C.; Kisty, E.A.; Maurais, A.J.; Weerapana, E. Profiling Cysteine Reactivity and Oxidation in the Endoplasmic Reticulum. *ACS Chem. Biol.* **2020**, *15*, 543–553. [CrossRef]
45. Topf, U.; Suppanz, I.; Samluk, L.; Wrobel, L.; Böser, A.; Sakowska, P.; Knapp, B.; Pietrzyk, M.K.; Chacinska, A.; Warscheid, B. Quantitative proteomics identifies redox switches for global translation modulation by mitochondrially produced reactive oxygen species. *Nat. Commun.* **2018**, *9*, 324. [CrossRef]
46. Menger, K.E.; James, A.M.; Cochemé, H.M.; Harbour, M.E.; Chouchani, E.T.; Ding, S.; Fearnley, I.M.; Partridge, L.; Murphy, M.P. Fasting, but Not Aging, Dramatically Alters the Redox Status of Cysteine Residues on Proteins in Drosophila melanogaster. *Cell Rep.* **2015**, *11*, 1856–1865. [CrossRef]
47. Abo, M.; Li, C.; Weerapana, E. Isotopically-Labeled Iodoacetamide-Alkyne Probes for Quantitative Cysteine-Reactivity Profiling. *Mol. Pharm.* **2017**, *15*, 743–749. [CrossRef]
48. Weerapana, E.; Wang, C.; Simon, G.M.; Richter, F.; Khare, S.; Dillon, M.B.D.; Bachovchin, D.A.; Mowen, K.; Baker, D.; Cravatt, B.F. Quantitative reactivity profiling predicts functional cysteines in proteomes. *Nature* **2010**, *468*, 790–795. [CrossRef]
49. Eng, J.K.; McCormack, A.L.; Yates, J.R. An approach to correlate tandem mass spectral data of peptides with amino acid sequences in a protein database. *J. Am. Soc. Mass Spectrom.* **1994**, *5*, 976–989. [CrossRef]
50. Tabb, D.L.; McDonald, W.H.; Yates, J.R.R. DTASelect and Contrast: Tools for Assembling and Comparing Protein Identifications from Shotgun Proteomics. *J. Proteome Res.* **2002**, *1*, 21–26. [CrossRef]
51. The UniProt Consortium. UniProt: The universal protein knowledgebase in 2021. *Nucleic Acids Res.* **2021**, *49*, D480–D489. [CrossRef] [PubMed]
52. Rath, S.; Sharma, R.; Gupta, R.; Ast, T.; Chan, C.; Durham, T.J.; Goodman, R.P.; Grabarek, Z.; Haas, M.E.; Hung, W.H.W.; et al. MitoCarta3.0: An updated mitochondrial proteome now with sub-organelle localization and pathway annotations. *Nucleic Acids Res.* **2021**, *49*, D1541–D1547. [CrossRef] [PubMed]
53. Mi, H.; Ebert, D.; Muruganujan, A.; Mills, C.; Albou, L.-P.; Mushayamaha, T.; Thomas, P.D. PANTHER version 16: A revised family classification, tree-based classification tool, enhancer regions and extensive API. *Nucleic Acids Res.* **2021**, *49*, D394–D403. [CrossRef] [PubMed]
54. Calvo, S.E.; Clauser, K.R.; Mootha, V.K. MitoCarta2.0: An updated inventory of mammalian mitochondrial proteins. *Nucleic Acids Res.* **2016**, *44*, D1251–D1257. [CrossRef] [PubMed]
55. Filadi, R.; Pendin, D.; Pizzo, P. Mitofusin 2: From functions to disease. *Cell Death Dis.* **2018**, *9*, 330. [CrossRef] [PubMed]
56. Thaher, O.; Wolf, C.; Dey, P.N.; Pouya, A.; Wüllner, V.; Tenzer, S.; Methner, A. The thiol switch C684 in Mitofusin-2 mediates redox-induced alterations of mitochondrial shape and respiration. *Neurochem. Int.* **2018**, *117*, 167–173. [CrossRef]
57. Wolf, C.; López Del Amo, V.; Arndt, S.; Bueno, D.; Tenzer, S.; Hanschmann, E.-M.; Berndt, C.; Methner, A. Redox Modifications of Proteins of the Mitochondrial Fusion and Fission Machinery. *Cells* **2020**, *9*, 815. [CrossRef]
58. McLain, A.L.; Szweda, P.A.; Szweda, L.I. α-Ketoglutarate dehydrogenase: A mitochondrial redox sensor. *Free. Radic. Res.* **2010**, *45*, 29–36. [CrossRef]
59. Mailloux, R.J.; Ayre, D.C.; Christian, S.L. Induction of mitochondrial reactive oxygen species production by GSH mediated S-glutathionylation of 2-oxoglutarate dehydrogenase. *Redox Biol.* **2016**, *8*, 285–297. [CrossRef]
60. Murray, C.I.; Kane, L.A.; Uhrigshardt, H.; Wang, S.-B.; Van Eyk, J.E. Site-Mapping of In Vitro S-nitrosation in Cardiac Mitochondria: Implications for Cardioprotection. *Mol. Cell. Proteom.* **2011**, *10*, M110.004721. [CrossRef]
61. Konovalova, S.; Liu, X.; Manjunath, P.; Baral, S.; Neupane, N.; Hilander, T.; Yang, Y.; Balboa, D.; Terzioglu, M.; Euro, L.; et al. Redox regulation of GRPEL2 nucleotide exchange factor for mitochondrial HSP70 chaperone. *Redox Biol.* **2018**, *19*, 37–45. [CrossRef] [PubMed]
62. Xiao, H.; Jedrychowski, M.P.; Schweppe, D.K.; Huttlin, E.L.; Yu, Q.; Heppner, D.E.; Li, J.; Long, J.; Mills, E.L.; Szpyt, J.; et al. A Quantitative Tissue-Specific Landscape of Protein Redox Regulation during Aging. *Cell* **2020**, *180*, 968–983.e24. [CrossRef] [PubMed]
63. Quinlan, C.L.; Gerencser, A.A.; Treberg, J.R.; Brand, M.D. The Mechanism of Superoxide Production by the Antimycin-inhibited Mitochondrial Q-cycle. *J. Biol. Chem.* **2011**, *286*, 31361–31372. [CrossRef] [PubMed]
64. De Silva, D.; Tu, Y.-T.; Amunts, A.; Fontanesi, F.; Barrientos, A. Mitochondrial ribosome assembly in health and disease. *Cell Cycle* **2015**, *14*, 2226–2250. [CrossRef] [PubMed]
65. Bonn, F.; Tatsuta, T.; Petrungaro, C.; Riemer, J.; Langer, T. Presequence-dependent folding ensures MrpL32 processing by the m-AAA protease in mitochondria. *EMBO J.* **2011**, *30*, 2545–2556. [CrossRef]
66. Nagai-Singer, M.A.; Morrison, H.A.; Allen, I.C. NLRX1 Is a Multifaceted and Enigmatic Regulator of Immune System Function. *Front. Immunol.* **2019**, *10*, 2419. [CrossRef]

67. De Simoni, S.; Linard, D.; Hermans, E.; Knoops, B.; Goemaere, J. Mitochondrial peroxiredoxin-5 as potential modulator of mitochondria-ER crosstalk in MPP$^+$-induced cell death. *J. Neurochem.* **2013**, *125*, 473–485. [CrossRef]
68. Seo, M.S.; Kang, S.W.; Kim, K.; Baines, I.C.; Lee, T.H.; Rhee, S.G. Identification of a New Type of Mammalian Peroxiredoxin That Forms an Intramolecular Disulfide as a Reaction Intermediate. *J. Biol. Chem.* **2000**, *275*, 20346–20354. [CrossRef]
69. Smeets, A.; Marchand, C.; Linard, D.; Knoops, B.; Declercq, J.-P. The crystal structures of oxidized forms of human peroxiredoxin 5 with an intramolecular disulfide bond confirm the proposed enzymatic mechanism for atypical 2-Cys peroxiredoxins. *Arch. Biochem. Biophys.* **2008**, *477*, 98–104. [CrossRef]
70. Szklarczyk, R.; Wanschers, B.F.; Nabuurs, S.B.; Nouws, J.; Nijtmans, L.G.; Huynen, M.A. NDUFB7 and NDUFA8 are located at the intermembrane surface of complex I. *FEBS Lett.* **2011**, *585*, 737–743. [CrossRef]
71. Fischer, M.; Horn, S.; Belkacemi, A.; Kojer, K.; Petrungaro, C.; Habich, M.; Ali, M.; Küttner, V.; Bien, M.; Kauff, F.; et al. Protein import and oxidative folding in the mitochondrial intermembrane space of intact mammalian cells. *Mol. Biol. Cell* **2013**, *24*, 2160–2170. [CrossRef] [PubMed]

Disclaimer/Publisher's Note: The statements, opinions and data contained in all publications are solely those of the individual author(s) and contributor(s) and not of MDPI and/or the editor(s). MDPI and/or the editor(s) disclaim responsibility for any injury to people or property resulting from any ideas, methods, instructions or products referred to in the content.

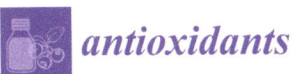

Article

Synthesis of Sulfides and Persulfides Is Not Impeded by Disruption of Three Canonical Enzymes in Sulfur Metabolism

Qamarul Hafiz Zainol Abidin [1,†], Tomoaki Ida [1,†], Masanobu Morita [1,*,†], Tetsuro Matsunaga [1,†], Akira Nishimura [1], Minkyung Jung [1], Naim Hassan [1], Tsuyoshi Takata [1], Isao Ishii [2], Warren Kruger [3], Rui Wang [4], Hozumi Motohashi [5], Masato Tsutsui [6,*] and Takaaki Akaike [1,*]

[1] Department of Environmental Medicine and Molecular Toxicology, Tohoku University Graduate School of Medicine, Sendai 980-8575, Japan
[2] Department of Health Chemistry, Showa Pharmaceutical University, Machida, Tokyo 194-8543, Japan
[3] Molecular Therapeutics Program, Fox Chase Cancer Center, Philadelphia, PA 19111-2497, USA
[4] Faculty of Science, York University, Toronto, ON M3J 1P3, Canada
[5] Department of Gene Expression Regulation, Institute of Development, Aging and Cancer, Tohoku University, Sendai 980-8575, Japan
[6] Department of Pharmacology, Graduate School of Medicine, University of the Ryukyus, Okinawa 903-0213, Japan
* Correspondence: morita@med.tohoku.ac.jp (M.M.); tsutsui@med.u-ryukyu.ac.jp (M.T.); takaike@med.tohoku.ac.jp (T.A.); Tel.: +81-22-717-8105 (M.M.); +81-98-895-1133 (M.T.); +81-22-717-8101 (T.A.); Fax: +81-22-717-8219 (M.M.); +81-98-895-1411 (M.T.); +81-22-717-8219 (T.A)
† These authors contributed equally to this work.

Abstract: Reactive sulfur species, or persulfides and polysulfides, such as cysteine hydropersulfide and glutathione persulfide, are endogenously produced in abundance in both prokaryotes and eukaryotes, including mammals. Various forms of reactive persulfides occur in both low-molecular-weight and protein-bound thiols. The chemical properties and great supply of these molecular species suggest a pivotal role for reactive persulfides/polysulfides in different cellular regulatory processes (e.g., energy metabolism and redox signaling). We demonstrated earlier that cysteinyl-tRNA synthetase (CARS) is a new cysteine persulfide synthase (CPERS) and is responsible for the in vivo production of most reactive persulfides (polysulfides). Some researchers continue to suggest that 3-mercaptopyruvate sulfurtransferase (3-MST), cystathionine β-synthase (CBS), and cystathionine γ-lyase (CSE) may also produce hydrogen sulfide and persulfides that may be generated during the transfer of sulfur from 3-mercaptopyruvate to the cysteine residues of 3-MST or direct synthesis from cysteine by CBS/CSE, respectively. We thus used integrated sulfur metabolome analysis, which we recently developed, with 3-MST knockout (KO) mice and CBS/CSE/3-MST triple-KO mice, to elucidate the possible contribution of 3-MST, CBS, and CSE to the production of reactive persulfides in vivo. We therefore quantified various sulfide metabolites in organs derived from these mutant mice and their wild-type littermates via this sulfur metabolome, which clearly revealed no significant difference between mutant mice and wild-type mice in terms of reactive persulfide production. This result indicates that 3-MST, CBS, and CSE are not major sources of endogenous reactive persulfide production; rather, CARS/CPERS is the principal enzyme that is actually involved in and even primarily responsible for the biosynthesis of reactive persulfides and polysulfides in vivo in mammals.

Keywords: cystathionine β-synthase; cystathionine γ-lyase; cysteine persulfide synthase; cysteinyl-tRNA synthetases; 3-mercaptopyruvate sulfurtransferase; reactive persulfides/polysulfides

Citation: Zainol Abidin, Q.H.; Ida, T.; Morita, M.; Matsunaga, T.; Nishimura, A.; Jung, M.; Hassan, N.; Takata, T.; Ishii, I.; Kruger, W.; et al. Synthesis of Sulfides and Persulfides Is Not Impeded by Disruption of Three Canonical Enzymes in Sulfur Metabolism. *Antioxidants* **2023**, *12*, 868. https://doi.org/10.3390/antiox12040868

Received: 31 January 2023
Revised: 24 March 2023
Accepted: 31 March 2023
Published: 3 April 2023

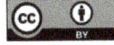

Copyright: © 2023 by the authors. Licensee MDPI, Basel, Switzerland. This article is an open access article distributed under the terms and conditions of the Creative Commons Attribution (CC BY) license (https://creativecommons.org/licenses/by/4.0/).

1. Introduction

Sulfides and persulfides/polysulfides (RSS_nH, RSS_nR, HSS_nH, $CysSS_nH$) are abundant endogenously produced metabolites in cells and tissues of mammals and humans [1–4].

Because of excess sulfurs on thiol moieties, persulfides possess strong antioxidant properties, which make persulfides superior metabolites compared with thiols. Furthermore, persulfides can manifest dual reactivity properties so that their deprotonated (RSS⁻) and protonated (RSSH) forms act as nucleophiles and electrophiles, respectively [5–8]. These unique properties make persulfides versatile reactive metabolites in biological signaling mechanisms, which were previously assigned to sulfides or hydrogen sulfide (H_2S) [9]. Increasing evidence indicates that persulfides play a significant role in cellular regulatory processes and are hypothesized to be as important as other reactive species (e.g., reactive oxygen species and reactive nitrogen species) [7,10–13].

Persulfides have important roles in various biological phenomena. For example, they were involved in cellular senescence pathways via their reduction/oxidation (redox) modification of 8-nitro-cGMP electrophilic signals [9,14]. Because of strong antioxidant properties, persulfides reportedly acted as excellent scavengers of electrophiles from exogenous sources, such as heavy metals (e.g., methylmercury), and from endogenous sources, such as oxidative/electrophilic stress [5,14–18]. Persulfidation of protein cysteine (CysSH) residues was also an important mechanism in regulating antioxidant responses and reducing processes, such as modification of the Keap1 protein in the Nrf2-Keap1 system and reduction of oxidized proteins, such as those in the thioredoxin (TRX) and peroxiredoxin systems [8,19,20]. Persulfides were recently hypothesized to be involved in electron cycles in the electron transport chain during mitochondrial energy metabolism [1,21,22]. Nevertheless, the primary biosynthesizer of persulfides at the cellular level is still being investigated, with various findings [1,2,7]. Despite these multiple findings, cysteine persulfide (CysSSH) is believed to be pivotal in the formation of persulfides/polysulfides.

The canonical pathway of sulfide and CysSSH production involves two CysSH synthesis/transsulfuration pathway enzymes—cystathionine β-synthase (CBS) and cystathionine γ-lyase (CSE)—and one CysSH metabolism pathway enzyme: 3-mercaptopyruvate sulfurtransferase (3-MST) [2,23,24]. Previously in our laboratory, we found that cysteinyl-tRNA synthetases (CARSs) involved in the synthesis of persulfides and mitochondrial CARS (CARS2) were responsible for the activity of cysteine persulfide synthases (CPERS) in producing CysSSH in mitochondria [1]. With regard to persulfide levels, we also discovered that HEK293T cells that had their expression of CBS and CSE silenced showed no significant reduction in CysSSH metabolites, whereas CysSSH reduction was substantial in the CARS2 knockout (KO) cell line [1]. We also determined that persulfide synthesis via the CBS/CSE pathway was inefficient because of the high K_m value of the reaction under normal physiological conditions [1,2]. Our previous results confirmed a significant reduction in persulfide synthesis in CARS2-KO cells but not in CBS and CSE knockdown cells, so these findings raise doubts about the importance of canonical sulfide-producing enzymes, such as CBS, CSE, and to some extent 3-MST, during persulfide synthesis. To assess the contribution of CBS, CSE, and 3-MST in persulfide production compared with the importance of CARS2, we generated triple-KO mice for CBS, CSE, and 3-MST and CARS2-deficient heterozygous mice ($Cars2^{+/-}$), and we quantitatively analyzed persulfide levels in various tissues of these KO and CARS2-deficient mice.

2. Materials and Methods

2.1. Materials

β-(4-Hydroxyphenyl)ethyl iodoacetamide (HPE-IAM) was obtained from ChemImpex (Wood Dale, IL, USA). Monobromobimane (Br-bimane) was obtained from Merck (Darmstadt, Germany). Liquid chromatography chemicals were obtained from FUJIFILM Wako Pure Chemical (Osaka, Japan). A Taq polymerase kit was obtained from Takara Bio (Shiga, Japan). A sequencing kit was obtained from Thermo Fisher Scientific (Waltham, MA, USA). For Western blotting, we used the ECL Prime Western Blotting Detection Reagent from GE Healthcare (Chicago, IL, USA), as well as antibodies such as anti-GAPDH (sc-25778) and anti-3-MST (sc-376168) obtained from Santa Cruz Biotechnology (Santa Cruz, CA, USA); anti-CBS (3E1) obtained from Abnova (Taipei, Taiwan); anti-CARS2 provided by

Prof. Hideshi Ihara (Osaka Prefecture University); and anti-CSE provided by Prof. Yoshito Kumagai (University of Tsukuba).

2.2. Animals

All experimental procedures were conducted according to the Regulations for Animal Experiments and Related Activities at Tohoku University, reviewed by the Institutional Laboratory Animal Care and Use Committee of Tohoku University, and approved by the President of Tohoku University. For the generation of 3-MST KO mice, we inserted a gene trap vector into the first intron of the mouse *3-MST* gene in mouse embryonic stem cell lines and generated chimera mice according to the standard protocol [25]. Single-heterozygous CBS mice ($Cbs^{+/-}$) [26], CSE mice ($Cth^{+/-}$) [27], and 3-MST mice ($Mpst^{+/-}$) were mated with each other to produce triple-heterozygous CBS/CSE/3-MST mice. The triple-heterozygous mice were then intercrossed, and CBS/CSE/3-MST triple-KO mice were generated (Figure 1A). Due to the lethality in KO CBS mice, triple-heterozygous KO mice were crossed with human CBS transgenic (Tg-hCBS) mice before the generation of triple-KO mice to avoid lethality in immature mice. The expression of human CBS in Tg-hCBS mice can be activated by supplying zinc water. Therefore, to ensure survivability of the mice to adulthood, zinc water was supplied and then stopped 2 weeks before the experiment [28]. Single CSE KO mice used in Figure S2 are a different strain from the CSE KO mice used to create the triple KO mice [29].

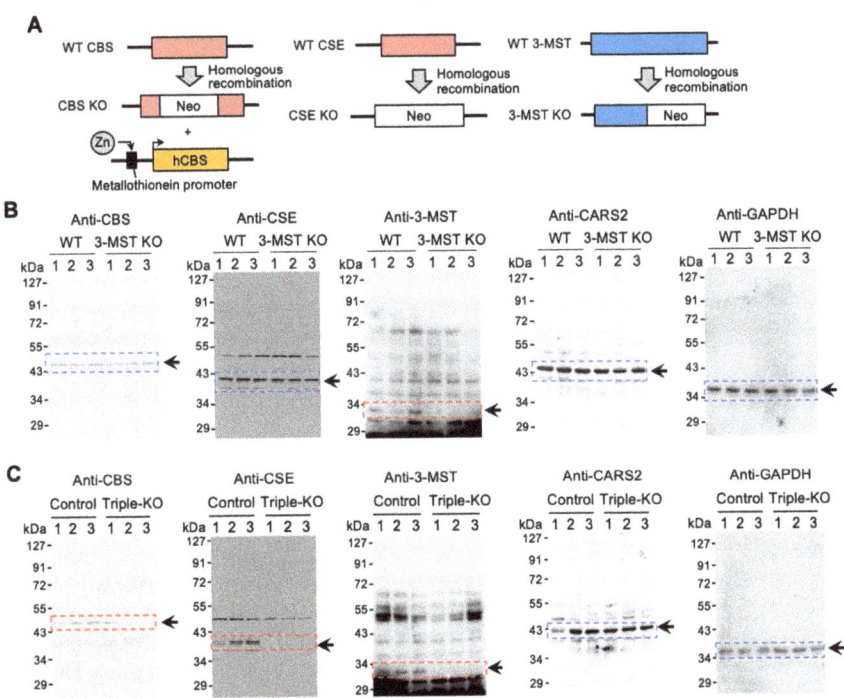

Figure 1. Generation of CBS/CSE/3-MST triple-KO mice. (**A**) CBS/CSE/3-MST triple-KO mice were generated by cross-breeding with single-KO CBS, CSE, and 3-MST mice. The triple-KO mice contained Tg-hCBS to prevent lethality in CBS KO mice. hCBS cDNA was conjugated to the metallothionein promoter controlled by zinc. Control mice had only Tg-hCBS along with wild-type (WT) CBS, CSE, and 3-MST. (**B**) Western blotting of CBS, CSE, 3-MST, and CARS2, obtained from the brains of control and 3-MST KO mice. (**C**) Western blotting of CBS, CSE, 3-MST, and CARS2, obtained from the brains of control and triple-KO mice. GAPDH was used as the internal control. The arrows and boxes outlined with dashed lines indicate the primary bands at the expected molecular weights.

CARS2-deficient heterozygous mice ($Cars2^{+/-}$) were from previously generated CARS2-deficient mice [1]. The genetic modifications of the mice were confirmed by using polymerase chain reaction (PCR) and direct sequencing. Briefly, genomic samples from mice were amplified by using the Taq polymerase PCR kit, with the PCR reaction as follows: initial denaturation at 94 °C for 1 min, followed by 95 °C for 30 s, 60 °C for 30 s, and 72 °C for 30 s for 35 cycles. Primers (0.4 µM) specific for the target genes were used. Resultant PCR fragments were processed via gel electrophoresis in 2% agar for confirmation and compared against known DNA size markers. Table S1 provides all primers used for the different genotypes.

2.3. Knockdown of CBS and CSE

For knockdown of CBS and CSE expression, we used small interfering RNAs: CBS, CBSHSS101428 (Invitrogen, Waltham, MA, USA), and CSE, CTHHSS102447 (Invitrogen, Waltham, MA, USA). We performed small interfering RNA transfection using Lipofectamine RNAiMAX (Invitrogen, Waltham, MA, USA) according to the manufacturer's instructions.

2.4. Measurement of Persulfides and Derivative Metabolites by Means of Br-Bimane Labeling

Liquid chromatography-electrospray ionization–tandem mass spectrometry (LC-ESI–MS/MS) combined with Br-bimane trapping was used to measure sulfur metabolites produced, according to our previous studies [2]. Metabolites from mouse tissue were extracted using a 5 mM Br-bimane with 100% methanol and then homogenized. Lysates were harvested and incubated at 37 °C for 15 min. After centrifugation, aliquots of the supernatants were diluted 10–100 times with distilled water containing known amounts of isotope-labeled internal standards. We used an Agilent 6430 Triple Quadrupole LC/MS (Agilent Technologies, Santa Clara, CA, USA) to perform LC-electrospray ionization–MS/MS. The ionization was achieved by using electrospray in the positive mode, and polysulfide derivatives were identified and quantified by means of multiple reaction monitoring. The MRM parameters and HPLC conditions for LC–MS/MS analysis using Br-bimane followed our report [2].

2.5. Measurement of Persulfides and Derivative Metabolites by Means of HPE-IAM Labeling

LC-ESI–MS/MS combined with HPE-IAM trapping was used to measure sulfur metabolites produced, according to our previous studies [1,30–32]. Metabolites were extracted using a solution containing 5 mM HPE-IAM with 70% methanol and then homogenized. Lysates were harvested and incubated at 37 °C for 20 min and then centrifuged at 15,000× g. After centrifugation, aliquots of the lysate supernatants were diluted 20–50 times with 0.1% formic acid containing known amounts of isotope-labeled internal standard (50–200 nM). Sulfide metabolites in each sample were quantified using the Nexera UHPLC system (Shimadzu, Kyoto, Japan) and LCMS-8060 (Shimadzu, Kyoto, Japan) LC-ESI–MS/MS. Samples were injected and separated by means of the YMC-Triart C18 column (50 × 2.0 mm inner diameter), eluted with a methanol mobile phase through a linear gradient (0–90%) for 15 min in the presence of 0.1% formic acid at a flow rate of 0.2 mL/min at 40 °C. CysSH, CysSSH, glutathione (GSH), glutathione persulfide (GSSH), glutathione disulfide (GSSG), homocysteine (homoCysSH), homocysteine persulfide (homoCysSSH), cystine, hydrogen sulfide anion (HS^-), hydrogen disulfide anion (HSS^-), and thiosulfate ($HS_2O_3^-$) were identified and quantified by multiple reaction monitoring (MRM) on the basis of their specific parameters (Table S2), as previously performed [1,2,31].

2.6. Statistical Analysis

Data are means ± s.d. of at least three independent experiments unless otherwise specified. We analyzed comparisons among multiple groups of mice or cell lines with a one-way ANOVA with Tukey's test, whereas we used Student's t-test for comparisons of continuous variables. We set p-values of less than 0.05 as significant. We used GraphPad Prism 9 (GraphPad Software) for statistical analysis.

3. Results

3.1. 3-MST Mice Demonstrated No Reduced CysSSH and GSSH

To determine the importance of canonical enzymes in persulfide synthesis, we used sulfur metabolome analysis to study 3-MST KO mice. We first generated 3-MST KO mice by inserting a gene trap vector into an intron in mouse 3-MST; we confirmed the absence of 3-MST protein expression using Western blotting (Figure 1A,B). The expression of CBS, CSE, and CARS2 was unchanged in 3-MST KO mice compared with wild-type mice. (Figure 1B). We therefore quantified CysSSH, GSSH, and other persulfides and their derivatives in liver, lung, and brain tissues and plasma from 3-MST KO mice using LC–MS/MS. We found no significant differences in the synthesis of CysSSH, GSSH, and other persulfides in all the samples that we examined (Figure 2). Although very few results showed some discrepancies, such as the increased level of CysSSH in the liver and the decreased level of HSS$^-$ in the plasma, the outcome of this experiment demonstrated that the synthesis of persulfides, including CysSSH, GSSH, and persulfide derivatives, does not depend on 3-MST activity. Section 4 provides a plausible explanation of these discrepancies.

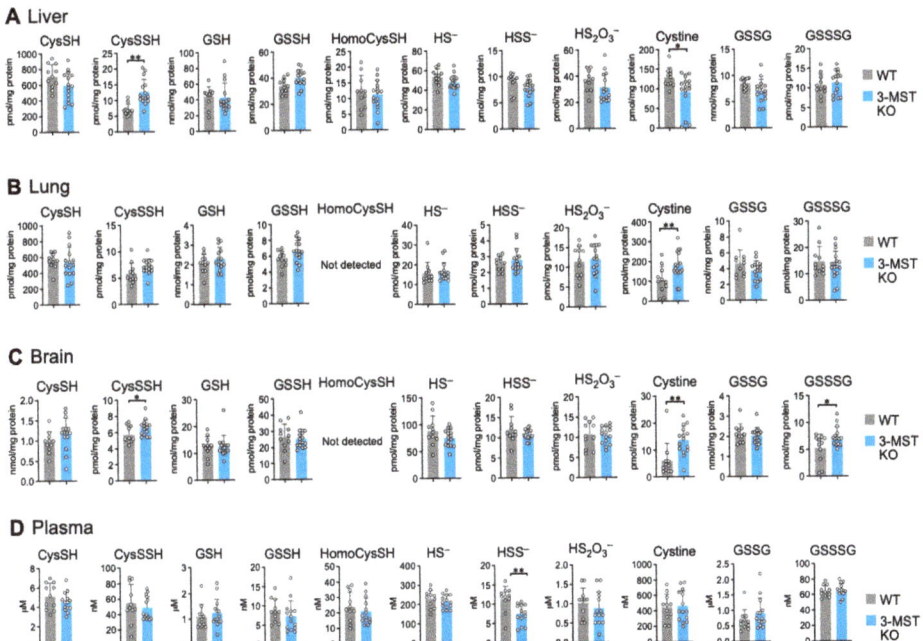

Figure 2. Sulfur metabolome analysis in 3-MST KO mice. Endogenous production of CysSSH, GSSH, and related compounds was identified by means of HPE-IAM labeling with LC–MS/MS analysis of the liver (**A**), lung (**B**), brain (**C**), and plasma (**D**) obtained from 8- to 10-week-old WT and 3-MST KO mice. Data are means ± s.d. n = 11 (WT) and 15 (3-MST KO). * $p < 0.05$; ** $p < 0.01$, as determined by Student's t-test.

3.2. Triple-KO Mice Showed No Reduced CysSSH and GSSH

To ascertain the importance of canonical enzymes in persulfide synthesis, single-KO CBS, CSE, and 3-MST mice were crossed to generate triple-heterozygous mice. These triple-heterozygous mice were then crossed to obtain triple-KO mice. CBS KO mice die within 5 weeks after birth [26]; therefore, Tg-hCBS mice containing a zinc-inducible metallothionein promoter that is activated by zinc were crossed with triple-heterozygous mice before the generation of triple-KO mice to avoid lethality in immature mice (Figure 1A) [28]. To ensure comparable results, both control mice and triple-KO mice had the Tg-hCBS expression cassette inserted, and CBS expression was controlled by supplying water containing zinc (Figure 1A). As Figure 1C shows, tissues of triple-KO mice manifested no expression of CBS, CSE, and 3-MST proteins when water without zinc was provided for 2 weeks.

To investigate persulfide synthesis in triple-KO mice, we used LC–MS/MS analysis to measure CysSSH and GSSH in various tissues from triple-KO and control mice. We also measured persulfides and their derivatives in plasma, the presence of which is an indicator of global physiology metabolites. Triple-KO mice demonstrated no significant differences when compared with control mice in terms of CysSSH synthesis in liver, lung, brain, and plasma tissues (Figure 3). The GSH level significantly decreased in livers of triple-KO mice (Figure 3A) but remained similar in lungs (Figure 3B), brains (Figure 3C), and plasma (Figure 3D) from both control and triple-KO mice. The GSSH level significantly increased in lungs (Figure 3B) and plasma (Figure 3D) of triple-KO mice compared with control mice, which were similar in liver (Figure 3A) and brain (Figure 3C) tissues. The discrepancies between these tissue GSSH metabolite levels may be due to various reasons, such as oxidative stress conditions caused by the generation of triple-KO mice and different gene expression levels of sulfide-metabolizing enzymes in the specific tissues; Section 4 addresses these issues. Nevertheless, our findings indicated that deletion of CBS, CSE, and 3-MST genes in mice did not affect persulfide synthesis. These results indicate that CARS2 functionally complements the three enzymes in the triple-KO mice.

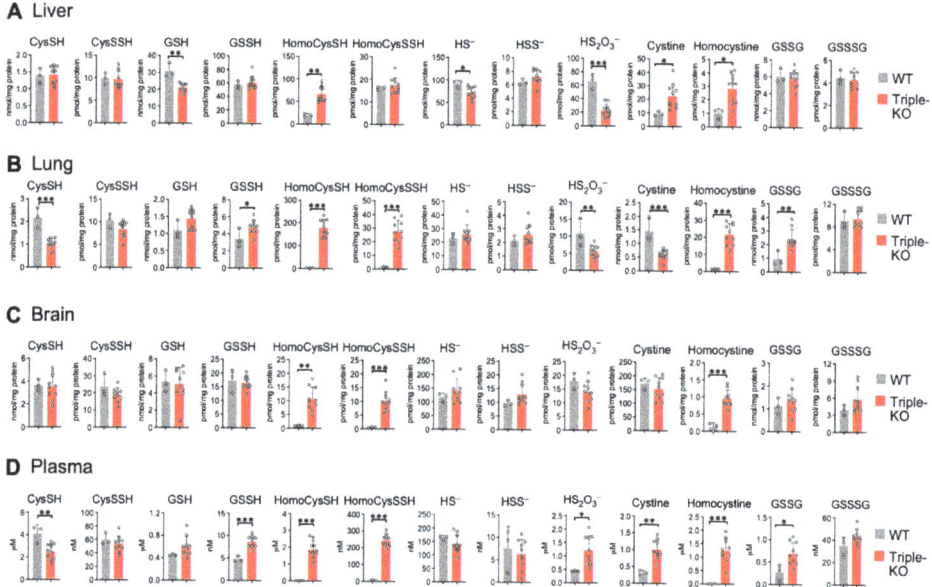

Figure 3. Sulfur metabolome analysis in triple-KO mice. Endogenous production of CysSSH, GSSH, and related compounds was identified by means of HPE-IAM labeling with LC–MS/MS analysis of the liver (**A**), lung (**B**), brain (**C**), and plasma (**D**) obtained from control and triple-KO mice. Mice were males, 14–16 weeks old. Data are means ± s.d. n = 3 (WT) and 10 (triple-KO). * p < 0.05; ** p < 0.01; *** p < 0.001, as determined by Student's t-test.

3.3. Triple-KO Mice Manifested Impaired CysSH Production and Aberrant Sulfide Metabolism

To determine the effects of KO genes in triple-KO mice, we also measured metabolites that are involved in the metabolic pathways for these genes. Since CBS and CSE are a part of the CysSH metabolic pathway [2,33,34], we measured CysSH using LC–MS/MS analysis. We found significantly reduced CysSH metabolite levels in lung tissues (Figure 3B) and plasma (Figure 3D) of triple-KO mice. We expected this finding because disruption of CBS and CSE enzymes reportedly prevented CysSH synthesis (Figure S2) [1,2]. To continue our investigation, we measured homoCysSH, which is an intermediate metabolite in the CysSH synthesis pathway via CBS and CSE, by means of LC–MS/MS analysis in triple-KO mice. We detected significantly elevated levels of homoCysSH in triple-KO mice. We found significantly increased homoCysSSH levels in lung (Figure 3B) and brain (Figure 3C) tissues, as well as in plasma, but not in liver (Figure 3A) tissues of triple-KO mice. Accumulations of homoCysSH may increase the chance of polysulfidation of homoCysSH, which would result in the formation of homoCysSSH [2,5,7,15,35]. Thus, our results for CysSH, homoCysSH, and homoCysSSH were related to the effects of CBS and CSE KO in triple-KO mice.

With regard to 3-MST in triple-KO mice, we utilized LC–MS/MS analysis to measure sulfide metabolites and their derivatives (HS$^-$, HSS$^-$, and thiosulfate). Levels of thiosulfate significantly decreased in liver and lung tissues (Figure 3A,B) but significantly increased in plasma (Figure 3D). The decrease in thiosulfate in lung tissues may be explained by a possible chemical reaction for thiosulfate to transfer its sulfur residue to homoCysSH and GSH to form their persulfide derivatives. This mechanism, in turn, may increase the production of homoCysSSH and GSSH in both lung tissues and plasma (Figure 3B,D). However, the thiosulfate level of brain and plasma was similar to or significantly higher than that in each control tissue, respectively, which indicates that sulfurtransferase activity was sustained by some potent sulfide biosynthesis pathways occurring in vivo even though all three genes were deleted. While it is possible that thiosulfate is derived via oxidative degradation of various hydropersulfides/polysulfides, a rhodanese family enzyme, named thiosulfate sulfurtransferase (TST), may possess sulfur transfer activity to generate thiosulfate similar to that of other canonical enzymes. Therefore, the varied levels of thiosulfate in our triple-KO mice may be because of compensatory activity of TST, as described in the Section 4.

3.4. CysSSH Synthesis Was Disrupted in Cars2$^{+/-}$ Mice

To clarify the importance of canonical enzymes in the persulfide synthesis pathway, we investigated another known persulfide synthesis pathway. We previously identified CARSs as serving as the principal CysSSH synthases in vivo [1]. Here, we used CARS2-deficient mice to highlight the importance of CARS2 in persulfide synthesis. Since deletion of the *Cars2* gene in mice proved to be embryonic lethal [1], we used previously generated *Cars2* heterozygous mice (*Cars2*$^{+/-}$) in this study. *Cars2*$^{+/-}$ mice had a 1-bp insertion in exon 3 of the *Cars2* gene, which led to impaired CARS2 protein and persulfide synthesis in *Cars2*$^{+/-}$ mice. Western blot assay results using tissues from *Cars2*$^{+/-}$ mice showed no change in protein expression level of 3-MST, CBS, and CSE between wild-type and Cars2-deficient mice [1]. This result indicates that there is no complementary increase in expression of the three canonical enzymes, at least under regular laboratory housing conditions. Since CARS2 protein uses CysSH as a substrate to synthesize CysSSH [1], and CysSH is subsequently utilized for the synthesis of other persulfides, we used LC–MS/MS analysis to measure CysSH and CysSSH in liver and lung tissues of *Cars2*$^{+/-}$ mice. Levels of CysSH were not significantly different in both wild-type (WT) and *Cars2*$^{+/-}$ mice, but CysSSH synthesis was significantly reduced to 56% and 55% in liver and lung tissues, respectively, in *Cars2*$^{+/-}$ mice (Figure 4). This finding was similar to results found in our previous experiment, in which the in vitro model using CARS2-KO HEK293T cells showed reduced CysSSH synthesis but no effects on the synthesis of CysSH [1] (Figure S1). Thus, reduced CysSSH synthesis here in *Cars2*$^{+/-}$ mice highlighted the CARS2 enzyme as the most important physiological CPERS.

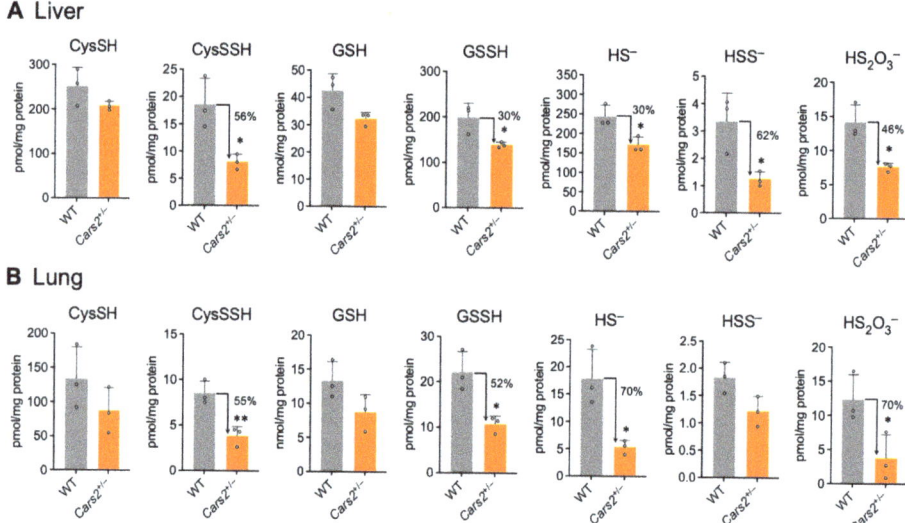

Figure 4. Sulfur metabolome analysis in $Cars2^{+/-}$ mice. Endogenous levels of sulfur metabolites were identified as those of HPE-IAM adducts by using LC–MS/MS analysis of liver (**A**) and lung (**B**) tissues of 10- to 16-week-old WT and $Cars2^{+/-}$ mice. Data are means ± s.d. $n = 3$. * $p < 0.05$; ** $p < 0.01$, determined by Student's t-test.

3.5. Persulfides and Their Derivatives Are Reduced in $Cars2^{+/-}$ Mice

We also used LC–MS/MS analysis to measure the production of persulfides such as GSSH and various sulfide metabolites, including HS$^-$, HSS$^-$, and thiosulfate in $Cars2^{+/-}$ mice. Measurement showed that levels of CysSSH, GSSH, and other derivative compounds were significantly reduced in the liver and lung tissues of $Cars2^{+/-}$ mice compared with those of WT mice. We observed reductions of 56% and 55% of CysSSH, and 30% and 52% of GSSH, respectively, in the liver and lung tissues of $Cars2^{+/-}$ mice, as well as reductions in other sulfide derivatives (Figure 4). However, levels of CysSH and GSH, precursors for the synthesis of each persulfide, showed no significant differences in $Cars2^{+/-}$ mice compared with WT mice (Figure 4A,B). These results indicate that the synthesis of persulfides, such as CysSSH, GSSH, and the sulfide derivatives (HS$^-$, HSS$^-$, and thiosulfate), depends on CARS2 in mouse tissues.

The present study shows that the canonical sulfide-producing enzymes—CBS, CSE, and 3-MST—are not essential for the synthesis of both sulfides and persulfides. Although CBS and CSE produce CysSSH by using cystine as substrate, our current study demonstrates that cysteinyl-tRNA synthetase (CARS) plays a major role in the synthesis of CysSSH in vivo.

4. Discussion

Our present study demonstrates that the absence of canonical H_2S-producing enzymes—CBS, CSE, and 3-MST—does not affect either sulfide or persulfide synthesis (Figure 5). To the best of our knowledge, this report presents the first in vivo study of the role of canonical H_2S-producing enzymes (CBS, CSE, and 3-MST) in the biosynthesis of persulfides using a mouse model in which all three genes were deleted. Until now, endogenous persulfides were thought to be produced via H_2S oxidation resulting from CBS, CSE, and 3-MST [2,24] enzymatic activities. In contrast to this earlier interpretation, significant reductions in persulfide metabolites were not observed for the triple-KO mice in this study. We previously showed, however, a significant decrease in CysSSH in CARS2-deficient mice [1], which we consistently observed in our current study. This finding thus supports CARS2 as the primary CPERS expressed in vivo.

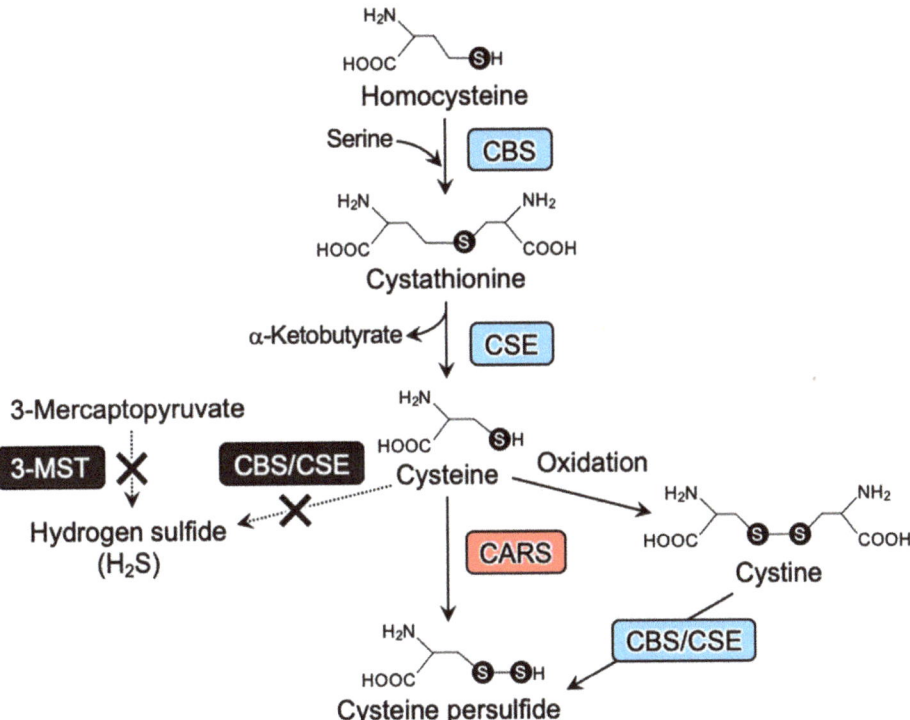

Figure 5. Canonical and true pathways for persulfide biosynthesis. The canonical pathway for persulfide production is composed of sulfurtransferase enzymes (e.g., CBS and CSE; bule boxes). CARS mediates the true and major pathway that mediates persulfide biosynthesis (red box). 3-MST, CBS/CSE may not be involved solely in the sulfide production (black box).

However, another finding that we obtained from our study is that CBS, CSE, and 3-MST regulated levels of metabolites related to persulfide metabolism in mouse tissues. In particular, CySSH, homoCySSH, and homoCySSSH levels were heavily affected by disruptions in CBS and CSE. CBS and CSE enzymes are involved in the synthesis of CySSH, with homoCySSH being the intermediate metabolite in the pathway of CySSH synthesis from methionine. Deletion of CBS and CSE genes increased homoCySSH and reduced CySSH levels in vivo, which was confirmed in our previous study with HEK293T cells [1] and in reports by others [26,28]. Although CBS and CSE may contribute to the synthesis of H_2S under physiological conditions, their substantial contributions depend on the activity levels of this enzyme expressed in different cells and tissues as well as under various cellular metabolic conditions [1,2,9,36–39]. For example, these canonical enzymes and Cars2 are known to be highly expressed in cancer tissues such as human Basal-like breast cancers and colorectal cancer tissues [40,41]. In the breast cancer tissues where CBS and CSE are highly expressed, CBS and CSE play important roles in sulfur metabolism and tumorigenesis [40]. Additionally, H_2S production by CSE reportedly increased under the oxidative conditions of hyperhomocysteinemia [36,38,39]. We found that, with the increased homoCySSH conditions in triple-KO mice, significantly higher accumulations of homocystine and homoCySSSH occurred in the tissues of triple-KO mice than those of WT mice (Figure 3). One plausible explanation for the homoCySSSH increase is the possible involvement of putative persulfide synthases yet to be identified, which may use homoCySH as a substrate to generate homoCySSH. In any case, our triple-KO mice study, showing increased homoCySSH in lung and brain tissues, indicates that CBS and CSE are, at the very least, not the primary regulators of endogenous persulfide production in vivo.

The accumulation of homoCySH and homoCySSH in triple-KO mice caused aberrant sulfur metabolism, which may explain the differences in the amounts of GSH, GSSH, and thiosulfate ($HS_2O_3^-$) in various tissues of these mice. In addition, the amino acid sequence of 3-MST had high homology with that of TST, with a conserved sulfurtransferase protein activity domain [42]. The gene structures of 3-MST and TST are close to each other, within 2 kb, so a bidirectional gene pair suggests that 3-MST and TST share a common enhancer/promoter region. Also, increased TST expression was noted in 3-MST KO mice [23]. This finding may indicate that both 3-MST and TST work in complementary ways in sulfur metabolism, as was observed for 3-MST KO mice for the triple-KO condition that we used here. In a recent report, it has been revealed that the 3-MST protein functions as a protein persulfidase, with the cytoplasmic form of CARS, known as CARS1, also expected to primarily operate in a similar capacity. Considering the potential for these canonical enzymes to collaborate as protein persulfidases [43]. Further research should be conducted to explore this possibility. Thus, studying the relationship between 3-MST, TST, and CARS in terms of sulfide metabolism and protein persulfidase would be interesting for future investigations.

CySSH was previously reported to be formed in an active center of a cysteine residue as an intermediate species during a sulfur transfer reaction catalyzed by 3-MST [24]. According to this potential catalytic scheme, CySSH formed in 3-MST may then react with GSH to produce GSSH. In contrast, other studies [1,2,35] suggested that the synthesis of CySSH via CBS and CSE mostly occurs under pathophysiological conditions such as oxidative stress. However, we found here that persulfide biosynthesis, at least as observed in triple-KO mice, is not likely to depend on CBS, CSE, and 3-MST (Figure 5).

The discrepancy between results of our study and those of others may be due to the different techniques used to measure sulfide and persulfides. For example, monobromobimane (MBB) and N-ethylmaleimide (NEM) are commonly utilized as polysulfide probes during high performance LC and LC–MS/MS measurement of persulfides [1,31]. MBB and NEM are harsh electrophiles that may participate in shifting the hydrolysis equilibrium by a nucleophilic attack on a sulfur residue of polysulfides, which would lead to polysulfide decomposition and result in artefactual sulfide determinations [1,6,30–32]. Such a technical flaw may be prevented by means of the polysulfide-stabilizing activity conferred by N-iodoacetyl l-tyrosine methyl ester (TME-IAM) and HPE-IAM [30–32]. In our study, therefore, we used HPE-IAM as a highly reliable reagent for sulfide/persulfide measurement via LC–MS/MS-based sulfur metabolome analysis, which allowed us to perform extremely accurate, quantitative, and reproducible measurements, as compared with the much less precise and classical approach via MBB and NEM derivatization.

5. Conclusions

Our current study exploited the novel and elegantly integrated animal model of CBS/CSE/3-MST triple-KO mice, which was, in fact, an efficient tool for investigating the sulfur metabolome, and it demonstrated that all three genes are not vital for CySSH biosynthesis in vivo under physiological conditions. We also confirmed the primary role of CBS and CSE genes in the CySH biosynthesis pathway rather than persulfide production. This study may also clarify the predominant role of CARS2/CPERS in the biosynthesis of persulfides and in sulfur metabolism as opposed to the role of three other canonical sulfide/persulfide-generating enzymes—CBS/CSE/3-MST. Moreover, our study may suggest a new study area of sulfur-based redox biology and medicine, in which reactive sulfur species and persulfides are potential therapeutic targets in various diseases that are associated with impaired endogenous persulfide production.

Supplementary Materials: The following supporting information can be downloaded at: https://www.mdpi.com/article/10.3390/antiox12040868/s1, Figure S1: Effect of CBS and CSE knockdown on CySSH, GSH, and related sulfide/persulfide metabolites formed in HEK293T cells with or without CARS2 expression; Figure S2: Sulfur metabolome analysis in CSE KO mice; Table S1: Primers used for different genotypes of KO mice; Table S2: MRM parameters used for LC-ESI-MS/MS analyses.

Author Contributions: Conceptualization, T.A.; funding acquisition, T.I., M.M, T.M., M.T. and T.A.; investigation, Q.H.Z.A., T.I., M.M., T.M., A.N., M.J., N.H., T.T. and M.T.; methodology, Q.H.Z.A., T.I., M.M., T.M., A.N., M.J., N.H., T.T., I.I., W.K. and R.W.; project administration, M.M., M.T. and T.A.; supervision, M.M., M.T. and T.A.; validation, Q.H.Z.A., T.I., M.M., T.M. and A.N.; visualization, T.I., M.M., T.M., A.N., M.J. and N.H.; writing—original draft, Q.H.Z.A., M.M., T.M., M.T. and T.A.; writing—review and editing, M.M., T.M., H.M., M.T. and T.A. All authors have read and agreed to the published version of the manuscript.

Funding: This study was supported in part by Natural Sciences and Engineering Research Council of Canada (RGPIN-2017-04392) to R.W. and Grants-in-Aid for Scientific Research [(S), (C)], Challenging Exploratory Research, Transformative Research Areas] from the Ministry of Education, Culture, Sports, Science and Technology (MEXT), Japan, to T.A. (18H05277, 21H05263 and 22K19707), M.T. (19K08657), M.M. (19K07341), T.I. (20K07306), and T.M. (19K07554 and 22K06893); Japan Science and Technology Agency (JST), CREST Grant Number JPMJCR2024, Japan, to T.A.; and AMED Grant Number JP21zf0127001, Japan, to T.A.

Institutional Review Board Statement: All animal protocols were reviewed by the Institutional Laboratory Animal Care and Use Committee of Tohoku University and approved by the President of Tohoku University (2019MdA-072-03).

Informed Consent Statement: Not applicable.

Data Availability Statement: The data are contained within the manuscript.

Acknowledgments: We thank J.B. Gandy for her editing of the manuscript and for evaluating the concepts and terminology of the paper with regard to understanding by non-specialist readers.

Conflicts of Interest: The authors declare no conflict of interest.

References

1. Akaike, T.; Ida, T.; Wei, F.; Nishida, M.; Kumagai, Y.; Alam, M.M.; Ihara, H.; Sawa, T.; Matsunaga, T.; Kasamatsu, S.; et al. Cysteinyl-tRNA synthetase governs cysteine polysulfidation and mitochondrial bioenergetics. *Nat. Commun.* **2017**, *8*, 1177. [CrossRef]
2. Ida, T.; Sawa, T.; Ihara, H.; Tsuchiya, Y.; Watanabe, Y.; Kumagai, Y.; Suematsu, M.; Motohashi, H.; Fujii, S.; Matsunaga, T.; et al. Reactive cysteine persulfides and S-polythiolation regulate oxidative stress and redox signaling. *Proc. Natl. Acad. Sci. USA* **2014**, *111*, 7606–7611. [CrossRef] [PubMed]
3. Numakura, T.; Sugiura, H.; Akaike, T.; Ida, T.; Fujii, S.; Koarai, A.; Yamada, M.; Onodera, K.; Hashimoto, Y.; Tanaka, R.; et al. Production of reactive persulfide species in chronic obstructive pulmonary disease. *Thorax* **2017**, *72*, 1074–1083. [CrossRef] [PubMed]
4. Khan, S.; Fujii, S.; Matsunaga, T.; Nishimura, A.; Ono, K.; Ida, T.; Ahmed, K.A.; Okamoto, T.; Tsutsuki, H.; Sawa, T.; et al. Reactive persulfides from *Salmonella* Typhimurium downregulate autophagy-mediated innate immunity in macrophages by inhibiting electrophilic signaling. *Cell Chem. Biol.* **2018**, *25*, 1403–1413. [CrossRef]
5. Bianco, C.L.; Akaike, T.; Ida, T.; Nagy, P.; Bogdandi, V.; Toscano, J.P.; Kumagai, Y.; Henderson, C.F.; Goddu, R.N.; Lin, J.; et al. The reaction of hydrogen sulfide with disulfides: Formation of a stable trisulfide and implications for biological systems. *Br. J. Pharmacol.* **2019**, *176*, 671–683. [CrossRef]
6. Sawa, T.; Takata, T.; Matsunaga, T.; Ihara, H.; Motohashi, H.; Akaike, T. Chemical biology of reactive sulfur species: Hydrolysis-driven equilibrium of polysulfides as a determinant of physiological functions. *Antioxid. Redox Signal.* **2021**, *36*, 327–336. [CrossRef]
7. Fukuto, J.M.; Ignarro, L.J.; Nagy, P.; Wink, D.A.; Kevil, C.G.; Feelisch, M.; Cortese-Krott, M.M.; Bianco, C.L.; Kumagai, Y.; Hobbs, A.J.; et al. Biological hydropersulfides and related polysulfides—A new concept and perspective in redox biology. *FEBS Lett.* **2018**, *592*, 2140–2152.
8. Jung, M.; Kasamatsu, S.; Matsunaga, T.; Akashi, S.; Ono, K.; Nishimura, A.; Morita, M.; Hamid, H.A.; Fujii, S.; Kitamura, H.; et al. Protein polysulfidation-dependent persulfide dioxygenase activity of ethylmalonic encephalopathy protein 1. *Biochem. Biophys. Res. Commun.* **2016**, *480*, 180–186. [CrossRef] [PubMed]
9. Nishida, M.; Sawa, T.; Kitajima, N.; Ono, K.; Inoue, H.; Ihara, H.; Motohashi, H.; Yamamoto, M.; Suematsu, M.; Kurose, H.; et al. Hydrogen sulfide anion regulates redox signaling via electrophile sulfhydration. *Nat. Chem. Biol.* **2012**, *8*, 714–724. [CrossRef]

10. Olson, K.R. Are reactive sulfur species the new reactive oxygen species? *Antioxid. Redox Signal.* **2020**, *33*, 1125–1142. [CrossRef]
11. Cortese-Krott, M.M.; Koning, A.; Kuhnle, G.G.C.; Nagy, P.; Bianco, C.L.; Pasch, A.; Wink, D.A.; Fukuto, J.M.; Jackson, A.A.; van Goor, H.; et al. The reactive species interactome: Evolutionary emergence, biological significance, and opportunities for redox metabolomics and personalized medicine. *Antioxid. Redox Signal.* **2017**, *27*, 684–712. [CrossRef] [PubMed]
12. Fujii, S.; Sawa, T.; Motohashi, H.; Akaike, T. Persulfide synthases that are functionally coupled with translation mediate sulfur respiration in mammalian cells. *Br. J. Pharmacol.* **2019**, *176*, 607–615. [CrossRef]
13. Kasamatsu, S.; Nishimura, A.; Morita, M.; Matsunaga, T.; Hamid, H.A.; Akaike, T. Redox signaling regulated by cysteine persulfide and protein polysulfidation. *Molecules* **2016**, *21*, 1721. [CrossRef]
14. Ihara, H.; Kasamatsu, S.; Kitamura, A.; Nishimura, A.; Tsutsuki, H.; Ida, T.; Ishizaki, K.; Toyama, T.; Yoshida, E.; Hamid, H.A.; et al. Exposure to electrophiles impairs reactive persulfide-dependent redox signaling in neuronal cells. *Chem. Res. Toxicol.* **2017**, *30*, 1673–1684. [CrossRef]
15. Millikin, R.; Bianco, C.L.; White, C.; Saund, S.S.; Henriquez, S.; Sosa, V.; Akaike, T.; Kumagai, Y.; Soeda, S.; Toscano, J.P.; et al. The chemical biology of protein hydropersulfides: Studies of a possible protective function of biological hydropersulfide generation. *Free Radic. Biol. Med.* **2016**, *97*, 136–147. [CrossRef] [PubMed]
16. Saund, S.S.; Sosa, V.; Henriquez, S.; Nguyen, Q.N.N.; Bianco, C.L.; Soeda, S.; Millikin, R.; White, C.; Le, H.; Ono, K.; et al. The chemical biology of hydropersulfides (RSSH): Chemical stability, reactivity and redox roles. *Arch. Biochem. Biophys.* **2015**, *588*, 15–24. [CrossRef]
17. Nishimura, A.; Shimoda, K.; Tanaka, T.; Toyama, T.; Nishiyama, K.; Shinkai, Y.; Numaga-Tomita, T.; Yamazaki, D.; Kanda, Y.; Akaike, T.; et al. Depolysulfidation of Drp1 induced by low-dose methylmercury exposure increases cardiac vulnerability to hemodynamic overload. *Sci. Signal.* **2019**, *12*, eaaw1920. [CrossRef] [PubMed]
18. Abiko, Y.; Yoshida, E.; Ishii, I.; Fukuto, J.M.; Akaike, T.; Kumagai, Y. Involvement of reactive persulfides in biological bis-methylmercury sulfide formation. *Chem. Res. Toxicol.* **2015**, *28*, 1301–1306. [CrossRef]
19. Dóka, É.; Pader, I.; Bíró, A.; Johansson, K.; Cheng, Q.; Ballagó, K.; Prigge, J.R.; Pastor-Flores, D.; Dick, T.P.; Schmidt, E.E.; et al. A novel persulfide detection method reveals protein persulfide- and polysulfide-reducing functions of thioredoxin and glutathione systems. *Sci. Adv.* **2016**, *2*, e1500968.
20. Dóka, É.; Ida, T.; Dagnell, M.; Abiko, Y.; Luong, N.C.; Balog, N.; Takata, T.; Espinosa, B.; Nishimura, A.; Cheng, Q.; et al. Control of protein function through oxidation and reduction of persulfidated states. *Sci. Adv.* **2020**, *6*, eaax8358. [CrossRef]
21. Marutani, E.; Morita, M.; Hirai, S.; Kai, S.; Grange, R.M.H.; Miyazaki, Y.; Nagashima, F.; Traeger, L.; Magliocca, A.; Ida, T.; et al. Sulfide catabolism ameliorates hypoxic brain injury. *Nat. Commun.* **2021**, *12*, 3108. [CrossRef] [PubMed]
22. Nishimura, A.; Nasuno, R.; Yoshikawa, Y.; Jung, M.; Ida, T.; Matsunaga, T.; Morita, M.; Takagi, H.; Motohashi, H.; Akaike, T. Mitochondrial cysteinyl-tRNA synthetase is expressed via alternative transcriptional initiation regulated by energy metabolism in yeast cells. *J. Biol. Chem.* **2019**, *294*, 13781–13788. [CrossRef] [PubMed]
23. Nagahara, N.; Tanaka, M.; Tanaka, Y.; Ito, T. Novel characterization of antioxidant enzyme, 3-mercaptopyruvate sulfurtransferase-knockout mice: Overexpression of the evolutionarily-related enzyme rhodanese. *Antioxidants* **2019**, *8*, 116. [CrossRef]
24. Hanaoka, K.; Sasakura, K.; Suwanai, Y.; Toma-Fukai, S.; Shimamoto, K.; Takano, Y.; Shibuya, N.; Terai, T.; Komatsu, T.; Ueno, T.; et al. Discovery and mechanistic characterization of selective inhibitors of H_2S-producing enzyme: 3-Mercaptopyruvate sulfurtransferase (3MST) targeting active-site cysteine persulfide. *Sci. Rep.* **2017**, *7*, 40227. [CrossRef]
25. Hogan, B.; Costantini, F.; Lacy, E. *Manipulating the Mouse Embryo: A Laboratory Manual*; Cold Spring Harbor Laboratory Press: New York, NY, USA, 1986.
26. Watanabe, M.; Osada, J.; Aratani, Y.; Kluckman, K.; Reddick, R.; Malinow, M.R.; Maeda, N. Mice deficient in cystathionine b-synthase: Animal models for mild and severe homocyst(e)inemia. *Proc. Natl. Acad. Sci. USA* **1995**, *92*, 1585–1589. [CrossRef]
27. Yang, G.; Wu, L.; Jiang, B.; Yang, W.; Qi, J.; Cao, K.; Meng, Q.; Mustafa, A.K.; Mu, W.; Zhang, S.; et al. H_2S as a physiologic vasorelaxant: Hypertension in mice with deletion of cystathionine γ-lyase. *Science* **2008**, *322*, 587–590. [CrossRef]
28. Wang, L.; Jhee, K.-H.; Hua, X.; DiBello, P.M.; Jacobsen, D.W.; Kruger, W.D. Modulation of cystathionine β-synthase level regulates total serum homocysteine in mice. *Circ. Res.* **2004**, *94*, 1318–1324. [CrossRef]
29. Ishii, I.; Akahoshi, N.; Yamada, H.; Nakano, S.; Izumi, T.; Suematsu, M. Cystathionine gamma-Lyase-deficient mice require dietary cysteine to protect against acute lethal myopathy and oxidative injury. *J. Biol. Chem.* **2010**, *285*, 26358–26368. [CrossRef]
30. Kasamatsu, S.; Ida, T.; Koga, T.; Asada, K.; Motohashi, H.; Ihara, H.; Akaike, T. High-precision sulfur metabolomics innovated by a new specific probe for trapping reactive sulfur species. *Antioxid. Redox Signal.* **2021**, *34*, 1407–1419. [CrossRef] [PubMed]
31. Takata, T.; Jung, M.; Matsunaga, T.; Ida, T.; Morita, M.; Motohashi, H.; Shen, X.; Kevil, C.G.; Fukuto, J.M.; Akaike, T. Methods in sulfide and persulfide research. *Nitric Oxide* **2021**, *116*, 47–64.
32. Hamid, H.A.; Tanaka, A.; Ida, T.; Nishimura, A.; Matsunaga, T.; Fujii, S.; Morita, M.; Sawa, T.; Fukuto, J.M.; Nagy, P.; et al. Polysulfide stabilization by tyrosine and hydroxyphenyl-containing derivatives that is important for a reactive sulfur metabolomics analysis. *Redox Biol.* **2019**, *21*, 101096. [CrossRef]
33. Brosnan, J.T.; Brosnan, M.E. The sulfur-containing amino acids: An overview. *Nutr. J.* **2006**, *136*, 1636S–1640S. [CrossRef]
34. Aitken, S.M.; Lodha, P.H.; Morneau, D.J.K. The enzymes of the transsulfuration pathways: Active-site characterizations. *Biochim. Biophys. Acta.* **2011**, *1814*, 1511–1517. [CrossRef]
35. Yadav, P.K.; Martinov, M.; Vitvitsky, V.; Seravalli, J.; Wedmann, R.; Filipovic, M.R.; Banerjee, R. Biosynthesis and reactivity of cysteine persulfides in signaling. *J. Am. Chem. Soc.* **2016**, *138*, 289–299. [CrossRef] [PubMed]

36. Maclean, K.N.; Sikora, J.; Kožich, V.; Jiang, H.; Greiner, L.S.; Kraus, E.; Krijt, J.; Crnic, L.S.; Allen, R.H.; Stabler, S.P.; et al. Cystathionine beta-synthase null homocystinuric mice fail to exhibit altered hemostasis or lowering of plasma homocysteine in response to betaine treatment. *Mol. Genet. Metab.* **2010**, *101*, 163–171. [CrossRef]
37. Kožich, V.; Ditrói, T.; Sokolová, J.; Křížková, M.; Krijt, J.; Ješina, P.; Nagy, P. Metabolism of sulfur compounds in homocystinurias. *Br. J. Pharmacol.* **2019**, *176*, 594–606. [CrossRef] [PubMed]
38. Kožich, V.; Schwahn, B.C.; Sokolová, J.; Křížková, M.; Ditroi, T.; Krijt, J.; Khalil, Y.; Křížek, T.; Vaculíková-Fantlová, T.; Stibůrková, B.; et al. Human ultrarare genetic disorders of sulfur metabolism demonstrate redundancies in H_2S homeostasis. *Redox Biol.* **2022**, *58*, 102517. [PubMed]
39. Ditrói, T.; Nagy, A.; Martinelli, D.; Rosta, A.; Kožich, V.; Nagy, P. Comprehensive analysis of how experimental parameters affect H_2S measurements by the monobromobimane method. *Free Radic. Biol. Med.* **2019**, *136*, 146–158. [CrossRef]
40. Erdélyi, K.; Ditrói, T.; Johansson, H.J.; Czikora, Á.; Balog, N.; Silwal-Pandit, L.; Ida, T.; Olasz, J.; Hajdú, D.; Mátrai, Z.; et al. Reprogrammed transsulfuration promotes basal-like breast tumor progression via realigning cellular cysteine persulfidation. *Proc. Natl. Acad. Sci. USA* **2021**, *118*, e2100050118. [CrossRef]
41. Chen, Z.; Mei, K.; Xiao, Y.; Xiong, Y.; Long, W.; Wang, Q.; Zhong, J.; Di, D.; Ge, Y.; Luo, Y.; et al. Prognostic Assessment of Oxidative Stress-Related Genes in Colorectal Cancer and New Insights into Tumor Immunity. *Oxid. Med. Cell. Longev.* **2022**, *2022*, 2518340. [CrossRef]
42. Nagahara, N.; Okazaki, T.; Nishino, T. Cytosolic mercaptopyruvate sulfurtransferase is evolutionarily related to mitochondrial rhodanese. *J. Biol. Chem.* **1995**, *270*, 16230–16235. [CrossRef]
43. Pedre, B.; Talwar, D.; Barayeu, U.; Schilling, D.; Luzarowski, M.; Sokolowski, M.; Glatt, S.; Dick, T.P. 3-Mercaptopyruvate sulfur transferase is a protein persulfidase. *Nat. Chem. Biol.* **2023**, *19*, 507–517. [CrossRef]

Disclaimer/Publisher's Note: The statements, opinions and data contained in all publications are solely those of the individual author(s) and contributor(s) and not of MDPI and/or the editor(s). MDPI and/or the editor(s) disclaim responsibility for any injury to people or property resulting from any ideas, methods, instructions or products referred to in the content.

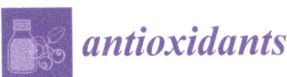

Article

Antiproliferative and Proapoptotic Effects of Erucin, a Diet-Derived H₂S Donor, on Human Melanoma Cells

Daniela Claudia Maresca, Lia Conte, Benedetta Romano, Angela Ianaro *,† and Giuseppe Ercolano *,†

Department of Pharmacy, School of Medicine and Surgery, University of Naples Federico II, 80131 Naples, Italy
* Correspondence: ianaro@unina.it (A.I.); giuseppe.ercolano@unina.it (G.E.);
Tel.: +39-081678663 (A.I.); +39-0816748428 (G.E.)
† These authors contributed equally to this work.

Abstract: Melanoma is the most dangerous form of skin cancer and is characterized by chemotherapy resistance and recurrence despite the new promising therapeutic approaches. In the last years, erucin (ERU), the major isothiocyanate present in *Eruca sativa*, commonly known as rocket salads, has demonstrated great efficacy as an anticancer agent in different in vitro and in vivo models. More recently, the chemopreventive effects of ERU have been associated with its property of being a H$_2$S donor in human pancreatic adenocarcinoma. Here, we investigated the effects of ERU in modulating proliferation and inducing human melanoma cell death by using multiple in vitro approaches. ERU significantly reduced the proliferation of different human melanoma cell lines. A flow cytometry analysis with annexin V/PI demonstrated that ERU was able to induce apoptosis and cell cycle arrest in A375 melanoma cells. The proapoptotic effect of ERU was associated with the modulation of the epithelial-to-mesenchymal transition (EMT)-related cadherins and transcription factors. Moreover, ERU thwarted the migration, invasiveness and clonogenic abilities of A375 melanoma cells. These effects were associated with melanogenesis impairment and mitochondrial fitness modulation. Therefore, we demonstrated that ERU plays an important role in inhibiting the progression of melanoma and could represent a novel add-on therapy for the treatment of human melanoma.

Keywords: hydrogen sulfide; melanoma; erucin; nutraceuticals; cancer therapy

Citation: Maresca, D.C.; Conte, L.; Romano, B.; Ianaro, A.; Ercolano, G. Antiproliferative and Proapoptotic Effects of Erucin, a Diet-Derived H₂S Donor, on Human Melanoma Cells. *Antioxidants* 2023, 12, 41. https://doi.org/10.3390/antiox12010041

Academic Editors: John Toscano and Vinayak Khodade

Received: 28 November 2022
Revised: 19 December 2022
Accepted: 21 December 2022
Published: 26 December 2022

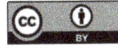

Copyright: © 2022 by the authors. Licensee MDPI, Basel, Switzerland. This article is an open access article distributed under the terms and conditions of the Creative Commons Attribution (CC BY) license (https://creativecommons.org/licenses/by/4.0/).

1. Introduction

Recognized as the most dangerous and fatal form of skin cancers, the incidence of melanoma is swiftly increasing in the entire world, and it mostly affects people with a median age of 57 years and with a fair phototype [1,2]. Melanoma is characterized by the dysfunctional proliferation of melanocytes, cells located in the basal layer of the epidermis which produce the melanin pigment, which are essential for skin protection from solar radiation. Excessive exposure to ultraviolet rays following sunbathing or tanning represents the major risk factor of melanoma [3]. Indeed, UVA and UVB rays cause DNA damage in skin cells which leads to specific mutations that, when accumulated or are in excess, may not be sheltered by DNA repair systems [4]. This triggers the development of genetic alterations, such as the tumor suppressor gene TP53 mutation, the CDK inhibitor gene CDKN2A mutation or the activating BRAF^{V600E} mutation [5,6]. The latter is not typically a UV-induced mutation although a potential sunlight-mediated origin has been described [7,8]. The BRAF^{V600E} mutation is harbored by more than 50% of melanoma patients, inducing uncontrolled cancer cell proliferation, migration and metastasis development [9]. In fact, BRAF inhibitors as well as the most recently approved anti-PDL1 and anti-CTLA-4 monoclonal antibodies represent the first line treatment for melanoma cancer patients. Nevertheless, an important percentage of patients become nonresponsive to these treatments, developing tumor resistance and exacerbation [10]. Therefore, there is an increasing interest in finding and characterizing new promising agents that can be proposed as novel therapeutic approaches for the treatment of melanoma in order to overcome tumor resistance and recurrence. In this context, the use of diet-derived phytochemicals has been proposed as an adjuvant therapeutic approach for cancer treatment. Different diet-derived compounds, such as resveratrol, curcumin, apigenin and capsaicin demonstrated potent bioactivities, showing anti-inflammatory, antibiotic and antitumoral effects [11]. In the last few years, plant and food research has been focused on cruciferous-vegetable-derived compounds. In particular, cruciferous vegetables, which include rocket salads, broccoli and cabbage, are rich in isothiocyanates, which are the hydrolysis products of glucosinolate. Importantly, isothiocyanates have been proposed as promising chemopreventive agents for modulating cancer development and progression as demonstrated by multiple in vitro and in vivo approaches [12,13]. 4-(methylthio) butyl isothiocyanate, commonly referred to as erucin (ERU), is the major component derived from rocket salad leaves and was demonstrated to affect the proliferation of different cancer cell lines through different mechanisms of action, such as apoptosis, autophagy, cell cycle arrest and antioxidant effects [14–17]. Importantly, Citi et al. recently demonstrated that the antiproliferative and proapoptotic effects of ERU in human pancreatic carcinoma cells are ascribed to the ability of ERU to release hydrogen sulfide (H_2S) [18,19]. Likewise, our own group, and others, showed that the H_2S pathway participates in melanoma progression and demonstrated that exogenous H_2S, by means of H_2S-releasing molecules, represents a promising therapeutic approach for the management of metastatic melanoma [20–25]. In this study, we characterized the therapeutic potential of ERU in human melanoma for the first time by evaluating its ability to modulate the proliferation, migration, ROS production and mitochondrial activity of human melanoma cells in vitro.

2. Materials and Methods

2.1. Reagents and Cell Culture

The human melanoma cells lines A375 were bought from Sigma–Aldrich (Milan, Italy). WM1862, WM983A and WM983B cell lines were purchased from Rockland (Limerick, Ireland). Human keratinocytes (HaCaT) were purchased from Lonza (Basel, Switzerland)). All cell lines were cultured in RPMI 1640 medium with GlutaMAXTM and were supplemented with 10% heat-inactivated fetal calf serum, 2 mmol/L L-glutamine, 100 U/mL penicillin, 100 µg/mL streptomycin and 10 mM HEPES buffer (all from Gibco; New York, NY, USA). Cells were grown at 37 °C in a humidified incubator under 5% CO_2. All cell lines used in this study were characterized by the cell bank where they were purchased. ERU was purchased from Cayman Chemicals (Michigan, CA, USA).

2.2. Proliferation Assay

Cell proliferation was measured with the 3-[4,5-dimethyltiazol2yl]-2,5 diphenyl tetrazolium bromide (MTT) assay. Different human melanoma cell lines (A375, WM1862, WM983A and WM983B) and normal keratinocytes (HaCaT) were seeded on 96-well plates (3×10^3/well) and were treated with different concentrations of ERU (5, 10, 20, 40 and 80 µM) for 48 h before adding 25 µL of MTT (Sigma, Milan, Italy) (5 mg/mL in saline). Thereafter, cells were incubated for 3 h at 37 °C and were then lysed in order to solubilize the dark blue crystals with a solution containing 50% (*vol/vol*) N,Ndimethylformamide and 20% (*wt/vol*) sodium dodecylsulfate with an adjusted pH of 4.5. The OD of each well was obtained by measuring the absorbance at 620 nm using Multiskan GO microplate reader (Thermo Fisher Scientific, Waltham, MA, USA).

2.3. Flow Cytometry Analysis

To assess cell proliferation, A375 cells were incubated with 5 µM carboxyfluorescein succinimidyl ester (CFSE, Thermo Fisher Scientific, Waltham, MA, USA) for 20 min and were either directly analyzed or grown for 48 h in the presence of 30 µM ERU before analyzing fluorescence intensity through flow cytometry.

Ki67 expression was evaluated through intracellular staining performed after fixation and permeabilization with Intracellular Fixation & Permeabilization Kit (eBioscience, Thermo Fisher Scientific Waltham, MA, USA) using APC antihuman Ki67 antibodies (REA183, Miltenyi, 2:50).

For live vs. dead status, 48 h ERU-treated A375 cells (30 µM) were labeled with the Zombie Green Fixable Viability Kit (BioLegend, San Diego, CA, USA) and washed as instructed by the manufacturer's instructions.

Apoptosis assay was performed by using the Annexin V-FITC Kit (BD Pharmingen, San Diego, CA, USA) according to the manufacturer's instructions. Briefly, A375 cells were seeded on a 6-well plate (3×10^5 cells/well) and were allowed to attach overnight. The day after, cells were treated with 30 µM ERU and were incubated for 48 h. Subsequently, cells were collected and stained for 10 min with FITC-conjugated annexin V. Then, the samples were washed and stained with propidium iodide before flow cytometry analysis.

Cell cycle analysis was performed using Cell Cycle Assay Solution Deep Red Kit (Dojindo, Kumamoto, Japan). The 24 h ERU-treated A375 cells (30 µM) were incubated with Cell Cycle Assay Solution (5 µL) in PBS for 15 min at 37 °C before flow cytometry analysis.

For E-CAD and N-CAD expression, 24 h ERU-treated A375 cells (30 µM) were incubated with the following antibodies: APC-Cy7 antihuman CD324 (E-CAD) (67A4, Biolegend, 1:50) and Alexa-Fluor 700 antihuman CD325 (N-CAD) (8C11, Biolegend, 2:50). Cells were stained with FACS buffer for 20 min at room temperature.

For ROS production and mitochondrial activity, 48 h ERU-treated A375 cells (1 µM) were stained with H2DCFDHA (D399 Thermo Fisher Waltham, MA, USA), MitoTracker Green (M7514 Thermo Fisher Waltham, MA, USA) and MitoTracker Deep Red (M22426, Thermo Fisher Waltham, MA, USA) as previously described [26].

Samples were acquired on BriCyte E6 flow cytometer (Mindray Medical Italy S.r.l., Milan, Italy), and data were analyzed using FlowJo software (TreeStar V.10; Carrboro, NC, USA). All the histograms were edited with modal option.

2.4. Caspase 3/9 Activity Assay

Activation of Caspase 3 and 9 in ERU-treated A375 cells (30 µM for 48 h) were determined with Caspase 3 and 9 Activity Colorimetric Assay Kits according to the manufacturer's instructions (Houston, Texas, 77079, USA).

2.5. RNA Extraction and Quantitative Real-Time PCR (qPCR)

Total RNA was isolated from A375 melanoma cells treated or not treated with 1 µM or 30 µM ERU for 6 h using the TRIZOL reagent (Invitrogen, Thermo Fisher Scientific Waltham, MA, USA) as previously described. RNA was quantified with Nanodrop and considered DNA- and protein-free if the ratio of readings at 260/280 nm was ≥ 1.7. Isolated mRNA was reverse-transcribed by iScript Reverse Transcription Supermix for RT-qPCR (Bio-Rad, Milan, Italy). qPCR was carried out in the Bio-Rad CFX384 real-time PCR detection system (Bio-Rad, Milan, Italy) with the following primers:

BCL-2 (Gene ID: 596)
5′-GGTGGGGTCATGTGTGTGG-3′;
5′-CGGTTCAGGTACTCAGTCATCC-3′
XIAP (Gene ID: 331)
5′-TATCAGACACCATATACCCGAGG-3′;
5′-TGGGGTTAGGTGAGCATAGTC-3′
CCNB1(Gene ID: 891)
5′-GACCTGTGTCAGGCTTTCTCTG-3′;
5′- GGTATTTTGGTCTGACTGCTTGC-3′
CDK1(Gene ID: 983)
5′-GGAAACCAGGAAGCCTAGCATC-3′;
5′-GGATGATTCAGTGCCATTTTGCC-3′
CDC25C (Gene ID: 995)

5′-TCTACGGAACTCTTCTCATCCAC-3′;
5′-TCCAGGA CAGGTTTAACATTTT-3′
SNAIL (Gene ID: 6615)
5′-ACTGCAACAAGGAATACCTCAG-3′;
5′-GCACTGGTACTTCTT GACATCTG-3′
SLUg (Gene ID: 6591)
5′-CGAACTGGACACACATACAGTG-3′;
5′-CTGAGGATCTCTGGTTGTGGT-3′
ZEB-1 (Gene ID: 6935)
5′-TTACACCTTTGCATACAGAACCC-3′;
5′-TTTACGAT TACACCCAGACTGC-3′
TWIST (Gene ID: 7291)
5′-GTCCGCAGTCTTACGAGGAG-3′;
5′-GCTTGAGGGTCTGAATCTTGCT-3′
GCLC (Gene ID: 2729)
5′GTTGGGGTTTGTCCTCTCCC-3′;
5′-GGGGTGACGAGGTGGAGTA-3′
GCLM (Gene ID: 2730)
5′-AGGAGCTTCGGGACTGTATCC-3′;
5′-GGGACATGGTGCATTCCAAAA-3′
HMOX-1(Gene ID: 3162)
5′-GCCGTGTAGATATGGTACAAGGA-3′;
5′-AAGCCGAGAATGCTGAGTTCA-3′
MITF (Gene ID:4286)
5′-TGGTTTTCCCACGAGCTATTTT-3′;
5′-GCACAGAG TCAATTTCCTGGT-3′
TYR (Gene ID: 7299)
5′-GCAAAGCATACCATCAGCTCA-3′;
5′-GCAGTGCATCCATTGACACAT-3′

The housekeeping gene ribosomal protein S16 (RPS16) was used as an internal control to normalize the Ct values using the $2^{-\Delta Ct}$ formula.

2.6. Migration Assay

A375 cells were plated in 12-well plates (2×10^5 cells/well) and were allowed to grow at confluence. Subsequently, a wound was created in the monolayer using a 200 µL pipette tip, and microscope photos were taken to mark the initial condition (time 0). Cells were treated with 1 µM ERU, and, after 24 and 48 h scratches were photographed. ImageJ's MRI Wound Healing Tool (MRI Redmine) was used to calculate the area of the cell-free gap.

2.7. Clonogenic Assay

A375 cells were plated in a 6-well plate (1×10^3 cells/well) and were treated with 1 µM ERU for 48 h. Next, fresh medium without ERU was changed every 2 days. After 14 days, colonies were formed, and the cells were washed with PBS, fixed with 4% paraformaldehyde and stained with 0.5% crystal violet. Colonies were manually counted, and images were acquired using a digital camera.

2.8. Invasion Assay

Boyden chambers with polycarbonate filters with a nominal pore size of 8 µm (Millipore, USA) were coated on the upper side with Matrigel (Becton Dickinson Labware, USA). The chambers were placed in a 24-well plate, and A375 cells (2.5×10^5 cells/mL) were plated in the upper chamber in the presence or absence of ERU (1 µM) in serum-free RPMI. At the end of the 16 h of incubation, the medium was removed, and the filters were fixed with 4% formaldehyde for 2 min, and, subsequently, the cells were permeabilized with 100% methanol for 20 min. The methanol was removed, and the chambers were stained with Giemsa for 15 min and then washed with PBS. The filters were removed, and the nonmigrating cells on the top of the filter were peeled off with the use of a cotton swab. Then, the filters were placed on a slide and were examined under a microscope. Cell invasion was determined by counting the number of cells stained on each filter in at least 4–5 randomly selected fields. The resulting data were presented as the average of the invaded cells ± SEM/microscopic field of three independent experiments.

2.9. Measurement of Melanin Content

A375 cells (3×10^5/well) were plated in a 6-well plate and treated with 1 µM ERU for 72 h. Thereafter, cell pellet was dissolved in NaOH 1N, and it was incubated for 90 min at 37 °C then centrifuged for 10 min at $10,000 \times g$. The optical density (OD) of supernatant was measured at 450 nm using Multiskan GO microplate reader (Thermo Fisher Scientific, Waltham, MA, USA).

2.10. Statistical Analysis

Statistical analysis was performed using GraphPad Prism software version 9 (San Diego, CA, USA). For comparison of two groups, a t test was used, and, for comparison of multiple groups ANOVA test was used. The data were shown as mean ± SEM. A p value < 0.05 was considered statistically significant and was labeled with *; p values < 0.01, 0.001 or 0.0001 were labeled with **, *** or ****, respectively.

3. Results

3.1. ERU Affected the Proliferation Rate of Human Melanoma Cell Lines

First, we assessed the antiproliferative effects of ERU on different human melanoma cell lines that featured the BRAF^{V600E} mutation. WM1862, WM983A, WM983B and A375 human melanoma cells were treated with an increasing concentration of ERU (0, 5, 10, 20, 40 and 80 µM) for 48 h prior to the evaluation of cell proliferation with an MTT analysis. As shown in Figure 1A, ERU significantly reduced the proliferation of all the melanoma cell lines that were tested. In particular, 80 µM ERU reduced the cell viability by about 50% in the WM983A and WM1862 cells ($p < 0.0001$ compared with the untreated cells) and by more than 70% in the A375 and WM983B cells ($p < 0.0001$ compared with the untreated cells). Conversely, a reduction of about 20% was observed for our negative control, which was represented by human keratinocytes (HaCaT) ($p < 0.01$ compared with the untreated cells). In fact, an IC50 analysis (Figure 1B) showed a value higher than 100 µM for the HaCaT cells, whilst, for the melanoma cancer cells, it was between 30 and 60 µM, suggesting that the antiproliferative effect of ERU at lower concentrations was specific to the cancer cell. Given that the MTT assay measures the cytotoxic effect by assessing the mitochondrial dehydrogenase activity, we decided to directly evaluate the antiproliferative effect of ERU by performing the carboxyfluorescein succinimidyl ester (CFSE) assay on the A375 melanoma cell lines that showed the lower IC50 values and displayed a more aggressive phenotype compared to the other melanoma cell lines that were tested [27]. As shown in Figure 1C,D, the CFSE fluorescence intensity was strongly reduced in the control cells at 48 h compared to the control cells at t0, confirming the high proliferation rate of the A375 melanoma cell line. Importantly, the CFSE fluorescence intensity was significantly higher in the ERU-treated cells compared to the control cells at 48 h, indicating that ERU reduced the proliferation rate of the A375 melanoma cells. To corroborate our findings, we evaluated the expression of Ki67, one of the key markers involved in cancer cell proliferation [28]. As shown in Figure 1E,F, the treatment with 30 µM ERU significantly reduced the expression levels of Ki67 as observed through the flow cytometry analysis. These results demonstrated that ERU at lower concentrations inhibited the proliferation rate of the human melanoma cells without affecting the proliferation rate of the healthy control cells.

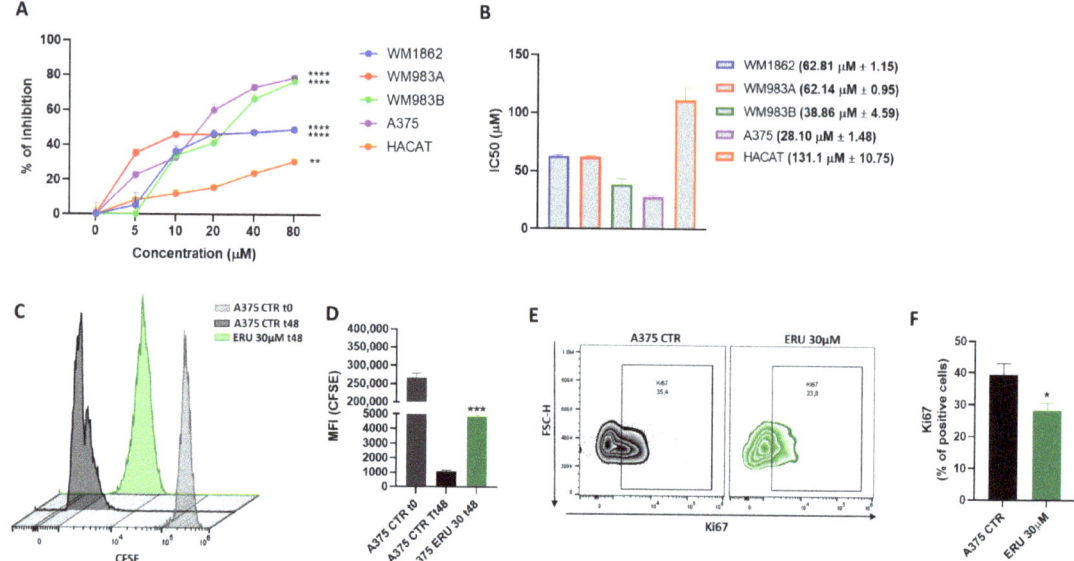

Figure 1. ERU affected the proliferation rate of human melanoma cell lines. (**A**) Antiproliferative effect of ERU (0–80 μM) was assessed with MTT assay in A375, WM1862, WM983A and WM983B melanoma cells and in normal human keratinocytes (HaCaT) at 48 h. (**B**) IC50 values for ERU-treated A375, WM1862, WM983A and WM983B melanoma cells and for HaCaT cells. (**C**) Representative example of flow cytometry analysis of CFSE staining in A375 cells after staining (grey histogram) and after 48 h of treatment (green histogram) or no treatment (black histogram) with 30 μM ERU. (**D**) CFSE quantification in terms of mean fluorescence intensity (MFI). (**E**) Representative example of flow cytometry analysis of A375-derived Ki67 upon treatment (green dot plot) or no treatment (black dot plot) with 30 μM ERU. (**F**) Frequency of Ki67 in A375 cells after treatment (green bar) or no treatment (black bar) with 30 μM ERU. Data were shown as mean ± SEM of at least three independent experiments (* $p < 0.05$, ** $p < 0.01$, *** $p < 0.001$ and **** $p < 0.0001$ vs. A375 CTRL).

3.2. ERU Induced Apoptosis and the Cell Cycle Arrest of Human Melanoma Cells

Next, we decided to evaluate whether the antiproliferative effect of ERU was due to the induction of cell death by apoptosis and/or necrosis. First, we assessed the live vs. dead status of the ERU-treated A375 melanoma cells using the fluorescent dye Zombie Green. As shown in Figure 2A,B, the ERU treatment for 48 h significantly induced cell death in the A375 melanoma cells compared to the control. Next, to define whether the A375 dead status was associated with apoptosis and/or necrosis, we performed an annexin V and PI double staining analysis (Figure 2C). A FACS analysis showed that ERU significantly induced the apoptosis of the A375 cells, confirming that cell death was mediated by apoptosis (Figure 2D). To support this finding, we monitored the activation of caspase 9 and 3, which are the key players in the upstream and downstream regulation of apoptotic signal transduction [29]. As expected, the 48 h treatment with 30 μM ERU significantly induced the activation of both caspase 9 and 3 (Figure 2E). In addition, we also assessed the expression of two antiapoptotic genes, the X-chromosome-linked inhibitor of the apoptosis protein (XIAP) and B-cell lymphoma gene 2 (Bcl-2). A qPCR analysis showed that ERU markedly decreased the expression of both antiapoptotic genes (Figure 2F) in the A375 human melanoma cells. Furthermore, we also performed a cell cycle assay to evaluate the cell cycle distribution of the A375 cells after a 24 h treatment with ERU (Figure 2G). The ERU treatment significantly increased the percentage of the A375 cells in the G2/M phase and reduced the percentage of the A375 cells in the G1 and S phases compared to the control (Figure 2H). To confirm this result, we also analyzed the expression of CCNB1, CDK1 and CDC25C, the most important cell cycle regulatory proteins involved in the regulation of G2/M progression [30]. As shown in Figure 2I, the mRNA levels of CCNB1, CDK1 and CDC25C were significantly decreased in the ERU-treated A375 cells compared to the control. These results demonstrated that ERU exerted a proapoptotic effect in the melanoma cells and induced their cell cycle arrest in the G2/M phase.

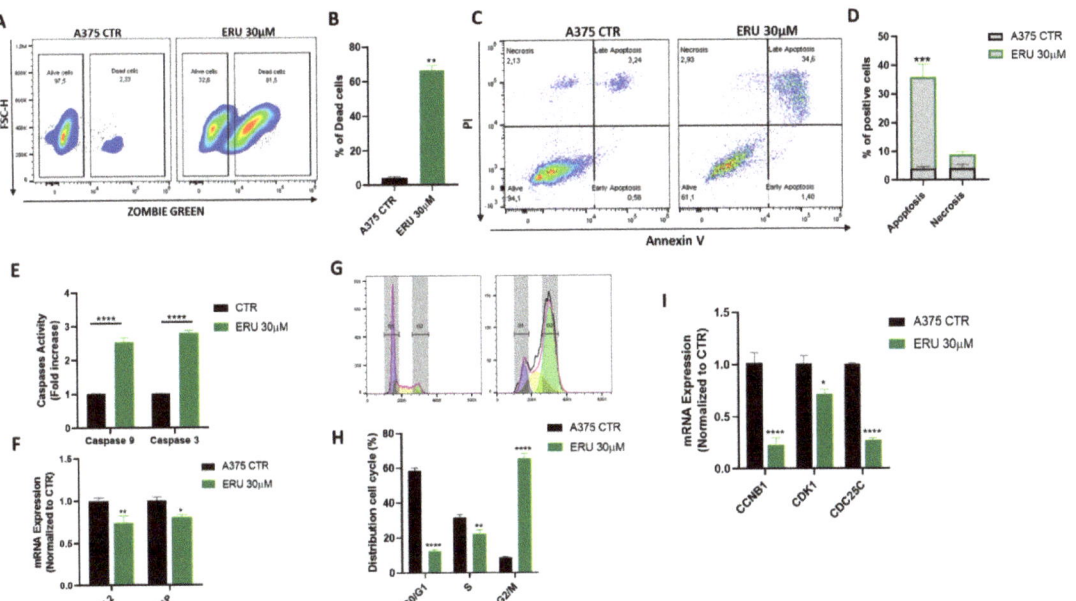

Figure 2. ERU induced apoptosis and cell cycle arrest of human melanoma cells. (**A**) Representative example of flow cytometry analysis of Zombie Green staining in A375 cells upon 48 h of treatment or no treatment with 30 μM ERU. (**B**) Frequency of dead cells after treatment (green bar) or no treatment (black bar) for 48 h with 30 μM ERU. (**C**) Representative example of annexin V/propidium iodide (PI) staining after 48 h of treatment or no treatment with 30 μM ERU. (**D**) Frequency of apoptotic cells after treatment (green bar) or no treatment (black bar) for 48 h with 30 μM ERU. (**E**) Activation of caspase 9 and 3 in A375 cells upon 48 h of treatment (green bar) or no treatment (black bar) with 30 μM ERU. (**F**) Expression of BCL2 and XIAP assessed with qPCR in A375 cells upon 6 h of treatment (green bar) or no treatment (black bar) with 30 μM ERU. (**G**) Representative example of cell cycle distribution in A375 cells upon 24 h of treatment or no treatment with 30 ERU. (**H**) Frequency of A375 cells in G0/G1, S and G2/M cell cycle distributions after treatment (green bar) or no treatment (black bar) for 24 h with 30 μM ERU. (**I**) Expression of CCNB1, CDK1 and CDC25C assessed with qPCR in A375 cells upon 6 h of treatment (green bar) or no treatment (black bar) with 30 μM ERU. Data were shown as mean ± SEM of at least three independent experiments (* $p < 0.05$, ** $p < 0.01$, *** $p < 0.001$ and **** $p < 0.0001$ vs. A375 CTRL).

3.3. ERU Modulated the Expression of Cadherins in Human Melanoma Cells

Apoptosis and the cell cycle are complex mechanisms that are finely tuned by different pathways. Among these, cadherins are key players involved in the phenomenon of the epithelial-to-mesenchymal transition (EMT) that favor cancer cell proliferation and invasion. In particular, the loss of E-cadherin (E-CAD) from cancer cells is associated with apoptosis inhibition, whilst the increase of N-cadherin (N-CAD) promotes cancer cell growth. Moreover, it has been also demonstrated that both N-CAD and E-CAD are associated with apoptosis given their ability to increase proapoptotic genes [31] or to interact with death receptors [32], respectively. Thus, we evaluated whether the expression of both E-CAD and N-CAD was modulated in the ERU-treated A375 melanoma cells. As shown in Figure 3A–C, ERU promoted the expression of the epithelial protein E-CAD and reduced the expression of the mesenchymal protein N-CAD after the 24 h treatment of A375 melanoma cells. Moreover, we analyzed the expression of transcription factors associated with the EMT and apoptosis resistance (e.g., SNAIL, SLUG, ZEB1 and TWIST) [33]. A qPCR analysis demonstrated that ERU significantly reduced the expression of all the transcription factors tested in the A375 melanoma cells (Figure 3D). These data further demonstrated that the proapoptotic effect of ERU was associated with the modulation of the EMT-related cadherins.

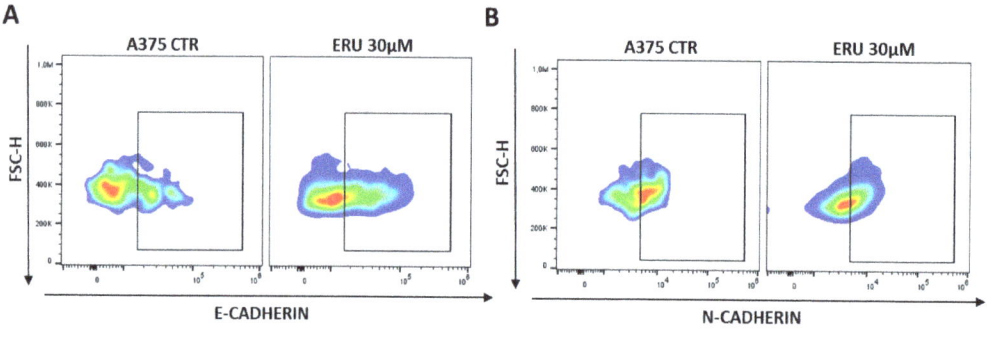

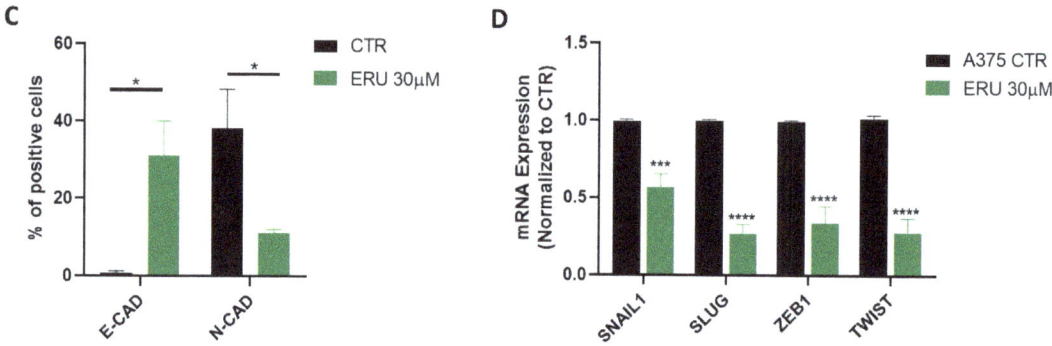

Figure 3. ERU modulated the expression of cadherins in human melanoma cells. (**A,B**) Representative example of flow cytometry analysis of A375-derived E-CAD and N-CAD upon treatment (green dot plot) or no treatment (black dot plot) with 30 µM ERU. (**C**) Frequency of Ki67 in A375 cells after treatment (green bar) or no treatment (black bar) with 30 µM ERU. (**D**) Expression of SNAIL1, SLUG, ZEB-1 and TWIST assessed with qPCR in A375 cells upon 6 h of treatment (green bar) or no treatment (black bar) with 30 µM ERU. Data were shown as mean ± SEM of at least three independent experiments (* $p < 0.05$, *** $p < 0.001$ and **** $p < 0.0001$ vs. A375 CTRL).

3.4. ERU at Low Concentrations Impaired Melanoma Cell Migration and Invasiveness

In line with the findings about cadherins, we decided to evaluate whether ERU at low concentrations below the IC50 value was able to affect the migration and invasion of the A375 melanoma cells. Thus, we decided to use the concentration of 1 µM which showed no cytotoxic effect on the A375 melanoma cells. First, we performed a migration assay on the A375 melanoma cells treated with 1 µM ERU. As shown in Figure 4A,B, ERU significantly reduced the migration of the A375 melanoma cells at both 24 and 48 h. Likewise, the colony formation assay confirmed that ERU reduced the number of the A375 colonies compared to the control (Figure 4C,D). In addition, the invasion assay demonstrated that ERU significantly reduced the invasiveness of the A375 melanoma cells (Figure 4E,F). Melanin production by cancer cells was reported to promote melanoma progression and metastasis development by affecting the different molecular mechanisms including the EMT [34]. Therefore, we hypothesized that ERU could modulate melanin production in the A375 cells. To address this point, we evaluated the melanin content in the ERU-treated A375 cells. As shown in Figure 4G, we found that ERU significantly reduced the melanin content in the A375 melanoma cells. To corroborate this finding, we evaluated the mRNA expression level of the microphthalmia-associated transcription factor (MITF) and the tyrosinase enzyme (TYR), the two most important genes involved in melanin synthesis and in melanoma development [35], with a qPCR analysis. As expected, 1 µM ERU significantly reduced the expression levels of both the MITF and TYR (Figure 4H). Taken together, our data suggested that ERU thwarted the migratory and invasive capacity of the melanoma cells by modulating their melanin production.

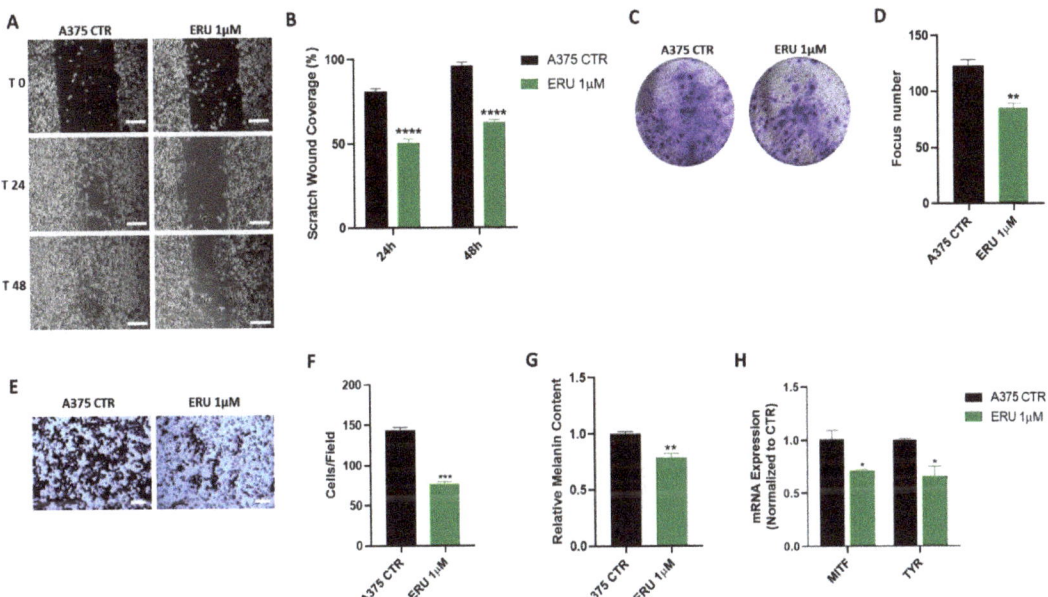

Figure 4. ERU at low concentrations impaired melanoma cell migration and invasiveness. (**A**) Representative example of wound healing assay of A375 cells after incubation with 1 µM ERU for 24 and 48 h (scale bar: 250 µm). (**B**) Quantification of the healed wound area at 24 and 48 h. (**C,D**) Representative example (**C**) and quantification (**D**) of clonogenic assays of A375 cells after incubation with 1 µM ERU. (**E**) Representative example of invasion assay of A375 cells after incubation with 1 µM ERU (scale bar: 200 µm). (**F**) Average number of invasive cells per field. (**G**) Melanin content in A375 melanoma cells upon treatment (green dot plot) or no treatment (black dot plot) with 1 µM ERU. (**H**) Expression of MITF and TYR assessed with qPCR in A375 cells upon 6 h of treatment (green bar) or no treatment (black bar) with 1 µM ERU. Data were shown as mean ± SEM of at least three independent experiments (* $p < 0.05$, ** $p < 0.01$, *** $p < 0.001$, and **** $p < 0.0001$ vs. A375 CTRL).

3.5. ERU Inhibited ROS Production in Melanoma Cells by Limiting Their Mitochondrial Function

It has been described that the presence of melanin inside melanoma cells triggers the production of important levels of reactive oxygen/nitrogen species (ROS/RNS), promoting melanoma progression [36]. To further dissect the mechanism underlying the antimigratory effects on the A375 cells, we evaluated the ability of ERU to modulate ROS production in the melanoma cells. Interestingly, the treatment for 48 h with ERU (1 µM) significantly suppressed ROS formation as demonstrated by the reduced fluorescence intensity of the DCF probe (Figure 5A). Next, we measured the mitochondrial mass and membrane potential of the ERU-treated A375 cells given the key role of the mitochondria in ROS production [37]. As shown in Figure 5B,C, both the Mitotracker Green and Deep Red dyes' uptakes were significantly decreased in the ERU-treated A375 cells, suggesting a reduced mitochondrial mass and mitochondrial membrane potential. To corroborate our data, we assessed the effect of ERU on the expression of different antioxidant enzymes such as GCLC and GCLM, the catalytic and modulatory subunits involved in the synthesis of glutathione, respectively, as well as the heme oxygenase-1 enzyme (HMOX-1). As expected, a qPCR analysis showed a significant increase in GCLC, GCLM and HMOX-1 after treatment of the A375 cells with 1uM ERU (Figure 5D). These findings indicated that the antimigratory effects of ERU correlated with a decline in the mitochondrial function, which, in turn, impaired ROS production and cellular fitness in the melanoma cancer cells.

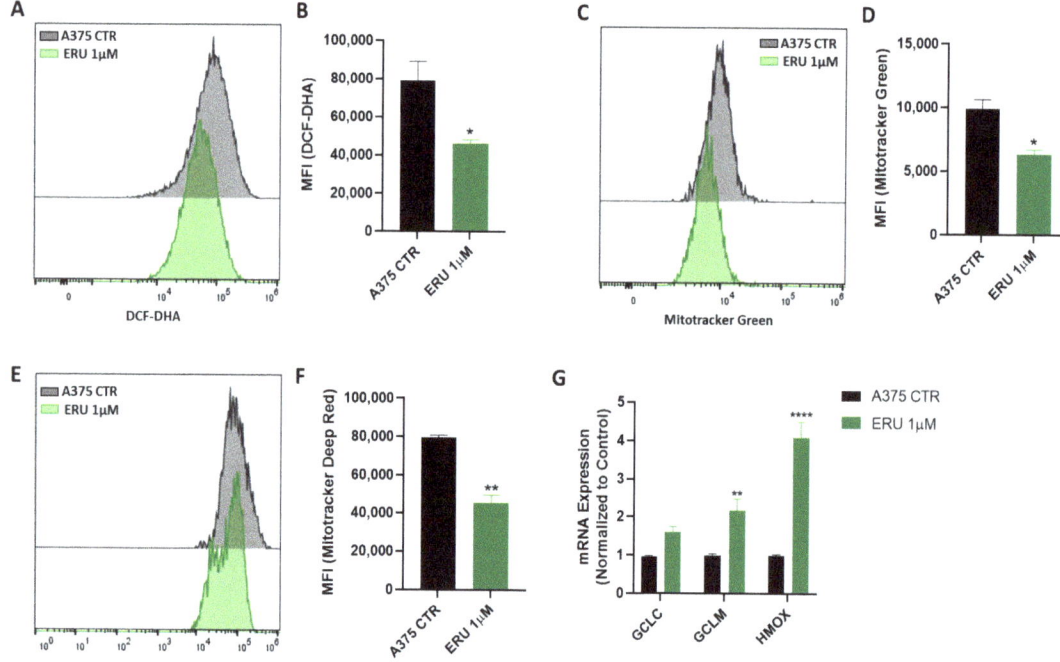

Figure 5. ERU inhibited ROS production in melanoma cells by limiting their mitochondrial function. (**A–F**) Representative examples of flow cytometry analysis of DCF-DHA. (**A**) MitoTracker Green (**C**) and MitoTracker Deep Red staining (**E**) in A375 cells that were untreated (black histograms) and those that underwent ERU treatment (green histograms) for 48 h with their respective quantification in terms of mean fluorescence intensity (MFI) (**B,D,F**). (**G**) Expression of GCLC, GCLM and HMOX assessed with qPCR analysis in A375 melanoma cells that were treated (green bar) or not treated (black bar) with 1 µM ERU. Data were shown as mean ± SEM of at least three independent experiments (* $p < 0.05$, ** $p < 0.01$ and **** $p < 0.0001$ vs. A375 CTRL).

4. Discussion

Natural products are emerging as promising tools in cancer therapy given their multitarget activity and their ability to modulate the tumor microenvironment. In particular, diet-derived compounds, such as coffee; tea; pomegranate; extra virgin olive oil; and brassicaceae vegetables, which include broccoli, brussels sprouts and rocket salads, have been widely demonstrated to prevent cancer development [11,38]. In fact, it has been reported that melanoma and nonmelanoma skin cancers' low incidence in Mediterranean populations might be associated with the intake of the vegetables, fish and fruit that constitute the traditional Mediterranean diet [39,40]. This is mainly due to the presence of different dietary antioxidant compounds, such as carotenoids, vitamins, polyphenols and isothiocyanates. Importantly, different data also suggested that these compounds may improve the efficacy of classic chemotherapeutics by exerting a synergistic effect on the one hand and by restraining chemoresistance on the other hand [41,42]. Particularly, the anticancer effects of isothiocyanates have been ascribed to their ability to release H_2S [19,43]. In fact, H_2S-releasing agents have been proposed as a promising therapeutic approach for the treatment of different types of cancer [44–47]. Likewise, ERU, the major isothiocyanate present in rocked salads with H_2S-releasing properties [48–53], demonstrated its anticancer activity in different tumor cell lines in vitro and in tumor-bearing mice in vivo [18,54–56]. In this study, we characterized the anticancer properties of ERU in human melanoma by using multiple in vitro approaches. We observed that ERU inhibited the proliferation of the different human melanoma cell lines in a time-dependent manner as has also been reported in pancreatic cancer cells [18]. Moreover, similarly to other diet-derived compounds [57–59], ERU modulated the expression of the proliferation marker Ki67 that has been proposed as a prognostic biomarker in cutaneous melanoma [60]. Our own group, and others, demonstrated that both natural and synthetic H_2S donors induce apoptosis in melanoma cells [20–22,24,25]. Likewise, we demonstrated that the antiproliferative effect of ERU was coupled with its ability to induce apoptosis in the A375 melanoma cells. In fact, we observed the activation of both caspase 3 and 9 and the downregulation of the proapoptotic genes BCL-2 and XIAP after 48 h of treatment with ERU. Moreover, ERU was able to induce cell cycle arrest in the G2/M phase as previously demonstrated in pancreatic and breast cancer cells [14,18]. E-CAD and N-CAD represented the two major proteins involved in the EMT phenomenon and was reported to orchestrate apoptosis [32,61]. ERU significantly increased the expression of the epithelial protein E-CAD, whilst it reduced the expression of the mesenchymal protein N-CAD. Melanoma progression and metastasis development were associated with the ability of melanoma cells to acquire aggressive properties, such as motility and invasion [62].

In fact, multiple diet-derived compounds were demonstrated to prevent tumor progression by modulating these parameters in different cancer cells [63–66]. In our study, we found that ERU at low concentrations below the IC50 value (1 μM) significantly reduced the migration, invasion and clonogenic potential of the A375 melanoma cells, which were parameters that reflected their ability to generate metastases in vivo. Emerging evidence demonstrated that the melanin secreted from the melanoma cells supported their progression and metastasis development, suppressing the immune response and promoting tumor angiogenesis [34,67]. Our results showed that ERU exerted an essential role in modulating the melanogenesis in the melanoma cells by inhibiting the melanin content and suppressing the expression of the MITF and TYR, which are the key factors that promote melanin synthesis [35,68]. Melanoma-cell-produced melanin also contributes to oxidative stress, which in turn promotes melanoma initiation and progression [69,70]. In our study, ERU reduced intracellular ROS generation in the A375 cells by modulating their mitochondrial activity. Moreover, ERU increased the expression of antioxidant target genes, such as GCLC, GCLM and HMOX-1, suggesting that the modulation of ROS production and the impairment of mitochondrial activity in the melanoma cells were among the contributing factors, which supported the antitumor activity of ERU.

5. Conclusions

This work widely characterized the anticancer properties of ERU in human melanoma in vitro. In fact, we demonstrated that, in the human melanoma cells, ERU (i) inhibited cell proliferation, (ii) induced apoptosis and cell cycle arrest and (iii) reduced the expression of cadherins and their related transcription factors. Moreover, a low concentration of ERU thwarted cell migration and invasion. This effect was associated with reduced levels of melanin and melanogenesis-associated genes. This is an important feature in melanoma progression since melanin production has been associated with the EMT and oxidative stress. Thus, ERU could represent a new promising diet-derived compound with anticancer properties, which are ascribed to its ability to release H_2S. However, translational in vivo studies are required to gain further insight into the antitumoral effects of ERU using murine models of cutaneous and metastatic melanoma.

Author Contributions: Conceptualization, G.E. and A.I.; methodology, D.C.M., B.R. and L.C.; software, D.C.M. and L.C.; data curation, G.E.; writing—original draft preparation, D.C.M. and L.C.; writing—review and editing, G.E. and A.I.; supervision, G.E.; funding acquisition, G.E. and A.I. All authors have read and agreed to the published version of the manuscript.

Funding: This work was supported by the Associazione Italiana per la Ricerca sul Cancro (AIRC) (MFAG No. 26002 to G.E.) and by Italian government grants (PRIN 2017 No. 2017BA9LM5 to A.I.).

Institutional Review Board Statement: Not applicable.

Informed Consent Statement: Not applicable.

Data Availability Statement: The data are contained within the manuscript.

Conflicts of Interest: The authors declare no conflict of interest.

References

1. Davis, L.E.; Shalin, S.C.; Tackett, A.J. Current state of melanoma diagnosis and treatment. *Cancer Biol. Ther.* **2019**, *20*, 1366–1379. [CrossRef] [PubMed]
2. Rastrelli, M.; Tropea, S.; Rossi, C.R.; Alaibac, M. Melanoma: Epidemiology, Risk Factors, Pathogenesis, Diagnosis and Classification. *In Vivo* **2014**, *28*, 1005–1011. [PubMed]
3. Sun, X.; Zhang, N.; Yin, C.; Zhu, B.; Li, X. Ultraviolet Radiation and Melanomagenesis: From Mechanism to Immunotherapy. *Front. Oncol.* **2020**, *10*, 951. [CrossRef] [PubMed]
4. Pfeifer, G.P. Mechanisms of UV-induced mutations and skin cancer. *Genome Instab. Dis.* **2020**, *1*, 99–113. [CrossRef]
5. Hocker, T.; Tsao, H. Ultraviolet radiation and melanoma: A systematic review and analysis of reported sequence variants. *Hum. Mutat.* **2007**, *28*, 578–588. [CrossRef]
6. Hainaut, P.; Pfeifer, G.P. Somatic TP53 Mutations in the Era of Genome Sequencing. *Cold Spring Harb. Perspect. Med.* **2016**, *6*, a026179. [CrossRef]
7. Thomas, N.E.; Berwick, M.; Cordeiro-Stone, M. Could BRAF mutations in melanocytic lesions arise from DNA damage induced by ultraviolet radiation? *J. Investig. Dermatol.* **2006**, *126*, 1693–1696. [CrossRef]
8. Besaratinia, A.; Pfeifer, G.P. Sunlight ultraviolet irradiation and BRAF V600 mutagenesis in human melanoma. *Hum. Mutat.* **2008**, *29*, 983–991. [CrossRef] [PubMed]
9. Davis, E.J.; Johnson, D.B.; Sosman, J.A.; Chandra, S. Melanoma: What do all the mutations mean? *Cancer* **2018**, *124*, 3490–3499. [CrossRef]
10. Thornton, J.; Chhabra, G.; Singh, C.K.; Guzman-Perez, G.; Shirley, C.A.; Ahmad, N. Mechanisms of Immunotherapy Resistance in Cutaneous Melanoma: Recognizing a Shapeshifter. *Front. Oncol.* **2022**, *12*, 880876. [CrossRef]
11. Langner, E.; Rzeski, W. Dietary derived compounds in cancer chemoprevention. *Contemp. Oncol.* **2012**, *16*, 394–400. [CrossRef] [PubMed]
12. Agagunduz, D.; Sahin, T.O.; Yilmaz, B.; Ekenci, K.D.; Duyar Ozer, S.; Capasso, R. Cruciferous Vegetables and Their Bioactive Metabolites: From Prevention to Novel Therapies of Colorectal Cancer. *Evid. Based Complement. Altern. Med.* **2022**, *2022*, 1534083. [CrossRef]
13. Veeranki, O.L.; Bhattacharya, A.; Tang, L.; Marshall, J.R.; Zhang, Y. Cruciferous vegetables, isothiocyanates, and prevention of bladder cancer. *Curr. Pharmacol. Rep.* **2015**, *1*, 272–282. [CrossRef]
14. Azarenko, O.; Jordan, M.A.; Wilson, L. Erucin, the major isothiocyanate in arugula (Eruca sativa), inhibits proliferation of MCF7 tumor cells by suppressing microtubule dynamics. *PLoS ONE* **2014**, *9*, e100599. [CrossRef] [PubMed]
15. Melchini, A.; Costa, C.; Traka, M.; Miceli, N.; Mithen, R.; De Pasquale, R.; Trovato, A. Erucin, a new promising cancer chemopreventive agent from rocket salads, shows anti-proliferative activity on human lung carcinoma A549 cells. *Food Chem. Toxicol.* **2009**, *47*, 1430–1436. [CrossRef] [PubMed]
16. Fimognari, C.; Nusse, M.; Iori, R.; Cantelli-Forti, G.; Hrelia, P. The new isothiocyanate 4-(methylthio)butylisothiocyanate selectively affects cell-cycle progression and apoptosis induction of human leukemia cells. *Investig. New Drugs* **2004**, *22*, 119–129. [CrossRef]
17. Melchini, A.; Traka, M.H. Biological profile of erucin: A new promising anticancer agent from cruciferous vegetables. *Toxins* **2010**, *2*, 593–612. [CrossRef] [PubMed]

18. Citi, V.; Piragine, E.; Pagnotta, E.; Ugolini, L.; Di Cesare Mannelli, L.; Testai, L.; Ghelardini, C.; Lazzeri, L.; Calderone, V.; Martelli, A. Anticancer properties of erucin, an H2 S-releasing isothiocyanate, on human pancreatic adenocarcinoma cells (AsPC-1). *Phytother. Res.* **2019**, *33*, 845–855. [CrossRef]
19. Martelli, A.; Citi, V.; Testai, L.; Brogi, S.; Calderone, V. Organic Isothiocyanates as Hydrogen Sulfide Donors. *Antioxid. Redox Signal.* **2020**, *32*, 110–144. [CrossRef] [PubMed]
20. De Cicco, P.; Panza, E.; Armogida, C.; Ercolano, G.; Taglialatela-Scafati, O.; Shokoohinia, Y.; Camerlingo, R.; Pirozzi, G.; Calderone, V.; Cirino, G.; et al. The Hydrogen Sulfide Releasing Molecule Acetyl Deacylasadisulfide Inhibits Metastatic Melanoma. *Front. Pharmacol.* **2017**, *8*, 65. [CrossRef] [PubMed]
21. De Cicco, P.; Panza, E.; Ercolano, G.; Armogida, C.; Sessa, G.; Pirozzi, G.; Cirino, G.; Wallace, J.L.; Ianaro, A. ATB-346, a novel hydrogen sulfide-releasing anti-inflammatory drug, induces apoptosis of human melanoma cells and inhibits melanoma development in vivo. *Pharmacol. Res.* **2016**, *114*, 67–73. [CrossRef] [PubMed]
22. Ercolano, G.; De Cicco, P.; Frecentese, F.; Saccone, I.; Corvino, A.; Giordano, F.; Magli, E.; Fiorino, F.; Severino, B.; Calderone, V.; et al. Anti-metastatic Properties of Naproxen-HBTA in a Murine Model of Cutaneous Melanoma. *Front. Pharmacol.* **2019**, *10*, 66. [CrossRef] [PubMed]
23. Xiao, Q.; Ying, J.; Qiao, Z.; Yang, Y.; Dai, X.; Xu, Z.; Zhang, C.; Xiang, L. Exogenous hydrogen sulfide inhibits human melanoma cell development via suppression of the PI3K/AKT/mTOR pathway. *J. Dermatol. Sci.* **2020**, *98*, 26–34. [CrossRef] [PubMed]
24. Cai, F.; Xu, H.; Cao, N.; Zhang, X.; Liu, J.; Lu, Y.; Chen, J.; Yang, Y.; Cheng, J.; Hua, Z.C.; et al. ADT-OH, a hydrogen sulfide-releasing donor, induces apoptosis and inhibits the development of melanoma in vivo by upregulating FADD. *Cell Death Dis.* **2020**, *11*, 33. [CrossRef]
25. Panza, E.; De Cicco, P.; Armogida, C.; Scognamiglio, G.; Gigantino, V.; Botti, G.; Germano, D.; Napolitano, M.; Papapetropoulos, A.; Bucci, M.; et al. Role of the cystathionine gamma lyase/hydrogen sulfide pathway in human melanoma progression. *Pigment. Cell Melanoma Res.* **2015**, *28*, 61–72. [CrossRef]
26. Ercolano, G.; Gomez-Cadena, A.; Dumauthioz, N.; Vanoni, G.; Kreutzfeldt, M.; Wyss, T.; Michalik, L.; Loyon, R.; Ianaro, A.; Ho, P.C.; et al. PPAR drives IL-33-dependent ILC2 pro-tumoral functions. *Nat. Commun.* **2021**, *12*, 2538. [CrossRef]
27. Widmer, D.S.; Cheng, P.F.; Eichhoff, O.M.; Belloni, B.C.; Zipser, M.C.; Schlegel, N.C.; Javelaud, D.; Mauviel, A.; Dummer, R.; Hoek, K.S. Systematic classification of melanoma cells by phenotype-specific gene expression mapping. *Pigment. Cell Melanoma Res.* **2012**, *25*, 343–353. [CrossRef]
28. Menon, S.S.; Guruvayoorappan, C.; Sakthivel, K.M.; Rasmi, R.R. Ki-67 protein as a tumour proliferation marker. *Clin. Chim. Acta* **2019**, *491*, 39–45. [CrossRef]
29. McIlwain, D.R.; Berger, T.; Mak, T.W. Caspase functions in cell death and disease. *Cold Spring Harb. Perspect. Biol.* **2013**, *5*, a008656. [CrossRef]
30. Wang, Y.; Ji, P.; Liu, J.; Broaddus, R.R.; Xue, F.; Zhang, W. Centrosome-associated regulators of the G(2)/M checkpoint as targets for cancer therapy. *Mol. Cancer* **2009**, *8*, 8. [CrossRef]
31. Lelievre, E.C.; Plestant, C.; Boscher, C.; Wolff, E.; Mege, R.M.; Birbes, H. N-cadherin mediates neuronal cell survival through Bim down-regulation. *PLoS ONE* **2012**, *7*, e33206. [CrossRef] [PubMed]
32. Lu, M.; Marsters, S.; Ye, X.; Luis, E.; Gonzalez, L.; Ashkenazi, A. E-cadherin couples death receptors to the cytoskeleton to regulate apoptosis. *Mol. Cell* **2014**, *54*, 987–998. [CrossRef] [PubMed]
33. Barrallo-Gimeno, A.; Nieto, M.A. The Snail genes as inducers of cell movement and survival: Implications in development and cancer. *Development* **2005**, *132*, 3151–3161. [CrossRef] [PubMed]
34. Cabaco, L.C.; Tomas, A.; Pojo, M.; Barral, D.C. The Dark Side of Melanin Secretion in Cutaneous Melanoma Aggressiveness. *Front. Oncol.* **2022**, *12*, 887366. [CrossRef] [PubMed]
35. Hartman, M.L.; Czyz, M. MITF in melanoma: Mechanisms behind its expression and activity. *Cell. Mol. Life Sci.* **2015**, *72*, 1249–1260. [CrossRef] [PubMed]
36. Napolitano, A.; Panzella, L.; Monfrecola, G.; d'Ischia, M. Pheomelanin-induced oxidative stress: Bright and dark chemistry bridging red hair phenotype and melanoma. *Pigment. Cell Melanoma Res.* **2014**, *27*, 721–733. [CrossRef]
37. Balaban, R.S.; Nemoto, S.; Finkel, T. Mitochondria, oxidants, and aging. *Cell* **2005**, *120*, 483–495. [CrossRef]
38. Ghazi, T.; Arumugam, T.; Foolchand, A.; Chuturgoon, A.A. The Impact of Natural Dietary Compounds and Food-Borne Mycotoxins on DNA Methylation and Cancer. *Cells* **2020**, *9*, 2004. [CrossRef]
39. Malagoli, C.; Malavolti, M.; Agnoli, C.; Crespi, C.M.; Fiorentini, C.; Farnetani, F.; Longo, C.; Ricci, C.; Albertini, G.; Lanzoni, A.; et al. Diet Quality and Risk of Melanoma in an Italian Population. *J. Nutr.* **2015**, *145*, 1800–1807. [CrossRef]
40. Arts, I.C.; Hollman, P.C. Polyphenols and disease risk in epidemiologic studies. *Am. J. Clin. Nutr.* **2005**, *81*, 317S–325S. [CrossRef]
41. Reitz, L.K.; Schroeder, J.; Longo, G.Z.; Boaventura, B.C.B.; Di Pietro, P.F. Dietary Antioxidant Capacity Promotes a Protective Effect against Exacerbated Oxidative Stress in Women Undergoing Adjuvant Treatment for Breast Cancer in a Prospective Study. *Nutrients* **2021**, *13*, 4324. [CrossRef] [PubMed]
42. Castaneda, A.M.; Melendez, C.M.; Uribe, D.; Pedroza-Diaz, J. Synergistic effects of natural compounds and conventional chemotherapeutic agents: Recent insights for the development of cancer treatment strategies. *Heliyon* **2022**, *8*, e09519. [CrossRef] [PubMed]
43. Lin, Y.; Yang, X.; Lu, Y.; Liang, D.; Huang, D. Isothiocyanates as H2S Donors Triggered by Cysteine: Reaction Mechanism and Structure and Activity Relationship. *Org. Lett.* **2019**, *21*, 5977–5980. [CrossRef] [PubMed]

44. Sakuma, S.; Minamino, S.; Takase, M.; Ishiyama, Y.; Hosokura, H.; Kohda, T.; Ikeda, Y.; Fujimoto, Y. Hydrogen sulfide donor GYY4137 suppresses proliferation of human colorectal cancer Caco-2 cells by inducing both cell cycle arrest and cell death. *Heliyon* **2019**, *5*, e02284. [CrossRef] [PubMed]
45. Chen, X.X.; Liu, X.W.; Zhou, Z.G.; Chen, X.Y.; Li, L.D.; Xiong, T.; Peng, L.; Tu, J. Diallyl disulfide inhibits invasion and metastasis of MCF-7 breast cancer cells in vitro by down-regulating p38 activity. *J. South. Med. Univ.* **2016**, *36*, 814–818.
46. Zheng, J.; Cheng, X.; Xu, S.; Zhang, L.; Pan, J.; Yu, H.; Bao, J.; Lu, R. Diallyl trisulfide induces G2/M cell-cycle arrest and apoptosis in anaplastic thyroid carcinoma 8505C cells. *Food Funct.* **2019**, *10*, 7253–7261. [CrossRef]
47. Yue, Z.; Guan, X.; Chao, R.; Huang, C.; Li, D.; Yang, P.; Liu, S.; Hasegawa, T.; Guo, J.; Li, M. Diallyl Disulfide Induces Apoptosis and Autophagy in Human Osteosarcoma MG-63 Cells through the PI3K/Akt/mTOR Pathway. *Molecules* **2019**, *24*, 2665. [CrossRef]
48. Testai, L.; Pagnotta, E.; Piragine, E.; Flori, L.; Citi, V.; Martelli, A.; Mannelli, L.D.C.; Ghelardini, C.; Matteo, R.; Suriano, S.; et al. Cardiovascular benefits of Eruca sativa mill. Defatted seed meal extract: Potential role of hydrogen sulfide. *Phytother. Res.* **2022**, *36*, 2616–2627. [CrossRef]
49. Martelli, A.; Piragine, E.; Gorica, E.; Citi, V.; Testai, L.; Pagnotta, E.; Lazzeri, L.; Pecchioni, N.; Ciccone, V.; Montanaro, R.; et al. The H(2)S-Donor Erucin Exhibits Protective Effects against Vascular Inflammation in Human Endothelial and Smooth Muscle Cells. *Antioxidants* **2021**, *10*, 961. [CrossRef]
50. Hu, X.; Xiao, Y.; Sun, J.; Ji, B.; Luo, S.; Wu, B.; Zheng, C.; Wang, P.; Xu, F.; Cheng, K.; et al. New possible silver lining for pancreatic cancer therapy: Hydrogen sulfide and its donors. *Acta Pharm. Sin. B* **2021**, *11*, 1148–1157. [CrossRef]
51. Martelli, A.; Piragine, E.; Citi, V.; Testai, L.; Pagnotta, E.; Ugolini, L.; Lazzeri, L.; Di Cesare Mannelli, L.; Manzo, O.L.; Bucci, M.; et al. Erucin exhibits vasorelaxing effects and antihypertensive activity by H(2) S-releasing properties. *Br. J. Pharmacol.* **2020**, *177*, 824–835. [CrossRef] [PubMed]
52. Sestito, S.; Pruccoli, L.; Runfola, M.; Citi, V.; Martelli, A.; Saccomanni, G.; Calderone, V.; Tarozzi, A.; Rapposelli, S. Design and synthesis of H(2)S-donor hybrids: A new treatment for Alzheimer's disease? *Eur. J. Med. Chem.* **2019**, *184*, 111745. [CrossRef] [PubMed]
53. Kashfi, K.; Olson, K.R. Biology and therapeutic potential of hydrogen sulfide and hydrogen sulfide-releasing chimeras. *Biochem. Pharmacol.* **2013**, *85*, 689–703. [CrossRef]
54. Kaur, H.; Kaur, K.; Singh, A.; Bedi, N.; Singh, B.; Alturki, M.S.; Aldawsari, M.F.; Almalki, A.H.; Haque, S.; Lee, H.J.; et al. Frankincense oil-loaded nanoemulsion formulation of paclitaxel and erucin: A synergistic combination for ameliorating drug resistance in breast cancer: In vitro and in vivo study. *Front. Pharmacol.* **2022**, *13*, 1020602. [CrossRef]
55. Awadelkareem, A.M.; Al-Shammari, E.; Elkhalifa, A.E.O.; Adnan, M.; Siddiqui, A.J.; Snoussi, M.; Khan, M.I.; Azad, Z.; Patel, M.; Ashraf, S.A. Phytochemical and In Silico ADME/Tox Analysis of Eruca sativa Extract with Antioxidant, Antibacterial and Anticancer Potential against Caco-2 and HCT-116 Colorectal Carcinoma Cell Lines. *Molecules* **2022**, *27*, 1409. [CrossRef] [PubMed]
56. Prelowska, M.; Kaczynska, A.; Herman-Antosiewicz, A. 4-(Methylthio)butyl isothiocyanate inhibits the proliferation of breast cancer cells with different receptor status. *Pharmacol. Rep.* **2017**, *69*, 1059–1066. [CrossRef] [PubMed]
57. Hell, T.; Dobrzynski, M.; Groflin, F.; Reinhardt, J.K.; Durr, L.; Pertz, O.; Hamburger, M.; Garo, E. Flavonoids from Ericameria nauseosa inhibiting PI3K/AKT pathway in human melanoma cells. *Biomed. Pharmacother.* **2022**, *156*, 113754. [CrossRef]
58. Zitek, T.; Bjelic, D.; Kotnik, P.; Golle, A.; Jurgec, S.; Potocnik, U.; Knez, Z.; Finsgar, M.; Krajnc, M.; Krajnc, I.; et al. Natural Hemp-Ginger Extract and Its Biological and Therapeutic Efficacy. *Molecules* **2022**, *27*, 7694. [CrossRef]
59. AlQathama, A.; Prieto, J.M. Natural products with therapeutic potential in melanoma metastasis. *Nat. Prod. Rep.* **2015**, *32*, 1170–1182. [CrossRef]
60. Gimotty, P.A.; Van Belle, P.; Elder, D.E.; Murry, T.; Montone, K.T.; Xu, X.; Hotz, S.; Raines, S.; Ming, M.E.; Wahl, P.; et al. Biologic and prognostic significance of dermal Ki67 expression, mitoses, and tumorigenicity in thin invasive cutaneous melanoma. *J. Clin. Oncol.* **2005**, *23*, 8048–8056. [CrossRef]
61. Loh, C.Y.; Chai, J.Y.; Tang, T.F.; Wong, W.F.; Sethi, G.; Shanmugam, M.K.; Chong, P.P.; Looi, C.Y. The E-Cadherin and N-Cadherin Switch in Epithelial-to-Mesenchymal Transition: Signaling, Therapeutic Implications, and Challenges. *Cells* **2019**, *8*, 1118. [CrossRef]
62. Arozarena, I.; Wellbrock, C. Targeting invasive properties of melanoma cells. *FEBS J.* **2017**, *284*, 2148–2162. [CrossRef] [PubMed]
63. Cheng, C.S.; Chen, J.X.; Tang, J.; Geng, Y.W.; Zheng, L.; Lv, L.L.; Chen, L.Y.; Chen, Z. Paeonol Inhibits Pancreatic Cancer Cell Migration and Invasion Through the Inhibition of TGF-beta1/Smad Signaling and Epithelial-Mesenchymal-Transition. *Cancer Manag. Res.* **2020**, *12*, 641–651. [CrossRef]
64. Allegra, M.; De Cicco, P.; Ercolano, G.; Attanzio, A.; Busa, R.; Cirino, G.; Tesoriere, L.; Livrea, M.A.; Ianaro, A. Indicaxanthin from Opuntia Ficus Indica (L. Mill) impairs melanoma cell proliferation, invasiveness, and tumor progression. *Phytomedicine* **2018**, *50*, 19–24. [CrossRef]
65. De Cicco, P.; Ercolano, G.; Tenore, G.C.; Ianaro, A. Olive leaf extract inhibits metastatic melanoma spread through suppression of epithelial to mesenchymal transition. *Phytother. Res.* **2022**, *36*, 4002–4013. [CrossRef] [PubMed]
66. De Cicco, P.; Busa, R.; Ercolano, G.; Formisano, C.; Allegra, M.; Taglialatela-Scafati, O.; Ianaro, A. Inhibitory effects of cynaropicrin on human melanoma progression by targeting MAPK, NF-kappaB, and Nrf-2 signaling pathways in vitro. *Phytother. Res.* **2021**, *35*, 1432–1442. [CrossRef] [PubMed]
67. Saud, A.; Sagineedu, S.R.; Ng, H.S.; Stanslas, J.; Lim, J.C.W. Melanoma metastasis: What role does melanin play? (Review). *Oncol. Rep.* **2022**, *48*, 1–10. [CrossRef]

68. Kawakami, A.; Fisher, D.E. The master role of microphthalmia-associated transcription factor in melanocyte and melanoma biology. *Lab. Investig.* **2017**, *97*, 649–656. [CrossRef]
69. Denat, L.; Kadekaro, A.L.; Marrot, L.; Leachman, S.A.; Abdel-Malek, Z.A. Melanocytes as instigators and victims of oxidative stress. *J. Investig. Dermatol.* **2014**, *134*, 1512–1518. [CrossRef]
70. Xing, X.; Dan, Y.; Xu, Z.; Xiang, L. Implications of Oxidative Stress in the Pathogenesis and Treatment of Hyperpigmentation Disorders. *Oxid. Med. Cell. Longev.* **2022**, *2022*, 7881717. [CrossRef]

Disclaimer/Publisher's Note: The statements, opinions and data contained in all publications are solely those of the individual author(s) and contributor(s) and not of MDPI and/or the editor(s). MDPI and/or the editor(s) disclaim responsibility for any injury to people or property resulting from any ideas, methods, instructions or products referred to in the content.

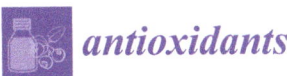

Article

Oral Administration of Glutathione Trisulfide Increases Reactive Sulfur Levels in Dorsal Root Ganglion and Ameliorates Paclitaxel-Induced Peripheral Neuropathy in Mice

Mariko Ezaka [1], Eizo Marutani [1], Yusuke Miyazaki [1], Eiki Kanemaru [1], Martin K. Selig [2], Sophie L. Boerboom [1], Katrina F. Ostrom [1], Anat Stemmer-Rachamimov [2], Donald B. Bloch [1,3], Gary J. Brenner [1], Etsuo Ohshima [4] and Fumito Ichinose [1,*]

[1] Anesthesia Center for Critical Care Research, Department of Anesthesia, Critical Care and Pain Medicine, Massachusetts General Hospital, Boston, MA 02114, USA
[2] Department of Pathology, Massachusetts General Hospital, Boston, MA 02114, USA
[3] Department of Medicine, Division of Rheumatology, Allergy and Immunology, Massachusetts General Hospital, Boston, MA 02114, USA
[4] Corporate Strategy Department, Kyowa Hakko Bio Co., Ltd., Tokyo 164-0001, Japan
* Correspondence: fichinose@mgh.harvard.edu; Tel.: +1-617-643-5757

Abstract: Peripheral neuropathy is a dose-limiting side effect of chemotherapy with paclitaxel. Paclitaxel-induced peripheral neuropathy (PIPN) is typically characterized by a predominantly sensory neuropathy presenting with allodynia, hyperalgesia and spontaneous pain. Oxidative mitochondrial damage in peripheral sensory neurons is implicated in the pathogenesis of PIPN. Reactive sulfur species, including persulfides (RSSH) and polysulfides (RS_nH), are strong nucleophilic and electrophilic compounds that exert antioxidant effects and protect mitochondria. Here, we examined the potential neuroprotective effects of glutathione trisulfide (GSSSG) in a mouse model of PIPN. Intraperitoneal administration of paclitaxel at 4 mg/kg/day for 4 days induced mechanical allodynia and thermal hyperalgesia in mice. Oral administration of GSSSG at 50 mg/kg/day for 28 days ameliorated mechanical allodynia, but not thermal hyperalgesia. Two hours after oral administration, ^{34}S-labeled GSSSG was detected in lumber dorsal root ganglia (DRG) and in the lumber spinal cord. In mice treated with paclitaxel, GSSSG upregulated expression of genes encoding antioxidant proteins in lumber DRG, prevented loss of unmyelinated axons and inhibited degeneration of mitochondria in the sciatic nerve. In cultured primary neurons from cortex and DRG, GSSSG mitigated paclitaxel-induced superoxide production, loss of axonal mitochondria, and axonal degeneration. These results indicate that oral administration of GSSSG mitigates PIPN by preventing axonal degeneration and mitochondria damage in peripheral sensory nerves. The findings suggest that administration of GSSSG may be an approach to the treatment or prevention of PIPN and other peripheral neuropathies.

Keywords: paclitaxel-induced peripheral neuropathy; glutathione trisulfide; persulfide; persulfidation

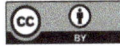

1. Introduction

In 2018, approximately 9.8 million cancer patients were treated with chemotherapy; the number of patients requiring cancer chemotherapy is expected to reach 15 million/year in 2040 [1]. Paclitaxel (PTX) is one of the most commonly used chemotherapeutic agents and is part of regimens to treat breast, ovarian, and prostate cancers. Paclitaxel-induced peripheral neuropathy (PIPN) is a dose-limiting side effect of paclitaxel, affecting 30% to 70% of treated patients [2]. PIPN manifests as allodynia, hyperalgesia and spontaneous pain, predominantly involving feet and hands [3]; PIPN generally develops during chemotherapy and often persists after cessation of paclitaxel [4]. PIPN worsens the quality of life of cancer survivors and can be severe enough to require discontinuation of chemotherapy. Unfortunately, other chemotherapeutic agents, including cisplatin and vincristine, can also cause peripheral neuropathy (termed "chemotherapy-induced peripheral neuropathy" (CIPN)). These chemotherapies may produce symptoms that are similar to those seen in patients with PIPN and are thought to act via similar pathogenetic mechanisms [5]. Because of the growing number of cancer survivors worldwide [1], the medico-economic impact of CIPN has increased significantly. Currently, there are few treatment options available for treating CIPNs, including PIPN.

While the precise pathogenesis of PIPN is unknown, the disease is thought to target peripheral sensory neuronal axons [6–8], which would explain why the longer axons of the hands and feet are predominantly affected. Impairment of Aβ fibers leads to mechanical allodynia, while hyperalgesia arises from damaged myelinated Aδ and unmyelinated C fibers [9]. The mechanism of action of paclitaxel as a chemotherapeutic agent is inhibition of cancer cell proliferation by stabilizing microtubule polymers, which need to disassemble during mitosis. In addition to this anti-tumor effect, paclitaxel causes mitochondrial dysfunction, which manifests as mitochondrial swelling [10], decreased mitochondrial membrane potential [11,12], increased levels of reactive oxygen species (ROS) [13], and impaired oxidative phosphorylation in peripheral neurons [14]. These off-target effects of paclitaxel have been implicated in the pathogenesis of PIPN. Nonetheless, no therapies have been developed to date that protect mitochondria in peripheral nerve sensory axons.

Reactive sulfur species, including persulfides and polysulfides, contain reactive sulfur that oxidizes or reduces other molecules. In particular, sulfane sulfur (S^0) atom has strong nucleophilicity that promotes persulfidation of protein thiols (cysteine residue). Thiol persulfidation competes with ROS-mediated thiol oxidation, thereby protecting proteins from irreversible oxidation. Endogenous persulfides, such as glutathione persulfide (GSSH) and cysteine persulfide (CysSSH), exert potent antioxidant effects, playing a key role in maintaining intracellular redox balance [15]. Nonetheless, the possible role of systemic administration of polysulfides to protect peripheral sensory neurons from paclitaxel injury by increasing local concentrations of reactive sulfur has not yet been examined. This study was designed to address this knowledge gap by examining the effects of a systemically administered stable formulation of glutathione trisulfide (GSSSG), an endogenous polysulfide, in a mouse model of PIPN. The structure of GSSSG contains a sulfane sulfur (Figure 1, arrow), and GSSSG is in equilibrium with GSSH as shown in the following equation [16].

$$\text{GSSSG} + \text{GSH} \leftrightarrow \text{GSSH} + \text{GSSG} \tag{1}$$

We hypothesized that systemic administration of GSSSG would increase the local concentration of reactive sulfur species in peripheral sensory nerves and ameliorate PIPN by protecting sensory nerve mitochondria. This study also examined whether GSSSG can attenuate PIPN without reducing the anti-tumor effects of paclitaxel.

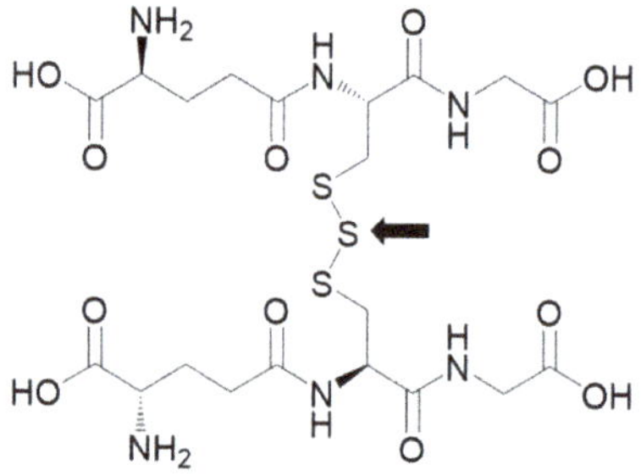

Figure 1. Structural formula of glutathione trisulfide (GSSSG). Purified GSSSG is white, odorless solid powder at 20 °C. Molecular weight is 644.7. It contains one sulfane sulfur (arrow).

2. Materials and Methods

2.1. Animals

All animal protocols were approved by the Massachusetts General Hospital Institutional Animal Care and Use Committee (protocol No. 2020N000126). Animals were cared for in accordance with the guidelines established by the NIH and the International Association for the Study of Pain [17]. Male C57BL/6J mice (6–7 weeks old) were purchased from the Jackson Laboratory (Bar Harbor, ME, USA). The mice were housed in a 12-h shift light-control environment from 7 a.m. to 7 p.m. with ad libitum access to food and water in our animal facility until the time of experiments.

2.2. Drugs and Animal Models

Paclitaxel (Sigma-Aldrich, St. Louis, MO, USA) was dissolved with ethanol and cremophor (1:1) and diluted with normal saline (1:4). Peripheral neuropathy was induced in mice by intraperitoneal (i.p.) administration of 4 mg/kg paclitaxel every other day for a total of 4 injections (cumulative dose of 16 mg/kg), according to a previously described protocol [18]. A stable, crystallized form of GSSSG was produced and provided by Kyowa Hakko Bio CO., Ltd. (Tokyo, Japan). GSSSG was pulverized and mixed in 0.5% methylcellulose. To evaluate the therapeutic effects of GSSSG in a model of PIPN, mice were randomly divided into three groups of 6. Mice were treated with: (1) paclitaxel alone; (2) paclitaxel and GSSSG; (3) or vehicle alone (control). Mice in groups 1 and 2 received paclitaxel as described above, while mice in the control group received the same volume of vehicle. The first dose of GSSSG was given within 1 h after the first PTX injection. Treatment was administered as oral gavage for 28 days with GSSSG at 50 mg/kg/day (group 2) or 0.5% methylcellulose (groups 1 and 3). The dose of GSSSG was determined based on pilot studies. To determine the effect of GSSSG on the development of PIPN, behavioral tests to assess allodynia and hyperalgesia were conducted on all mice on days −1 (baseline), 7, 14, 21, and 28 after paclitaxel administration. Behavioral tests were performed by an investigator who was blinded to the treatment groups, as described in the next section.

To determine the tissue distribution of orally administered GSSSG, ^{34}S-labelled GSSSG was administered by gavage to each of four mice. ^{34}S-labelled GSSSG was synthesized and provided by Kyowa Hakko Bio Co., Ltd. (Tokyo, Japan). Two hours after a single dose of ^{34}S-GSSSG, DRG, lumber spinal cord, brain, liver, and plasma were obtained and snap frozen for later analysis.

2.3. Behavior Testing

2.3.1. Measurement of Mechanical Allodynia—Von Frey Filament Test

To assess allodynia, mechanical withdrawal thresholds were measured by the manual von Frey filament test. Before testing, mice were habituated for 3–4 days and acclimated in the test apparatus (a plastic cage on a wire mesh floor) for 30 min for 3 consecutive days. An investigator who was blinded to treatment group stimulated the mid-plantar surface of their hind paws with von Frey filaments (Ugo Basile, Gemonio, Italy) in the range from 0.04 g force (g) to 2.0 g. Filaments were applied with constant speed until they bent. Behavioral responses, withdrawal and licking of their paws, were considered reactive. The stimulation of the same size filament was repeated up to 2 times if the mouse did not react. Mice were initially tested with a 0.6 g filament and subsequent filament size was determined based the response. A smaller filament was used after a positive response and a larger filament was used after a negative response. Filaments were applied up to a total of 9 times. The 50% threshold of a paw withdrawal response was calculated using the Up-down Reader (an open-source program, ver. 2.0) [19] based on the up and down method [20]. This behavior test was conducted weekly for 4 weeks.

2.3.2. Measurement of Thermal Hyperalgesia—Hot Plate Test

To assess thermal hyperalgesia, the heat threshold was determined by the hot plate test [21]. Mice were placed on the hot plate (Hot/Cold Plate NG, Ugo Basile, Gemonio,

Italy) warmed to 52 °C. Response latency was the time required to exhibit nociceptive behavior, including hind paw withdrawal or licking, stamping, and jumping. The test was repeated 2 times after 5 min interval by a blinded examiner, and the average time was calculated. For each test, the ratio of change from baseline was determined, based on the difference in the latency response time from the baseline divided by the baseline time. This test was conducted weekly for 4 weeks.

2.4. Immunohistochemistry Staining of Intraepidermal Nerve Fibers

The density of intraepidermal nerve fibers (fibers/mm) in the hind paws was calculated to evaluate peripheral nerve fiber damage by paclitaxel. Mice were deeply anesthetized with Isoflurane (4%) and euthanized by exsanguination on week 1 or week 4 after paclitaxel treatment. Mice were perfused with cold 4% paraformaldehyde in PBS through the left ventricle. Skin from the hind paws was harvested and fixed in 4% paraformaldehyde overnight, then cryoprotected in 20% sucrose solution at 4 °C until they sank and then in 30% sucrose solution overnight at 4 °C. Tissue blocks were then submerged in optimal cutting temperature medium, frozen at −80 °C, and sectioned using a cryostat (25 μm thickness). The sections were then incubated with 0.3% hydrogen peroxide for 10 min and with blocking solution (5% donkey serum; Sigma-Aldrich, St. Louis, MO, USA, 0.3% Triton-114) for one-hour. Sections were then incubated overnight at 4 °C with anti-protein gene product (PGP) 9.5 antibody (1:100, rabbit, Abcam, Cambridge, UK) and anti-collagen IV antibody (1:400, goat, SouthernBiotech, AL, USA). Sections were subsequently incubated with secondary antibodies (1:300, donkey anti-rabbit, Abcam, Cambridge, UK; donkey anti-goat, Abcam) for one-hour at room temperature and covered with fluoroshield mounting medium with DAPI (Sigma-Aldrich, St. Louis, MO, USA). Ten images per mouse (6 mice per group) were taken by fluorescence microscopy (Nikon Eclipse 80i, Nikon Instruments, Inc., Melville, NY, USA), and four of the ten images were randomly selected. The density (fibers/mm basement membrane) was calculated as the number of intraepidermal nerve fiber divided by the length of basement membrane, in accordance with published guidelines [22].

2.5. Histological Evaluation of Sciatic Nerves

2.5.1. Toluidine Blue Staining

Four weeks after paclitaxel treatment, sciatic nerves were evaluated by toluidine blue staining as described previously [23]. Briefly, mice were deeply anesthetized and placed in a prone position to facilitate exposure of the sciatic nerves. Sciatic nerves were covered with Trump's fixative (Quimigen, Madrid, Spain) for 10 min. Subsequently, nerves were harvested and fixed in the same fixative for one week changing fixative every other day. Samples were immersed in 2% osmium tetroxide (TGI, Dallas, TX, USA) for 2 h and embedded in Resin-Epoxy medium (Sigma-Aldrich, St. Louis, MO, USA) overnight at 60 °C by following the protocol provided by the manufacturer. The embedded nerve block was sectioned at 1 μm by an ultramicrotome (Reichert-Jung, Ultracut E, Vienna, Austria) and stained in 1% toluidine blue (Sigma-Aldrich, St. Louis, MO, USA). Two images per mouse (6 mice per group) were taken by light microscopy (Nikon Eclipse 80i, Nikon Instruments, Inc., Melville, NY, USA) and analyzed by ImageJ. Thickness of myelin was evaluated using the G-ratio, which compares the size of the inner radius and outer radius. G-ratio was calculated using GRatio for ImageJ, an ImageJ (ver. 1.53, NIH, Bethesda, MD, USA) plugin available online (http://gratio.efil.de/ (accessed on 1 April 2021)) that converts inner and outer perimeter of myelin to the radius. Counting the number of axons and measuring the size of each axon was performed by an examiner who was blinded to the treatment of mice.

2.5.2. Transmission Electron Microscopy

To evaluate unmyelinated axons and mitochondria, we examined sciatic nerve axons by transmission electron microscopy. Resin-embedded nerve blocks were sectioned at 50 nm using an ultramicrotome. Sections were examined with an FEI Morgagni transmission electron microscope (FEI, Lausanne, Switzerland). Low (×2200) and high (×11,000) magnification of images were captured with an AMT 2K charge-coupled device camera (Advanced Microscopy Techniques, Woburn, MA, USA). Unmyelinated axons were quantified using 9 low magnified images per group (3 mice per group). The percentage of unmyelinated axons was calculated by dividing unmyelinated axons by the total number of axons. The cross-sectional area of mitochondria (μm^2) in unmyelinated axons was quantified in 18 to 20 high magnified images per group (3 mice per group). In total, 80 to 100 mitochondrion per group were evaluated. Quantification was conducted by a blinded examiner, and the images were evaluated by a pathologist (A.S.-R.) who was also blinded to the identity of samples.

2.6. Real-Time Quantitative Polymerase Chain Reaction (qPCR)

Paclitaxel alone- and paclitaxel and GSSSG-induced changes in gene expression in lumber dorsal root ganglions (DRG) were examined using real-time qPCR after a single administration of paclitaxel with or without GSSSG. We simultaneously administered 16 mg/kg paclitaxel by i.p. injection and 50 mg/kg GSSSG by oral gavage and determined the level of mRNA 2 h later. Lumbar DRG were isolated from mice as described previously [24]. DRG were immersed in "RNA later" (Invitrogen, Waltham, MA, USA) at 4 °C overnight. After retrieval from RNA later, samples were stored at −80 °C. DRGs were homogenized in TRIzol reagent (Thermo Scientific Scientific, Waltham, MA, USA) and mixed with chloroform. After centrifugation at 14,000× g at 4 °C for 15 min, the transparent top layer was transferred to a new tube. The samples were mixed with 400 µL of isopropanol and incubated at −20 °C for 20 min. After centrifugation at 14,000× g at 4 °C for 15 min, the pellets were collected, mixed with 70% ethanol, and centrifuged at 14,000× g at 4 °C for 10 min. The pellets were dried for 10 min and incubated with 50 µL of nuclease-free water. Complementary DNA was synthesized using the cDNA Reverse Transcription Kit (Applied Biosystems, Waltham, MA, USA) and quantitative PCR was performed using SYBR green (Applied Biosystems, Waltham, MA, USA). Primers are listed in Appendix A Table A1. Relative quantification of gene expression was performed via $2^{-\Delta\Delta CT}$ method.

2.7. Mass Spectrometry to Detect GSSSG Administered by Oral Gavage

We used liquid chromatography with tandem mass spectrometry (LC-MS/MS) to determine whether GSSSG, administered via oral gavage, reaches the peripheral nervous system. Fifty mg/kg of ^{34}S-labeled GSSSG (in which the middle sulfur, that is a sulfane sulfur, was replaced to ^{34}S; G-^{32}S-^{34}S-^{32}S-G) was orally administered to mice. Two hours after administration, plasma and tissue from liver, brain, lumbar spinal cord, and lumbar DRG (L1 to L6) were collected and immediately frozen at −80 °C. Tissues were homogenized with 5 mM β-(4-hydroxyphenyl)ethyl iodoacetamide (HPE-IAM) (Santa Cruz, Dallas, TX, USA) and incubated for 20 min at 37 °C to promote the HPE-IAM reaction, which stabilizes persulfide residues [25]. Proteins were removed by centrifugation at 15,000× g for 10 min at 4 °C, and total protein concentration was measured by BCA assay. The supernatant was diluted by 0.1% formic acid for LC-MS/MS analysis. The amount of ^{34}S-labeled GSSSG was quantified in selective reaction monitoring (SRM) with precursor ion (647.14 m/z), product ion (389.1 m/z), and HCD (21 v) and normalized by protein concentration. The ratio of ^{34}S-labeled reactive sulfur species to endogenous (^{32}S) reactive sulfur species (GSSH, CySSH, and CySSSCys) was calculated from their peak areas, measured by Dionex UltiMate 3000 RS UPLC-Orbitrap Exploris 480 mass spectrometer (Thermo Scientific Scientific, Waltham, MA, USA). In brief, samples were subjected to the UPLC system with a Hypersil Gold C-18 (100 × 2.1 mm, 3.0 µm, Thermo Fisher Scientific) column and components were eluted using a linear methanol gradient of the mobile phase (0–90%, 15 min) in the presence of 0.1% formic acid at a flow rate of 0.2 mL/min at 40 degrees. The raw data were obtained by Compound Discoverer software 3.3 (Thermo Scientific Scientific, Waltham, MA, USA).

The molecular weight of reactive sulfur species combined with HPE-IAM were reported in previous studies [26,27].

2.8. In Vitro Studies

2.8.1. Primary DRG Neuron Isolation and Histological Evaluation

Primary DRG neurons were prepared from 8 to 10-week old mice as described previously [28]. Briefly, lumber DRG (L1 to L6) were isolated from mice and incubated with Dispase-II Solution (Sigma-Aldrich, St. Louis, MO, USA) and collagenase type II (Worthington, Columbus, OH, USA) for 70 min and with 0.25% trypsin for 5 min. DRG were triturated using a frame polished glass pipet, and neurons were seeded on a 12-well plate with 15 mm coverslip. Cells were incubated in Neurobasal A-medium with 2% B27 supplement (Gibco, Waltham, MA, USA), 1% penicillin/streptomycin, 1% Glutamax (Gibco, Waltham, MA, USA), and nerve growth factor (Sigma Aldrich, St. Louis, MO, USA) for 24 h. Cells were then exposed to 100 nM of paclitaxel, with or without GSSSG (500 nM), for one-hour and with MitoTracker (50 nM) (Invitrogen, Waltham, MA, USA) for 30 min. After fixing in 4% paraformaldehyde for 10 min at room temperature, cells were immersed in 0.2% Triton X-100 in PBS for 7 min and washed with PBS. Cells were then incubated with anti-NF200 antibody (1:400, mouse, Sigma-Aldrich, St. Louis, MO, USA) overnight at 4 °C and with the secondary antibody (1:1000, donkey anti-mouse, Abcam, Cambridge, UK) for one-hour at room temperature. After being covered with fluoroshield mounting medium with DAPI (Sigma-Aldrich, St. Louis, MO, USA), 9–10 cells per group (3 mice per group) were imaged using confocal microscopy (ZEISS LSM 800, Carl Zeiss, Thornwood, NY, USA) with a $63\times$ oil immersion objectives lens with 1024×1024 pixels image size.

2.8.2. Primary Cortical Neuron Isolation and ROS Assay

Primary cortical neurons were prepared from mice on embryonic day 15, as described previously [29]. In brief, each embryo's cortex was isolated in Hanks' balanced salt solution and centrifuged at $176\times g$ (1000 rpm) for 3 min. After aspirating the solution, cells were incubated with 0.25% trypsin for 15 min and cells were seeded at a density of 20,000 cells/well in a 96-well plate coated with the poly-D-lysine (Gibco, Waltham, MA, USA). Cells were incubated in Neurobasal medium (Gibco, Waltham, MA, USA) with 2% B27 supplement (Gibco, Waltham, MA, USA), 1% penicillin/streptomycin, and 1% Glutamax (Gibco, Waltham, MA, USA) until day 11, when they were used in experiments.

To examine whether GSSSG reduces ROS generated by paclitaxel, we conducted a dihydroethidium (DHE) assay (Abcam, Cambridge, UK) that is sensitive to superoxide. The experiment was performed according to the protocol provided by the manufacturer. Briefly, primary cortical neurons were incubated in DHE reagent with or without 10 and 30 µM of GSSSG for 30 min. Cells were subsequent treated with paclitaxel (100 nM) for one-hour. Fluorescence of DHE was measured at 490 nm of excitation and 585 nm of emission wavelength.

2.9. Cancer Cell Line and Viability Assay

To examine whether administration of GSSSG affects anti-tumor effects of paclitaxel, we conducted experiments using the human breast cancer cell line MDA-MB-231 (HTB-26, ATCC). Cells were cultured in medium consisting of 90% RPMI1640 (Corning, Corning, NY, USA), 10% FBS, and 1% penicillin/streptomycin. After being seeded into a 96-well plate at the density of 20,000 cells/well and cultured overnight, cells were exposed to different concentrations of paclitaxel (0.125 µM, 0.25 µM, 0.5 µM, 1 µM, and 2 µM) and incubated for 24 h. Cell viability was evaluated using the LDH Cytotoxicity Detection Kit (Roche, Basel, Switzerland). Cells were washed with PBS and incubated with 100 µL of 1% Triton X-100 at 37 °C for 30 min. After mixing with assay enzyme for 30 min at 25 °C, absorbance was measured at wavelength 492 nm to determine cell viability. The half-maximal inhibitory concentration (IC_{50}) of paclitaxel was determined. Using the IC_{50} of paclitaxel, we determined the effect of GSSSG on the anti-tumor effect of paclitaxel using the trypan blue exclusion assay. MDA-MB-231 cells were seeded at $5.6 \times 10,000$ cells/well in a 6-well plate and incubated overnight. The cells were treated with paclitaxel (at the IC_{50} concentration), with or without GSSSG (10 µM) for 24 h. After suspension using 0.25% trypsin, cells were treated with 0.04% trypan blue and the percentage of cells that retained the ability to exclude blue dye was determined. Five wells were evaluated per group.

2.10. Statistical Analysis

Sample sizes for behavior tests were chosen based on a previous study [30]. All values are expressed as mean ± standard deviation (SD). Behavior test results were analyzed in the mixed effect model because the behavior was measured repeatedly five times in each animal, and individual differences at baseline were confirmed in the preliminary study. Bonferroni correction was applied to correct for multiple comparisons in the mixed effect model. Parametric data were analyzed by one-way analysis of variance (ANOVA) with Dunnett's multiple comparisons test. Non-parametric data were analyzed by Kruskal–Wallis test with Dunn's multiple comparisons test. DRG morphology was analyzed by two-way repeated measures ANOVA with Dunnett's multiple comparisons test. Anti-tumor effect of paclitaxel with GSSSG was analyzed by equivalence test using two one-sided t-tests. The margin of equivalence was defined as 10% difference in cell count. Probability (p) value less than 0.05 was considered significant. Statistical analyses were performed using GraphPad Prism 9.1 (GraphPad Software Inc., La Jolla, CA, USA).

3. Results

3.1. GSSSG Prevented Paclitaxel-Induced Mechanical Allodynia

Male adult mice were treated with 4 mg/kg paclitaxel i.p. on days 0, 2, 4, and 6. Starting on day 7 and continuing through week 4, paclitaxel-treated mice demonstrated mechanical allodynia as assessed using von Frey testing of the hind paw (Figure 2A closed circles, $p = 0.0014$). Paclitaxel also induced thermal hyperalgesia as measured using the hot plate test (Figure 2B, closed circles, $p < 0.0001$). Oral administration of GSSSG at 50 mg/kg/day mitigated mechanical allodynia over the experimental period (Figure 2A, black squares, $p = 0.003$). In contrast, thermal hyperalgesia was not altered by GSSSG administration (Figure 2B, black squares).

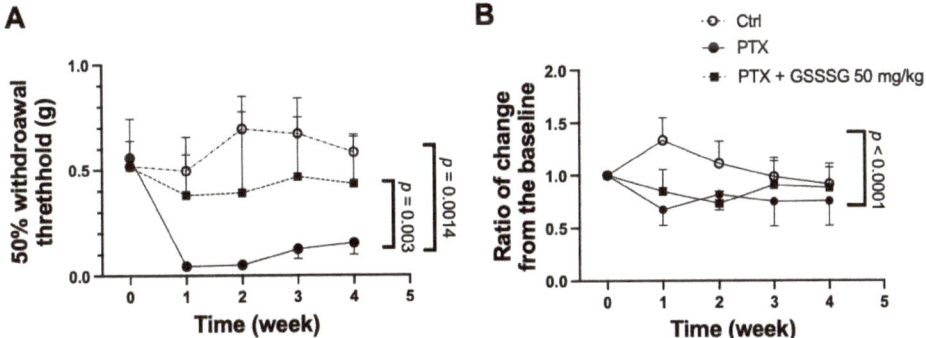

Figure 2. GSSSG prevented mechanical allodynia evoked by paclitaxel-induced peripheral neuropathy. (**A**) Mechanical withdrawal threshold by the von Frey test for 4 weeks after paclitaxel treatment with or without co-treatment of GSSSG. 50 mg/kg of GSSSG prevented mechanical allodynia over the experimental period. (**B**) Relative change of response time compared to the baseline in hot plate test for 4 weeks. PTX induced thermal hyperalgesia. Data are analyzed by mixed effect model and adjusted by Bonferroni correction. Data are shown as the mean ± SD, $n = 6$ mice per group. PTX, paclitaxel.

3.2. GSSSG Prevented Loss of Intraepidermal Nerve Fibers Induced by Paclitaxel

We evaluated degeneration of unmyelinated nerve endings by determining the density of intraepidermal nerve fibers, which is a widely used indicator of peripheral neuropathy. The density of the intraepidermal nerve fibers in the planter surface skin of hind paws of mice was calculated as the number of intraepidermal nerve fibers (Figure 3A, yellow arrowheads) divided by the length of epidermal basement membrane (Figure 3A, white dashed line). Paclitaxel decreased the density of intraepidermal nerve fibers at 4 weeks, but not at 1 week, after starting paclitaxel (Figure 3B,C). Daily oral administration of 50 mg/kg GSSSG prevented paclitaxel-induced loss of intraepidermal nerve fibers at 4 weeks after starting paclitaxel ($p = 0.0024$).

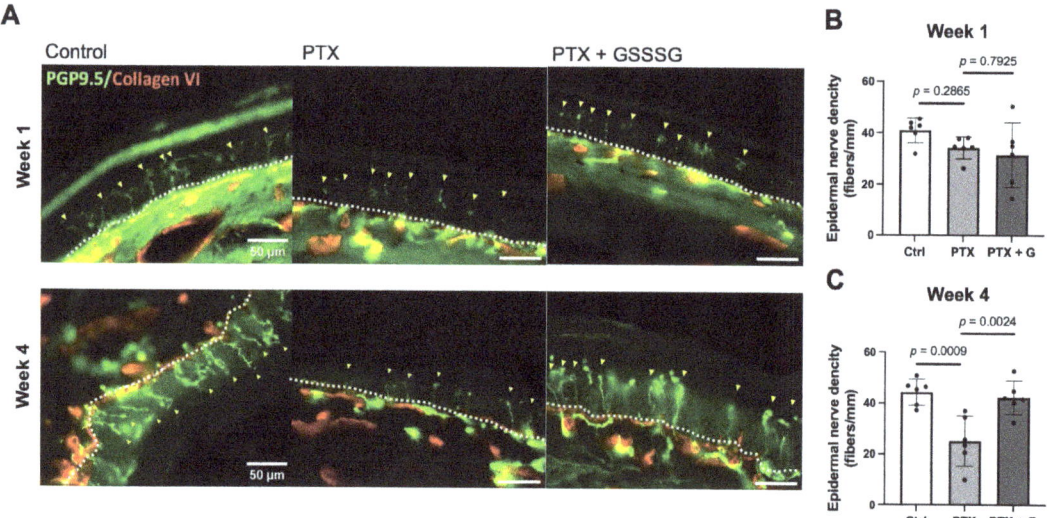

Figure 3. (**A**) Representative immunofluorescence images of intraepidermal nerve fibers (stained by PGP9.5, shown by yellow arrowheads) and basement membrane (stained by Collagen IV, white dashed lines) in hind paw at 1 week and 4 weeks after paclitaxel treatment. Quantification of unmyelinated fiber density calculated by dividing number of intraepidermal nerve fibers by basement membrane at 1 week (**B**) and at 4 weeks (**C**). Data were analyzed by one-way ANOVA with Dunnett's multiple comparisons test. Individual data (black dots) are shown with mean ± SD, $n = 6$ mice per group. PTX, paclitaxel; G, GSSSG.

3.3. GSSSG Prevented the Paclitaxel-Induced Loss of Unmyelinated Axons in the Sciatic Nerve

To evaluate the impact of paclitaxel on myelinated and unmyelinated axons, we counted the number of axons in the sciatic nerve at 4 weeks after starting paclitaxel. The number of myelinated axons was similar between control, paclitaxel, and paclitaxel with GSSSG groups (Figure 4A,B). The thickness of myelin, calculated using the G-ratio (a ratio of the inner and outer radius), was not affected by paclitaxel either without or with GSSSG (Figure 4C,D). We also examined transmission electron microscopy images (low magnification, ×2200) to determine the number of unmyelinated axons in the sciatic nerve. Unmyelinated (Figure 5A, arrows) and myelinated axons (Figure 5A, arrowheads) were counted and divided by a total number of axons. Paclitaxel tended to decrease unmyelinated axons compared to control mice ($p = 0.0695$) and showed disruption of architecture in the nerve fascicle (Figure 5A, double arrow), indicating axonal degeneration. Compared to mice that received paclitaxel alone, mice that received paclitaxel and GSSSG had a larger ratio of unmyelinated axons in the sciatic nerve (Figure 5A,B, $p = 0.0153$). These results suggest that GSSSG prevents axonal loss of unmyelinated neurons after paclitaxel treatment.

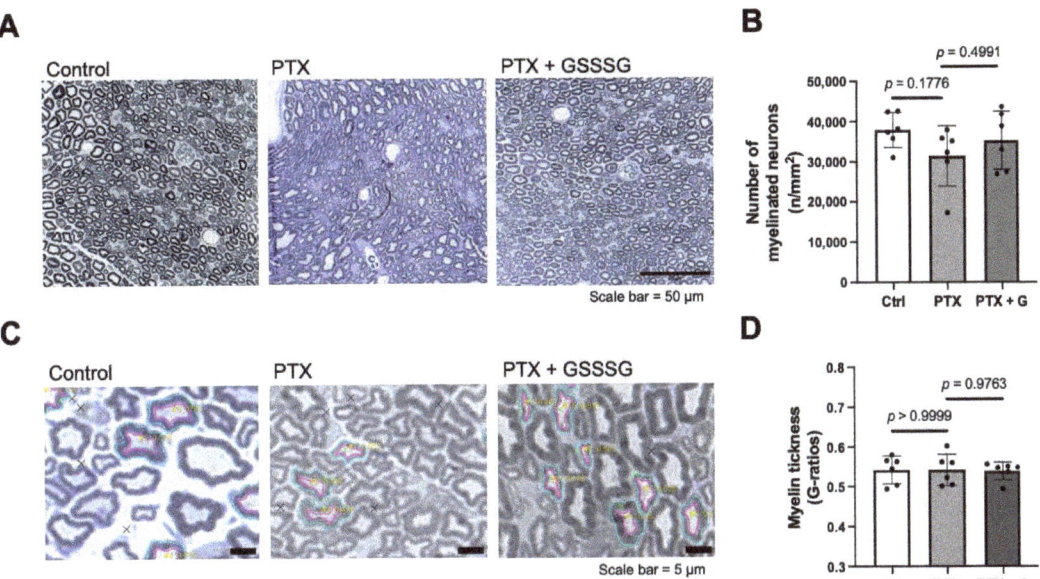

Figure 4. Neither PTX nor GSSSG changed number of myelinated axons. (**A**) Representative microscopic images of sciatic nerve at 4 weeks after PTX treatment stained with toluidine blue. (**B**) Quantification of total myelinated neurons axons in sciatic nerve. (**C**) Representative high magnification images of myelinated neurons axons to measure thickness of myelin. The thickness of myelin was calculated by GRatio software, an ImageJ plugin in ten neurons per image randomly selected by cross marks generated by GRatio. (**D**) Quantification of G-ratios. Neither PTX nor GSSSG did not change thickness of myelin. Data were analyzed by one-way ANOVA with Dunnett's multiple comparisons test. Individual data (black dots) are shown with mean ± SD, $n = 6$ mice per group. PTX, paclitaxel; G, GSSSG.

3.4. GSSSG Prevented Mitochondrial Swelling in Unmyelinated Sciatic Nerve Axons

To explore the mechanisms by which paclitaxel induces degeneration of unmyelinated axons, we examined mitochondrial morphology in unmyelinated sciatic nerve axons 4 weeks after starting paclitaxel. Mitochondria appeared to be larger and swollen in the unmyelinated axons of paclitaxel-treated mice (Figure 6A, arrowheads) compared to control mice and mice treated with paclitaxel and GSSSG. The cross-sectional area of mitochondria in unmyelinated axons in paclitaxel-treated mice was significantly larger than those in control mice (Figure 6B, $p < 0.0001$) and mice treated with paclitaxel and GSSSG (Figure 6B, $p = 0.001$). These results suggest that the beneficial effects of GSSSG on paclitaxel-induced axonal degeneration are mediated by protection of mitochondrial integrity.

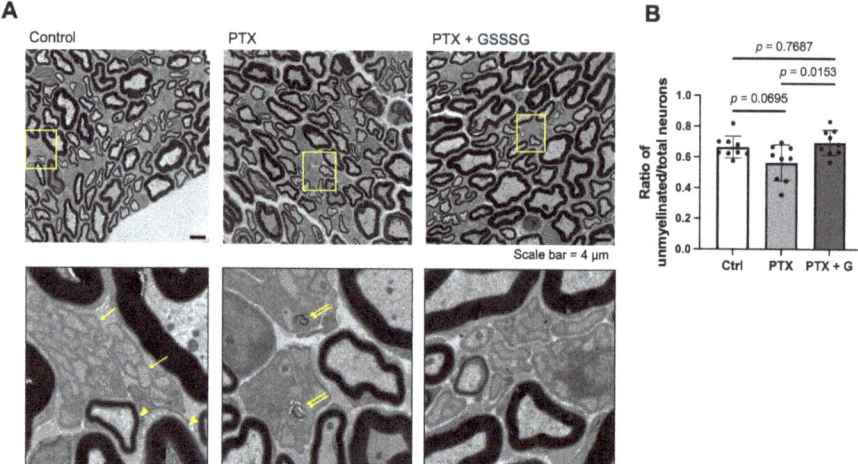

Figure 5. GSSSG prevented loss of unmyelinated axons in sciatic nerve. (**A**) Representative transmission electron microscopy images of sciatic nerve at 4 weeks. Images in the second row are magnified images of the area indicated by yellow frames in the first row image of respective column. Number of unmyelinated axons (yellow arrows) and myelinated axons (yellow arrowheads) were counted. (**B**) Ratio of the number of unmyelinated axons of the total number of axons in sciatic nerve at 4 weeks. Data were analyzed by one-way ANOVA with Tukey's multiple comparisons test. Individual data (black dots) are shown with mean ± SD, n = 3 mice per group. PTX, paclitaxel. G, GSSSG.

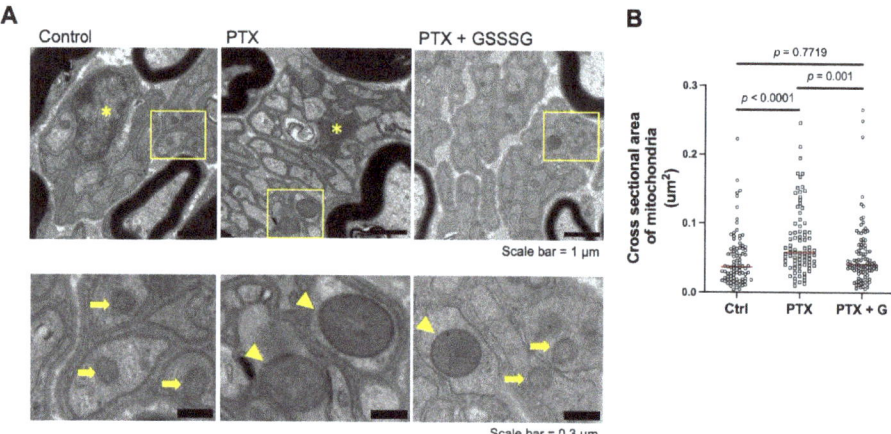

Figure 6. GSSSG prevented degeneration of mitochondria. (**A**) Representative transmission electron microscopy images of sciatic nerve at 4 weeks after paclitaxel treatment. Images in the second row are magnified images of the area indicated by yellow frames in the first row image of respective column. Asterisks show Schwann cell, arrows indicate mitochondria and arrowheads indicate swollen mitochondria. (**B**) Quantification of mitochondria area in unmyelinated neuron. The median area of mitochondria in control, paclitaxel, and paclitaxel with GSSSG were 0.036 μm^2, 0.057 μm^2, and 0.041 μm^2, respectively. Red bars indicate median values of each group. Data were analyzed by Kruskal–Wallis test with Dunn's multiple comparisons test. Four high (×11,000) magnification images from each mouse were examined. n = 3 mice per group. PTX, paclitaxel; G, GSSSG.

3.5. ^{34}S-Labeled GSSSG Was Detected in DRG, Spinal Cord, Brain, and Liver after Oral Administration

To study the pharmacokinetics of orally administered GSSSG, we used ^{34}S-labelled GSSSG to determine the distribution of GSSSG and its metabolites in central and peripheral nervous systems. Lumber DRG, lumber spinal cord, brain, liver, and plasma were harvested 2 h after oral administration of ^{34}S-labelled GSSSG at 50 mg/kg, and the levels of ^{34}S-labelled GSSSG in each tissue were determined by liquid chromatography-tandem mass spectrometry (LC-MS/MS). While endogenous GSSSG was not detected, the average concentration of administered ^{34}S-labelled GSSSG was 415, 518, 142, and 158 pmol/mg protein in lumber DRG, lumber spinal cord, brain, and liver, respectively (Figure 7A). The plasma level of GSSSG was 58 pmol/mL. We also determined the ratio of exogenous (containing ^{34}S) to endogenous (containing ^{32}S) reactive sulfur species: GSSH, CysSSH, and CysSSSCys, in these 4 tissues (Figure 7B–D, respectively). The concentration of ^{34}S-labelled GSSH, CysSSH, and CysSSSCys was more than 10-fold higher than the endogenous levels of GSSH, CysSSH, and CysSSSCys in all four tissues. These observations indicate that orally administered GSSSG was absorbed from the gastrointestinal tract, entered the central and peripheral nervous systems and was partially metabolized to other reactive sulfur species.

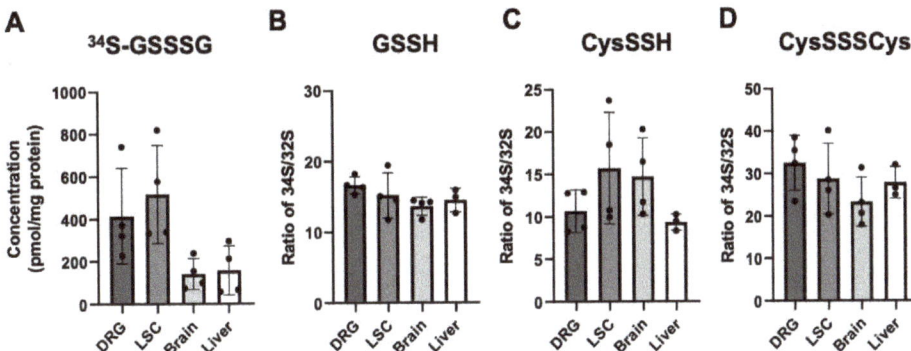

Figure 7. ^{34}S-labeled GSSSG and related polysulfides were detected in peripheral tissues 2 h after oral administration of ^{34}S-labeled GSSSG. Quantification of GSSSG and reactive sulfur species by LC-MS/MS. (**A**) ^{34}S-labeled GSSSG concentration in 4 tissues that were obtained 2 h after oral administration. Relative ratio of ^{34}S-laveled reactive sulfur species to endogenous reactive sulfur species (^{32}S-) were calculated. The ratios of ^{34}S-laveled to endogenous glutathione persulfide (GSSH) (**B**), cysteine persulfide (CysSSH) (**C**), cysteine trisulfide (CysSSSCys) (**D**) in lumber DRG, lumber spinal cord, brain, and liver were reported. Individual data (black dots) are shown with mean ± SD, n = 4 per group; DRG, dorsal root ganglion; LSC, lumber spinal cord.

3.6. GSSSG Prevented Paclitaxel-Induced Axonal Degeneration and Fragmentation of Mitochondria in Cultured Primary DRG Neurons

The effects of GSSSG on axonal integrity were examined in cultured murine primary DRG neurons treated with paclitaxel. Neurons that were incubated with paclitaxel (100 nM) for one-hour showed bulbed axonal endings compared to untreated neurons (Figure 8A arrowheads). The number and morphology of neurons (length, and branching of neurites), were assessed using the Sholl analysis, using ImageJ [31]. The Sholl analysis plugin draws equally spaced circles from the soma and counts the number of intersections between neurites and circles to quantify neuronal morphology (Figure 8B). Incubation with paclitaxel for one-hour inhibited the elongation of axons while co-administration of GSSSG restored axonal elongation (Figure 8A,C). The number of neurites greater than 160 μm from the soma in paclitaxel and GSSSG treated cells was significantly larger than the number in neurites treated with paclitaxel alone ($p < 0.05$). Incubation with paclitaxel also decreased the ratio of the total mitochondria length to axonal length and the number of mitochondria in axons, which are signs of increased mitochondrial fragmentation (Figure 9A). GSSSG prevented the paclitaxel-induced decrease in the ratio of mitochondrial to axonal length (Figure 9B, $p < 0.0001$) and the number of mitochondria (Figure 9C, $p = 0.0017$). These results suggest that the beneficial effects of GSSSG on PIPN are mediated by prevention of axonal degeneration via preservation of mitochondrial integrity in peripheral neural axons.

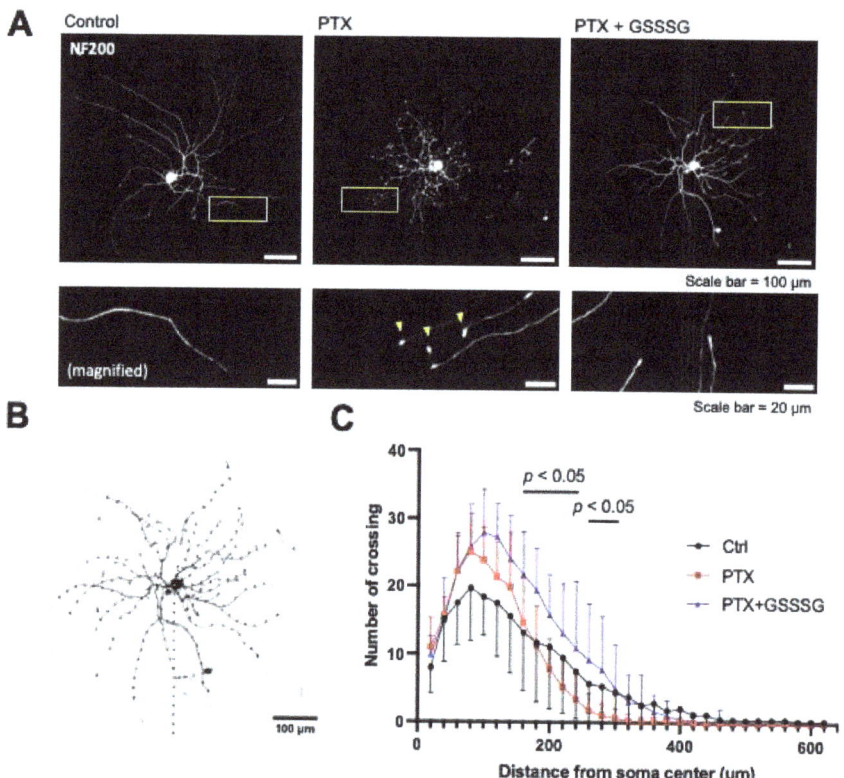

Figure 8. GSSSG prevented axon degeneration in primary DRG neurons. (**A**) Representative immunofluorescence images of primary DRG neurons stained by NF200. Neurons were cultured for 24 h and incubated by paclitaxel with or without GSSSG for one hour. (**B**) Sholl circles of cultured neuron. The interval between Sholl circles is 10 μm. (**C**) Analysis of neuronal intersections with Sholl circles. Data were analyzed by repeated ANOVA with Dunnett's multiple comparisons test. p values are shown to indicate the comparison between paclitaxel and paclitaxel + GSSSG. Data are shown as the mean ± SD, $n = 3$ mice per group, 9–10 neurons per group. PTX, paclitaxel.

3.7. GSSSG Attenuated Paclitaxel-Induced Increase of Superoxide Levels in Primary Cortical Neurons

To consider the possibility that GSSSG protects axons via an antioxidant effect [15], we examined the change in intracellular ROS in primary cortical neurons. After incubating primary cortical neurons with paclitaxel (100 nM) for one-hour, intracellular levels of superoxide were measured using the Dihydroethidium (DHE). The levels of superoxide increased after incubation with paclitaxel (Figure 10, $p = 0.01$, paclitaxel vs. control). Co-incubation with GSSSG (10 μM) prevented the paclitaxel-induced increase in intracellular superoxide ($p = 0.0114$, paclitaxel vs. paclitaxel + GSSSG). These results suggest that GSSSG attenuates ROS production induced by paclitaxel.

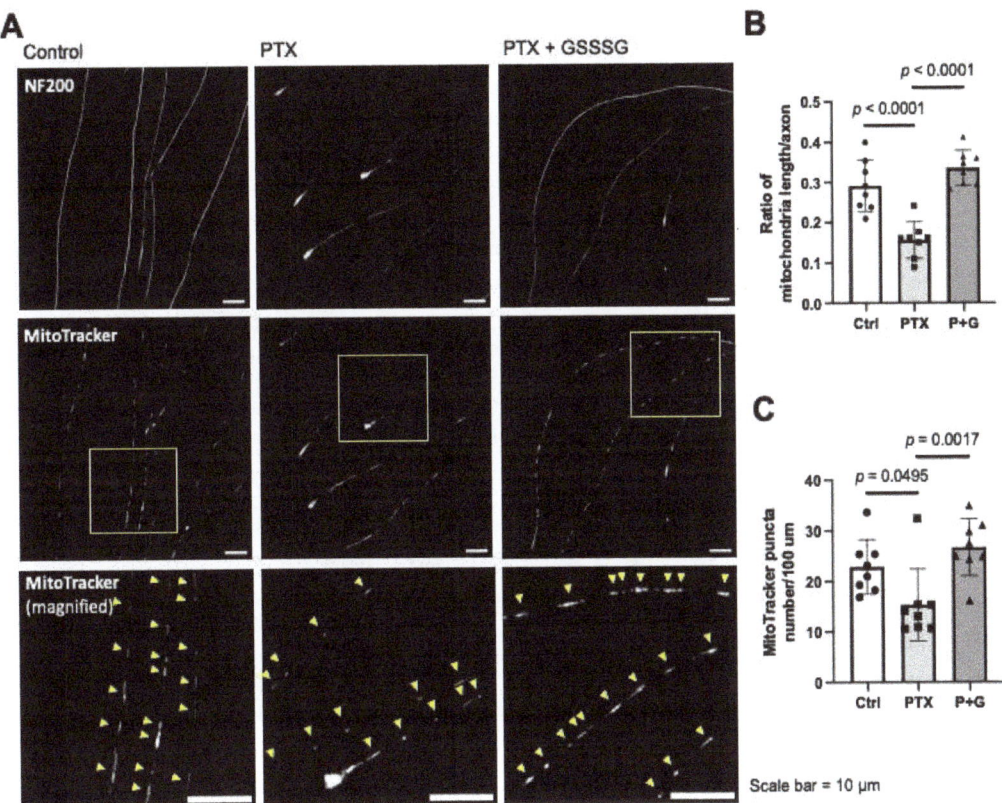

Figure 9. GSSSG protected mitochondria in axon of primary DRG neurons. (**A**) Representative images of neural axons stained by NF200 with axonal mitochondria stained by MitoTracker. Images in the second row are magnified images of the area indicated by yellow frames in the first row image of respective column. The number and length of mitochondria (yellow arrowheads) in axon was measured manually. (**B**) Ratio of the total mitochondria length to the total axonal length and (**C**) The number of MitoTracker puncta per 100 μm of axon. Data were analyzed by one-way ANOVA with Dunnett's multiple comparison. Individual data (black dots) are shown with mean ± SD, n = 3 mice per group, 8 images per group, and 450–790 mitochondria per group. PTX, paclitaxel; G, GSSSG.

3.8. GSSSG Upregulated Antioxidant Signaling in DRG

To further characterize the effects of GSSSG on PIPN, we used real-time qPCR to measure the levels of mRNA encoding antioxidant proteins in lumber DRG, 2 h after a single paclitaxel injection (16 mg/kg) with or without 50 mg/kg GSSSG. Treatment with either paclitaxel or paclitaxel and GSSSG increased Nrf2 mRNA levels (Figure 11A, p = 0.0008 control vs. paclitaxel, p < 0.0001 control vs. paclitaxel and GSSSG). The levels of mRNAs encoding enzymes that are downstream of Nrf2, including Heme Oxygenase 1 (HO1, Figure 11B), NAD(P)H Quinone Dehydrogenase 1 (NQO1, Figure 11C) and Glutamate-Cysteine Ligase Catalytic Subunit (GCLC, Figure 11D), were increased only in mice that received paclitaxel and GSSSG (p = 0.0127, 0.0024 and 0.0038, respectively, control vs. paclitaxel and GSSSG). These results suggest that GSSSG enhances Nrf2-dependent antioxidant signaling in DRG after paclitaxel treatment.

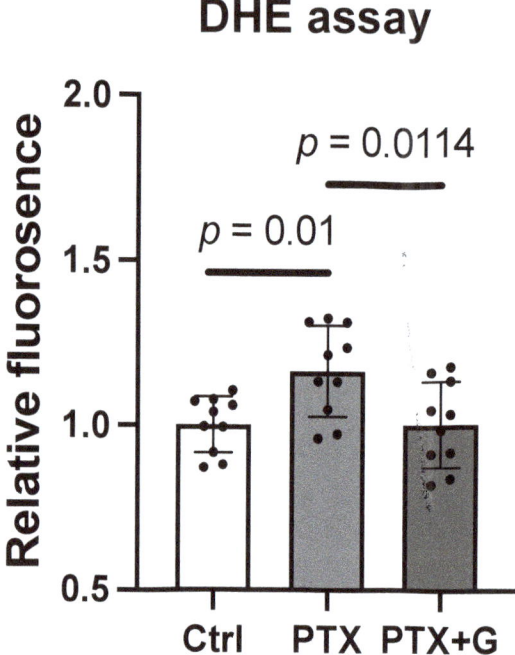

Figure 10. GSSSG treatment blocked increase of superoxide. Relative fluorescence change of Dihydroethidium (DHE) 30 min incubation of GSSSG and 60 min after paclitaxel exposure. Data were analyzed by one-way ANOVA with Dunnett's multiple comparisons test. Individual data (black dots) are shown with mean ± SD, n = 8 per group. PTX, paclitaxel; G, GSSSG.

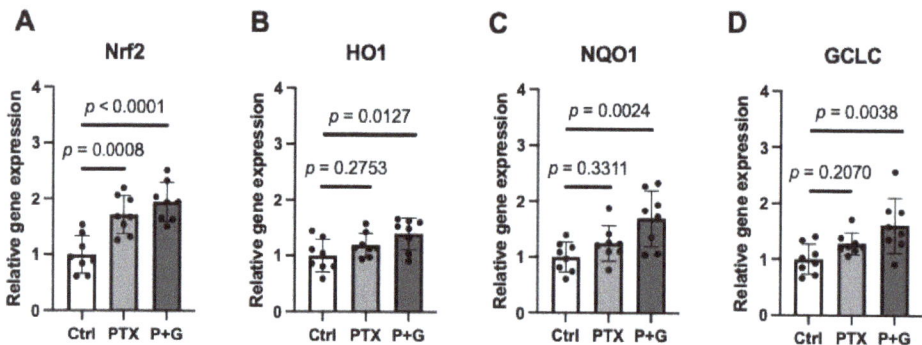

Figure 11. GSSSG upregulated antioxidant signaling in DRG. Relative gene expression of Nrf2 (**A**), HO1 (**B**), NQO1 (**C**), and GCLC (**D**) in DRG tissue at 2 h after single 16 mg/kg paclitaxel with or without 50 mg/kg GSSSG treatment. Data were analyzed by one-way ANOVA with Dunnett's multiple comparisons test. Data are shown as the mean ± SD, n = 8 mice per group. PTX, paclitaxel; G, GSSSG; Nrf2, Nuclear factor-erythroid factor 2-related factor 2; HO1, Heme Oxygenase 1; NQO1, NAD(P)H Quinone Dehydrogenase 1; GCLC, Glutamate-Cysteine Ligase Catalytic Subunit.

3.9. GSSSG Did Not Affect the Anti-Tumor Effects of Paclitaxel in a Human Breast Cancer Cell Line

Because several studies showed that enhanced antioxidant effects contribute to the resistance of cancer cells to chemotherapy [32,33], we assessed whether GSSSG affects the anti-tumor effect of paclitaxel. We examined the in vitro effect of paclitaxel on MDA-MB-231 human breast cancer cell viability. After incubation with paclitaxel for 24 h, the viability of MDA-MB-231 cells was assessed using the LDH Cytotoxicity Detection assay (Figure 12A). The IC_{50} of paclitaxel for MDA-MB-231 cells was 1.66 µM. Based on these results, we applied paclitaxel (2 µM) and GSSSG (10 µM) to MDA-MB-231 cells for 24 h to determine whether co-administration of GSSSG alters the cytotoxic effects of paclitaxel on MDA-MB-231 cells. After 24 h of incubation with paclitaxel alone or paclitaxel with GSSSG, the percentage of viable MDA-MB-231 cells (compared to untreated cells) was 44.9% and 48.3%, respectively, (Figure 12B). The statistical test did not show a difference more than defined 10% margin (mean difference: 0.034, 90% confidence interval: −0.280 to 0.357). These results demonstrate that GSSSG does not inhibit that ability of paclitaxel to kill MDA-MB-231 cells.

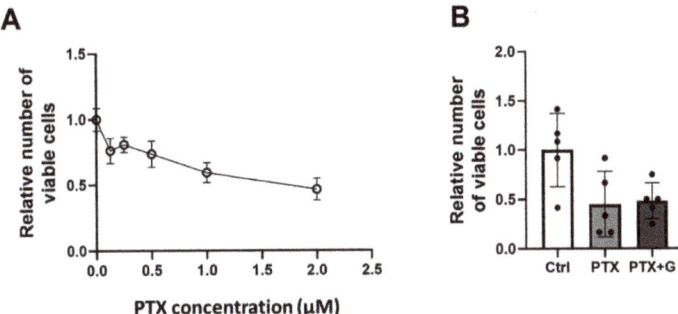

Figure 12. Co-administration of GSSSG did not inhibit anti-tumor effect of paclitaxel. (**A**) Cell viability of human breast cancer cell line, MDA-MB-231 measured by LDH assay at 24 h after PTX with/without 10 µM of GSSSG. (**B**) Relative viable numbers of MDA-MB-231 cells 24 h after 2 µM of PTX with/without 10 µM of GSSSG. Data were analyzed by two one-sided *t*-tests. The margin of equivalence was defined as 10% difference in cell count. Data are shown as the mean ± SD, *n* = 5 per group; LDH, lactate dehydrogenase, PTX, paclitaxel; G, GSSSG.

4. Discussion

The current study revealed that GSSSG, a polysulfide, has the potential to mitigate paclitaxel-induced peripheral neuropathy by protecting mitochondria in the axons of peripheral neurons. This conclusion is based on the following results: (1) daily oral administration of GSSSG attenuated mechanical allodynia in the hind paw of mice treated with paclitaxel; (2) orally administered GSSSG was absorbed and increased reactive sulfur levels in lumbar DRG and spinal cord (both regions which contain the primary sensory neurons that innervate the hind paw); (3) GSSSG inhibited axonal degeneration and prevented mitochondrial swelling in paclitaxel treated mice treated and maintained the number of axonal mitochondria in paclitaxel-exposed cultured primary DRG neurons; and (4) GSSSG attenuated the increase in superoxide levels in primary cortical neurons incubated with paclitaxel. Taken together, these results suggest GSSSG ameliorates PIPN. The beneficial effects of GSSSG were associated with protection of mitochondrial integrity in peripheral nervous system axons.

In the current study, we observed that oral administration of GSSSG at 50 mg/kg/day for 4 weeks ameliorated paclitaxel-induced mechanical allodynia and ^{34}S-labeled GSSSG was detected in lumber DRG and lumber spinal cord 2 h after single oral administration. The results show that GSSSG is well absorbed from the gastrointestinal tract and readily taken up by central and peripheral nervous tissues [34]. We also observed that the concentrations of related polysulfides and persulfides containing ^{34}S were more than 10-fold greater than those of respective endogenous polysulfides and persulfides 2 h after ^{34}S-labeled GSSSG administration. These observations suggest that GSSSG is in dynamic equilibrium with other reactive sulfur species. To the best of our knowledge, this is the first study demonstrating an association between neuroprotective effects and increased levels of polysulfides in the peripheral nervous system after systemic administration of a polysulfide donor.

Impairment of mitochondria and increased oxidative stress play crucial roles in PIPN [35]. Mitochondria are a main source of cellular ROS but are also important targets of ROS. Normal mitochondria release low levels of ROS, as small amounts of electrons leak from complex I, III, and IV of the electron transport chain (ETC) and bind with molecular oxygen to produce superoxide. When electron transport is impaired, more electrons leak from ETC complexes to produce more ROS. Increased ROS production by dysfunctional mitochondria further impairs mitochondrial function, eventually leading to collapse of the mitochondrial membrane potential. Defective mitochondria are degraded and replaced by quality control mechanisms, such as mitophagy. Because neurons predominantly rely on oxidative phosphorylation in mitochondria to produce ATP, mitochondrial dysfunction causes degeneration of neuronal axons [36].

Reactive sulfur species are thought to protect mitochondria through several mechanisms: (1) supporting bioenergetics [37]; (2) scavenging ROS [15]; (3) activating superoxide dismutase (SOD) [38]; (4) preventing fission of mitochondria by inhibiting Drp1 activity [37]; and (5) upregulating the Nrf2/Keap1 pathway by persulfidation of Keap1 [39]. In the current study, administration of GSSSG attenuated paclitaxel-induced ROS production and prevented swelling and loss of mitochondria in peripheral neural axons. These observations suggest that GSSSG has anti-oxidative effects and that GSSSG may support bioenergetics. Our results in primary DRG neurons suggest that GSSSG prevents not only mitochondria fragmentation (or fission) induced by paclitaxel, but also loss of mitochondria in neural axons. As reported previously, redox balance and glutathione oxidation in neural axons partly regulate mitochondrial transportation from cell body to axon [40], and loss of axonal mitochondria results in axonal degeneration [41] and neuropathy [42]. Our observations support that GSSSG attenuates PIPN via protecting mitochondria by regulating redox balance in peripheral neurons. Interestingly, paclitaxel, without or with GSSSG, upregulated Nrf2 a master regulator of cellular homeostasis, redox balance, and inflammation [43], suggesting that paclitaxel triggers an antioxidant defense mechanism. However, we observed that GSSSG with paclitaxel, but not paclitaxel alone, upregulated expression of HO1, NQO1 and GCLC, which are the downstream genes of Nrf2. One possible reason why GSSSG upregulates genes that are downstream of Nrf2 is that GSSSG induces persulfidation of Keap1, a Nrf2 binding protein. Persulfidation of Keap1 promotes activation of Nrf2, thereby upregulating the downstream genes and exerting an antioxidative effect [39]. In addition to the Nrf2 pathway, GSSSG may exert protective effects on peripheral neurons via multiple antioxidant mechanisms.

We recognize several limitations in our current study. First, there is a discrepancy that GSSSG mitigates only mechanical allodynia (a sign of Aβ fiber impairment) but not thermal hyperalgesia (a sign of altered Aδ and C fiber function) whereas it protects unmyelinated fibers (C fibers). This discrepancy was also reported in previous studies [44,45]. While several mechanisms have been proposed to explain the discrepancy between mechanical allodynia and thermal hyperalgesia, one conceivable mechanism is phenotypic switch in which, following injury (in this case chemotherapeutic-induced), Aβ function is altered leading to mechanical allodynia via central secretion of pro-nociceptive compounds [46]. Second, in this study, we used LC-MS/MS to demonstrate that GSSSG is absorbed and distributed in the DRG. However, we did not measure levels of reactive sulfur species, GSH, and cysteine after administration of paclitaxel and/or GSSSG. Dynamic changes in the levels of reactive sulfur species and intracellular thiols in peripheral neurons under paclitaxel-induced oxidative stress remain to be determined. Third, all mice in the current study were male. Although previous studies showed that mechanical allodynia induced by paclitaxel was not affected by gender [47], this was not confirmed in the present study. Lastly, we used qPCR to measure the levels of mRNA encoding proteins involved in the anti-oxidative response. The small size of murine lumbar DRG made it difficult to measure the level of proteins in this pathway.

5. Conclusions

In conclusion, the current study showed that oral administration of GSSSG ameliorated paclitaxel-induced mechanical allodynia in a mouse model of PIPN. After oral administration, GSSSG reached DRG and prevented impairment of mitochondria and axonal degeneration in peripheral neurons. We also found that GSSSG upregulated Nrf2-dependent antioxidant signaling pathway in vivo and diminished ROS levels in vitro. Because impairment of mitochondria is a common feature of diverse forms of peripheral neuropathy [42], these results imply potential therapeutic effects of GSSSG, not only for CIPN, but also for other forms of peripheral neuropathy caused by mitochondrial dysfunction, such as diabetic neuropathy.

Author Contributions: Conceptualization, F.I., E.O. and M.E.; methodology, M.E., E.M., Y.M., E.K., M.K.S. and G.J.B.; validation, M.E., A.S.-R., S.L.B. and K.F.O.; writing—original draft preparation, M.E.; writing—review and editing, F.I, D.B.B. and G.J.B.; supervision, F.I.; funding acquisition, F.I. All authors have read and agreed to the published version of the manuscript.

Funding: This study was supported by a sponsored research agreement from Kyowa Hakko Bio Co., Ltd. (Tokyo, Japan) to Fumito Ichinose.

Institutional Review Board Statement: All animal protocols were approved by the Massachusetts General Hospital Institutional Animal Care and Use Committee (protocol No. 2020N000126).

Informed Consent Statement: Not applicable.

Data Availability Statement: The data presented in this study are available on request from the corresponding author.

Acknowledgments: GSSSG and ^{34}S-labeled GSSSG were provided by Kyowa Hakko Bio Co., Ltd. (Tokyo, Japan). HPE-IAM LC-MS/MS sulfide metabolite analysis was performed by the Center for Redox Biology and Cardiovascular Disease at LSU Health Shreveport supported by an Institutional Development Award (IDeA) from the National Institutes of General Medical Sciences of the NIH under grant number GM121307.

Conflicts of Interest: Etsuo Ohshima is an employee of Kyowa Hakko Bio. Fumito Ichinose receives research funding from Kyowa-Hakko Bio. Mariko Ezaka, Eizo Marutani, Eiki Kanemaru, Etsuo Ohshima, and Fumito Ichinose are listed as inventors of patents filed by MGH related to GSSSG.

Appendix A

Table A1. List of primer sequences for quantitative polymerase chain reaction.

Gene		Sequence
Nrf2	Forward	5′-TCCTCAGCAGAACAGGAACAG-3′
	Reverse	5′-CCTCCAAAGGATGTCAATCAA-3′
HO1	Forward	5′-AAGCCGAGAATGCTGAGTTC-3′
	Reverse	5′-GCCGTGTAGATATGGTACAAGGA-3′
NQO1	Forward	5′-AGGATGGGAGGTACTCGAATC-3′
	Reverse	5′-AGGCGTCCTTCCTTATATGCTA-3′
GCLC	Forward	5′-GGACAAACCCCAACCATCC-3′
	Reverse	5′-GTTGAACTCAGACATCGTTCCTC-3′
18S	Forward	5′-CGGCTACCACATCCAAGGAA-3′
	Reverse	5′-GCTGGAATTACCGCGGCT-3′

Abbreviations: GCLC, Glutamate-Cysteine Ligase Catalytic Subunit; HO1, Heme Oxygenase 1; NQO1, NAD(P)H Quinone Dehydrogenase 1; Nrf2, Nuclear factor-erythroid factor 2-related factor 2.

References

1. Wilson, B.E.; Jacob, S.; Yap, M.L.; Ferlay, J.; Bray, F.; Barton, M.B. Estimates of global chemotherapy demands and corresponding physician workforce requirements for 2018 and 2040: A population-based study. *Lancet. Oncol.* **2019**, *20*, 769–780. [CrossRef]
2. Seretny, M.; Currie, G.L.; Sena, E.S.; Ramnarine, S.; Grant, R.; MacLeod, M.R.; Colvin, L.A.; Fallon, M. Incidence, prevalence, and predictors of chemotherapy-induced peripheral neuropathy: A systematic review and meta-analysis. *Pain* **2014**, *155*, 2461–2470. [CrossRef] [PubMed]
3. Scripture, C.D.; Figg, W.D.; Sparreboom, A. Peripheral neuropathy induced by paclitaxel: Recent insights and future perspectives. *Curr. Neuropharmacol.* **2006**, *4*, 165–172. [CrossRef] [PubMed]
4. Dougherty, P.M.; Cata, J.P.; Cordella, J.V.; Burton, A.; Weng, H.-R. Taxol-induced sensory disturbance is characterized by preferential impairment of myelinated fiber function in cancer patients. *Pain* **2004**, *109*, 132–142. [CrossRef] [PubMed]
5. Colvin, L.A. Chemotherapy-induced peripheral neuropathy: Where are we now? *Pain* **2019**, *160*, S1–S10. [CrossRef]
6. Yang, I.H.; Siddique, R.; Hosmane, S.; Thakor, N.; Höke, A. Compartmentalized microfluidic culture platform to study mechanism of paclitaxel-induced axonal degeneration. *Exp. Neurol.* **2009**, *218*, 124–128. [CrossRef]
7. Pease-Raissi, S.E.; Pazyra-Murphy, M.F.; Li, Y.; Wachter, F.; Fukuda, Y.; Fenstermacher, S.J.; Barclay, L.A.; Bird, G.H.; Walensky, L.D.; Segal, R.A. Paclitaxel Reduces Axonal Bclw to Initiate IP3R1-Dependent Axon Degeneration. *Neuron* **2017**, *96*, 373–386.e6. [CrossRef]
8. Chine, V.B.; Au, N.P.B.; Kumar, G.; Ma, C.H.E. Targeting Axon Integrity to Prevent Chemotherapy-Induced Peripheral Neuropathy. *Mol. Neurobiol.* **2018**, *56*, 3244–3259. [CrossRef]
9. Koltzenburg, M. Neural Mechanisms of Cutaneous Nociceptive Pain. *Clin. J. Pain* **2000**, *16*, S131–S138. [CrossRef]
10. Flatters, S.J.; Bennett, G.J. Studies of peripheral sensory nerves in paclitaxel-induced painful peripheral neuropathy: Evidence for mitochondrial dysfunction. *Pain* **2006**, *122*, 245–257. [CrossRef]
11. Xiao, W.H.; Zheng, H.; Zheng, F.Y.; Nuydens, R.; Meert, T.F.; Bennett, G.J. Mitochondrial abnormality in sensory, but not motor, axons in paclitaxel-evoked painful peripheral neu-ropathy in the rat. *Neuroscience* **2011**, *199*, 461–469. [CrossRef]
12. McCormick, B.; Lowes, D.A.; Colvin, L.; Torsney, C.; Galley, H.F. MitoVitE, a mitochondria-targeted antioxidant, limits paclitaxel-induced oxidative stress and mito-chondrial damage in vitro, and paclitaxel-induced mechanical hypersensitivity in a rat pain model. *Br. J. Anaesth.* **2016**, *117*, 659–666. [CrossRef]
13. Duggett, N.A.; Griffiths, L.A.; McKenna, O.E.; Santis, V.; Yongsanguanchai, N.; Mokori, E.B.; Flatters, S.J.L. Oxidative stress in the development, maintenance and resolution of paclitaxel-induced painful neurop-athy. *Neuroscience* **2016**, *333*, 13–26. [CrossRef]
14. Zheng, H.; Xiao, W.H.; Bennett, G.J. Functional deficits in peripheral nerve mitochondria in rats with paclitaxel- and oxaliplatin-evoked painful peripheral neuropathy. *Exp. Neurol.* **2011**, *232*, 154–161. [CrossRef]
15. Ida, T.; Sawa, T.; Ihara, H.; Tsuchiya, Y.; Watanabe, Y.; Kumagai, Y.; Suematsu, M.; Motohashi, H.; Fujii, S.; Matsunaga, T. Reactive cysteine persulfides and Spolythiolation regulate oxidative stress and redox signaling. *Proc. Natl. Acad. Sci. USA* **2014**, *111*, 7606–7611. [CrossRef]
16. Benchoam, D.; Semelak, J.A.; Cuevasanta, E.; Mastrogiovanni, M.; Grassano, J.S.; Ferrer-Sueta, G.; Zeida, A.; Trujillo, M.; Möller, M.N.; Estrin, D.A. Acidity and nucleophilic reactivity of glutathione persulfide. *J. Biol. Chem.* **2020**, *295*, 15466–15481. [CrossRef]
17. Wall, P.D. Vigilance in defense of animal welfare. International Association for the Study of Pain. *Pain* **1993**, *54*, 239. [CrossRef]
18. Chen, L.-H.; Yeh, Y.-M.; Chen, Y.-F.; Hsu, Y.-H.; Wang, H.-H.; Lin, P.-C.; Chang, L.-Y.; Lin, C.-C.K.; Chang, M.-S.; Shen, M.-R. Targeting interleukin-20 alleviates paclitaxel-induced peripheral neuropathy. *Pain* **2020**, *161*, 1237–1254. [CrossRef]
19. Gonzalez-Cano, R.; Boivin, B.; Bullock, D.; Cornelissen, L.; Andrews, N.; Costigan, M. Up–Down Reader: An Open Source Program for Efficiently Processing 50% von Frey Thresholds. *Front. Pharmacol.* **2018**, *9*, 433. [CrossRef]
20. Chaplan, S.R.; Bach, F.W.; Pogrel, J.W.; Chung, J.M.; Yaksh, T.L. Quantitative assessment of tactile allodynia in the rat paw. *J. Neurosci. Methods* **1994**, *53*, 55–63. [CrossRef]
21. Bannon, A.W.; Malmberg, A.B. Models of nociception: Hot-plate, tail-flick, and formalin tests in rodents. *Curr. Protoc. Neurosci.* **2007**, *8*, 8–9. [CrossRef] [PubMed]
22. Lauria, G.; Hsieh, S.-T.; Johansson, O.; Kennedy, W.R.; Leger, J.M.; Mellgren, S.I.; Nolano, M.; Merkies, I.S.J.; Polydefkis, M.; Smith, A.G.; et al. European Federation of Neurological Societi es/Peripheral Nerve Society Guideline on the use of skin biopsy in the diagnosis of small fiber neuropathy. Report of a joint task force of the European Fe-deration of Neurological Societies and the Peripheral Ne. *Eur. J. Neurol.* **2010**, *17*, 903–912, e44-9. [CrossRef] [PubMed]
23. Ghnenis, A.B.; Czaikowski, R.E.; Zhang, Z.J.; Bushman, J.S. Toluidine Blue Staining of Resin-Embedded Sections for Evaluation of Peripheral Nerve Morphology. *J. Vis. Exp.* **2018**, e58031. [CrossRef] [PubMed]
24. Sleigh, J.N.; West, S.J.; Schiavo, G. A video protocol for rapid dissection of mouse dorsal root ganglia from defined spinal levels. *BMC Res. Notes.* **2020**, *13*, 302. [CrossRef] [PubMed]
25. Hamid, H.A.; Tanaka, A.; Ida, T.; Nishimura, A.; Matsunaga, T.; Fujii, S.; Morita, M.; Sawa, T.; Fukuto, J.M.; Nagy, P.; et al. Polysulfide stabilization by tyrosine and hydroxyphenyl-containing derivatives that is important for a reactive sulfur metabolomics analysis. *Redox. Biol.* **2019**, *21*, 101096. [CrossRef]
26. Zhang, T.; Ono, K.; Tsutsuki, H.; Ihara, H.; Islam, W.; Akaike, T.; Sawa, T. Enhanced Cellular Polysulfides Negatively Regulate TLR4 Signaling and Mitigate Lethal Endotoxin Shock. *Cell. Chem. Biol.* **2019**, *26*, 686–698.e4. [CrossRef]
27. Takata, T.; Jung, M.; Matsunaga, T.; Ida, T.; Morita, M.; Motohashi, H.; Shen, X.; Kevil, C.G.; Fukuto, J.M.; Akaike, T. Methods in sulfide and persulfide research. *Nitric. Oxide* **2021**, *116*, 47–64. [CrossRef]

28. Perner, C.; Sokol, C.L. Protocol for dissection and culture of murine dorsal root ganglia neurons to study neuropeptide release. *STAR Protoc.* **2021**, *2*, 100333. [CrossRef]
29. Marutani, E.; Kosugi, S.; Tokuda, K.; Khatri, A.; Nguyen, R.; Atochin, D.N.; Kida, K.; Van Leyen, K.; Arai, K.; Ichinose, F. A Novel Hydrogen Sulfide-releasing N-Methyl-d-Aspartate Receptor Antagonist Prevents Ischemic Neuronal Death. *J. Biol. Chem.* **2012**, *287*, 32124–32135. [CrossRef]
30. Gadgil, S.; Ergün, M.; Heuvel, S.A.V.D.; Van Der Wal, S.E.; Scheffer, G.J.; Hooijmans, C.R. A systematic summary and comparison of animal models for chemotherapy induced (peripheral) neuropathy (CIPN). *PLoS ONE* **2019**, *14*, e0221787. [CrossRef]
31. Ferreira, T.A.; Blackman, A.V.; Oyrer, J.; Jayabal, S.; Chung, A.J.; Watt, A.J.; Sjöström, P.J.; Van Meyel, D.J. Neuronal morphometry directly from bitmap images. *Nat. Methods* **2014**, *11*, 982–984. [CrossRef]
32. Homma, S.; Ishii, Y.; Morishima, Y.; Yamadori, T.; Matsuno, Y.; Haraguchi, N.; Kikuchi, N.; Satoh, H.; Sakamoto, T.; Hizawa, N.; et al. Nrf2 Enhances Cell Proliferation and Resistance to Anticancer Drugs in Human Lung Cancer. *Clin. Cancer Res.* **2009**, *15*, 3423–3432. [CrossRef]
33. Cho, J.-M.; Manandhar, S.; Lee, H.-R.; Park, H.-M.; Kwak, M.-K. Role of the Nrf2-antioxidant system in cytotoxicity mediated by anticancer cisplatin: Implication to cancer cell resistance. *Cancer Lett.* **2008**, *260*, 96–108. [CrossRef]
34. Szabó, C. Hydrogen sulphide and its therapeutic potential. *Nat. Rev. Drug. Discov.* **2007**, *6*, 917–935. [CrossRef]
35. Trecarichi, A.; Flatters, S.J.L. Mitochondrial dysfunction in the pathogenesis of chemotherapy-induced peripheral neuropathy. *Int. Rev. Neurobiol.* **2019**, *145*, 83–126.
36. Cirrincione, A.; Pellegrini, A.D.; Dominy, J.R.; Benjamin, M.E.; Utkina-Sosunova, I.; Lotti, F.; Jergova, S.; Sagen, J.; Rieger, S. Paclitaxel-induced peripheral neuropathy is caused by epidermal ROS and mitochondrial damage through conserved MMP-13 activation. *Sci. Rep.* **2020**, *10*, 1–12. [CrossRef]
37. Akaike, T.; Ida, T.; Wei, F.; Nishida, M.; Kumagai, Y.; Alam, M.M.; Ihara, H.; Sawa, T.; Matsunaga, T.; Kasamatsu, S.; et al. Cysteinyl-tRNA synthetase governs cysteine polysulfidation and mitochondrial bioenergetics. *Nat. Commun.* **2017**, *8*, 1177. [CrossRef]
38. de Beus, M.D.; Chung, J.; Colon, W. Modification of cysteine 111 in Cu/Zn superoxide dismutase results in altered spectroscopic and biophysical properties. *Protein. Sci.* **2004**, *13*, 1347–1355. [CrossRef]
39. Shinkai, Y.; Abiko, Y.; Ida, T.; Miura, T.; Kakehashi, H.; Ishii, I.; Nishida, M.; Sawa, T.; Akaike, T.; Kumagai, Y. Reactive Sulfur Species-Mediated Activation of the Keap1-Nrf2 Pathway by 1,2-Naphthoquinone through Sulfenic Acids Formation under Oxidative Stress. *Chem. Res. Toxicol.* **2015**, *28*, 838–847. [CrossRef]
40. Smith, G.A.; Lin, T.-H.; Sheehan, A.E.; Naters, W.V.D.G.V.; Neukomm, L.J.; Graves, H.K.; Bis-Brewer, D.M.; Züchner, S.; Freeman, M.R. Glutathione S-Transferase Regulates Mitochondrial Populations in Axons through Increased Glutathione Oxidation. *Neuron* **2019**, *103*, 52–65.e6. [CrossRef]
41. Ding, C.; Wu, Y.; Hammarlund, M. Activation of the CaMKII-Sarm1-ASK1-p38 MAP kinase pathway protects against axon degeneration caused by loss of mitochondria. *Elife* **2022**, *11*, e73587. [CrossRef] [PubMed]
42. Baloh, R.H. Mitochondrial Dynamics and Peripheral Neuropathy. *Neuroscientist* **2007**, *14*, 12–18. [CrossRef] [PubMed]
43. Cuadrado, A.; Manda, G.; Hassan, A.; Alcaraz, M.J.; Barbas, C.; Daiber, A.; Ghezzi, P.; León, R.; López, M.G.; Oliva, B.; et al. Transcription Factor NRF2 as a Therapeutic Target for Chronic Diseases: A Systems Medicine Approach. *Pharmacol. Rev.* **2018**, *70*, 348–383. [CrossRef] [PubMed]
44. Bessaguet, F.; Danigo, A.; Bouchenaki, H.; Duchesne, M.; Magy, L.; Richard, L.; Sturtz, F.; Desmoulière, A.; Demiot, C. Neuroprotective effect of angiotensin II type 2 receptor stimulation in vincristine-induced mechanical allodynia. *Pain* **2018**, *159*, 2538–2546. [CrossRef] [PubMed]
45. Mo, M.; Erdelyi, I.; Szigeti-Buck, K.; Benbow, J.H.; Ehrlich, B.E. Prevention of paclitaxel-induced peripheral neuropathy by lithium pretreatment. *FASEB J.* **2012**, *26*, 4696–4709. [CrossRef]
46. Todd, A.J. Neuronal circuitry for pain processing in the dorsal horn. *Nat. Rev. Neurosci.* **2010**, *11*, 823–836. [CrossRef]
47. Hwang, B.-Y.; Kim, E.-S.; Kim, C.-H.; Kwon, J.-Y.; Kim, H.-K. Gender differences in paclitaxel-induced neuropathic pain behavior and analgesic response in rats. *Korean J. Anesthesiol.* **2012**, *62*, 66–72. [CrossRef]

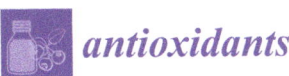

Article

Metabolic and Structural Insights into Hydrogen Sulfide Mis-Regulation in *Enterococcus faecalis*

Brenna J. C. Walsh [1], Sofia Soares Costa [2], Katherine A. Edmonds [1], Jonathan C. Trinidad [1], Federico M. Issoglio [2,3], José A. Brito [2,*] and David P. Giedroc [1,4,*]

[1] Department of Chemistry, Indiana University, Bloomington, IN 47405-7102, USA
[2] Instituto de Tecnologia Química e Biológica António Xavier, Universidade Nova de Lisboa, 2780-157 Oeiras, Portugal
[3] Instituto de Química Biológica de la Facultad de Ciencias Exactas y Naturales (IQUIBICEN)-CONICET and Departamento de Química Biológica, Universidad de Buenos Aires, Buenos Aires C1428EHA, Argentina
[4] Department of Molecular and Cellular Biochemistry, Indiana University, Bloomington, IN 47405-7003, USA
* Correspondence: jbrito@itqb.unl.pt (J.A.B.); giedroc@indiana.edu (D.P.G.); Tel.: +351-214-469-760 (J.A.B.); +1-812-856-3178 (D.P.G.)

Citation: Walsh, B.J.C.; Costa, S.S.; Edmonds, K.A.; Trinidad, J.C.; Issoglio, F.M.; Brito, J.A.; Giedroc, D.P. Metabolic and Structural Insights into Hydrogen Sulfide Mis-Regulation in *Enterococcus faecalis*. *Antioxidants* 2022, 11, 1607. https://doi.org/10.3390/antiox11081607

Academic Editors: John Toscano and Vinayak Khodade

Received: 9 July 2022
Accepted: 17 August 2022
Published: 19 August 2022

Publisher's Note: MDPI stays neutral with regard to jurisdictional claims in published maps and institutional affiliations.

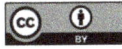

Copyright: © 2022 by the authors. Licensee MDPI, Basel, Switzerland. This article is an open access article distributed under the terms and conditions of the Creative Commons Attribution (CC BY) license (https://creativecommons.org/licenses/by/4.0/).

Abstract: Hydrogen sulfide (H_2S) is implicated as a cytoprotective agent that bacteria employ in response to host-induced stressors, such as oxidative stress and antibiotics. The physiological benefits often attributed to H_2S, however, are likely a result of downstream, more oxidized forms of sulfur, collectively termed reactive sulfur species (RSS) and including the organic persulfide (RSSH). Here, we investigated the metabolic response of the commensal gut microorganism *Enterococcus faecalis* to exogenous Na_2S as a proxy for H_2S/RSS toxicity. We found that exogenous sulfide increases protein abundance for enzymes responsible for the biosynthesis of coenzyme A (CoA). Proteome S-sulfuration (persulfidation), a posttranslational modification implicated in H_2S signal transduction, is also widespread in this organism and is significantly elevated by exogenous sulfide in CstR, the RSS sensor, coenzyme A persulfide (CoASSH) reductase (CoAPR) and enzymes associated with de novo fatty acid biosynthesis and acetyl-CoA synthesis. Exogenous sulfide significantly impacts the speciation of fatty acids as well as cellular concentrations of acetyl-CoA, suggesting that protein persulfidation may impact flux through these pathways. Indeed, CoASSH is an inhibitor of *E. faecalis* phosphotransacetylase (Pta), suggesting that an important metabolic consequence of increased levels of H_2S/RSS may be over-persulfidation of this key metabolite, which, in turn, inhibits CoA and acyl-CoA-utilizing enzymes. Our 2.05 Å crystallographic structure of CoA-bound CoAPR provides new structural insights into CoASSH clearance in *E. faecalis*.

Keywords: hydrogen sulfide toxicity; reactive sulfur species; persulfide; persulfidation profiling; coenzyme A persulfide; X-ray structure; fatty acids

1. Introduction

Recent studies based on seminal work [1] suggest that H_2S may be a clinically relevant bacterial adaptive response to host-derived oxidative stress and antibiotics during infections [2–7]. These cytoprotective properties attributed to H_2S may well be the result of downstream, more oxidized sulfur species, collectively termed reactive sulfur species (RSS) [8]. One of these RSS is the organic persulfide (RSSH), which has enhanced nucleophilicity compared to its thiol counterpart and readily reacts with infection-relevant oxidants and β-lactam antibiotics [8–11]. Although much of the work on RSS has focused on mammalian systems [8], RSS biogenesis has been shown to be present in a number of bacteria [7,12–14].

The beneficial impact of H_2S and RSS can only be accessed when the negative impact of sulfide poisoning [15] and over-persulfidation of the thiol metabolome and proteome can be limited [7,16] in a process we call H_2S/RSS homeostasis. Maintaining H_2S/RSS homeostasis may be particularly important in the sulfide-rich environment of the gastrointestinal tract, where H$_2$S has been documented to be physiologically beneficial [17–19] and linked to several gut-derived human diseases at elevated concentrations [20–22]. Sulfide has been estimated to range from ~0.2 to 2.4 mM in this niche derived from both host- and microbially-derived sulfate reduction [23]. Furthermore, a recent study suggested that taurine, an organosulfonate produced by the host during infections, enables the host to resist colonization by pathogens by increasing endogenous H$_2$S production from taurine by resident microbiota [24]. This suggests that organisms, both commensals and pathogens, that inhabit this niche must evolve ways to sense and detoxify H$_2$S and consequential downstream oxidized sulfur species [25].

All bacteria encode RSS-sensing transcriptional regulators that control the expression of genes that encode enzymes that are known or projected to be involved in the biogenesis and clearance of H$_2$S/RSS [25]. Previously, we identified and characterized the *cst*-like operon in the human pathogen and commensal member of the gut microbiota *Enterococcus faecalis* [12]. This operon is transcriptionally regulated by the RSS-sensing transcriptional repressor CstR [26–28]. The *cst*-like operon consists of two sulfurtransferases, RhdA and RhdB, which possess thiosulfate sulfurtransferase (TST) activity; however, their in-cell sulfur donors and acceptors are not yet known. Additionally, CstR regulates *coaP*, which encodes the coenzyme A (CoA) persulfide (CoASSH) reductase (CoAPR), which reduces CoASSH to the free thiol and H$_2$S [12]. The biogenesis of H$_2$S by CoAPR combined with its specificity toward CoASSH over other low molecular weight (LMW) persulfides implies that RSS, specifically CoASSH, confers a greater physiological impact relative to H$_2$S in this organism. The fate of CoAPR-generated H$_2$S is not known, nor is the mechanism by which *E. faecalis* generates LMW persulfides, although these species are readily detected and quantitated in soluble cell lysates [12].

Here, we sought to investigate the physiological response of *E. faecalis* to conditions of sulfide mis-regulation by adding exogenous Na$_2$S as a probe of a pathophysiological response to elevated H$_2$S. A proteomic analysis revealed an increased cellular abundance of CoA- and acyl-CoA requiring enzymes, including CoAPR, with the latter anticipated on the basis of regulation by CstR [12]. Protein *S*-sulfuration (persulfidation) profiling reveals that ≈13% of the proteome is persulfidated and identifies potential regulatory targets of H$_2$S/RSS signaling, including enzymes involved in de novo fatty acid biosynthesis and the acetyl-CoA-producing enzyme phosphotransacetylase (Pta). As anticipated, both CstR and CoAPR are heavily persulfidated in cells consistent with their proposed mechanisms of action [12,27,28]. In addition, the spectrum of fatty acids changes significantly following the addition of exogenous sulfide; this is coupled with a significant increase in cellular acetyl-CoA, the major cellular fate of which is fatty acid biosynthesis. We demonstrate that CoASSH is a potent inhibitor of *E. faecalis* Pta, which suggests that CoASSH poisoning of CoA- and acyl-CoA-requiring enzymes [29] may underscore the metabolic burden of H$_2$S toxicity in this organism. Finally, our crystallographic structure and molecular dynamics simulations of CoA-bound *E. faecalis* CoAPR provide new mechanistic insights into CoASSH clearance.

2. Materials and Methods

2.1. Growth of Enterococcus faecalis

Unless otherwise noted, all cultures were grown microaerophilically, defined here as static cultures in sealed culture tubes at 37 °C with minimal head-space. *E. faecalis* strain OG1RF (wild-type, WT) was grown overnight in tryptic soy broth (TSB) medium, supplemented with 0.25% (*w/v*) glucose. Overnight cultures were diluted into fresh medium at an OD$_{600}$ ≈ 0.007 and grown until ≈0.1 as a preculture. Precultures were then diluted into fresh medium to an OD$_{600}$ of ≈0.007 and grown until OD$_{600}$ ≈ 0.2, at which time cells were treated as described for each experiment below.

2.2. Proteomic Analysis of Wild Type E. faecalis before and after the Addition of Exogenous Na$_2$S

Quadruplicate 15 mL cultures of wild type *E. faecalis* were collected by centrifugation for untreated cells or treated with 0.2 mM Na$_2$S for 30 min followed by centrifugation. All cells were washed with ice-cold PBS and stored at −80 °C. Pellets were thawed on ice and resuspended in 600 µL lysis buffer (25 mM HEPES, pH 7.4, 150 mM NaCl, 5 mM tris(2-carboxyethyl) phosphine hydrochloride (TCEP), EDTA-free protease-inhibitor cocktail [1:500] dilution). Resuspended cells were transferred to Lysing matrix B tubes and lysed in a bead beater with a rate of 6 m/s for 45 s, three times, with 5 min cooling on ice in between runs. Samples were centrifuged at 13,200 rpm for 15 min at 4 °C. The supernatant was transferred to a new 1.5 mL tube and the protein concentration was quantified by a Bradford assay using a standard protocol. A total of 25 µg of protein was dried down in a SpeedVac™ concentrator (Thermo Fisher Scientific, Waltham, MA, USA) and resuspended in 8 M urea in 100 mM ammonium bicarbonate. To these solutions, 5 mM TCEP and 50 mM iodoacetamide was added for 45 min at room temperature to reduce and alkylate cysteine residues. Proteins were then precipitated by 20% (*v*/*v*) trichloroacetic acid and allowed to sit at −20 °C for 1 h. Samples were then centrifuged at 15,000 rpm for 20 min at 4 °C, with the supernatant removed. Pellets were washed with cold methanol and centrifuged at 15,000 rpm for 20 min at 4 °C twice. Samples were dried in a SpeedVac™ concentrator, resuspended in 10 µL 8 M urea in 100 mM ammonium bicarbonate, diluted to 1 M urea with 100 mM ammonium bicarbonate, and digested overnight at 37 °C, with the addition of 1:100 (*w/w*) ratio of trypsin. Peptides were desalted by a C18 Omix Tip (Agilent Technologies, Santa Clara, CA, USA) by a standard protocol and analyzed as described below.

2.3. Enrichment and Identification of S-Sulfurated Proteins in E. faecalis

This analysis was carried out essentially as previously described [7,30]. Wild-type *E. faecalis* was grown in 300 mL cultures as described above, and the experiment was performed in biological triplicate. At OD$_{600}$ ≈ 0.2, cultures were collected by centrifugation for untreated cells or treated with 0.2 mM Na$_2$S for 30 min followed by centrifugation. All cells were washed with ice-cold PBS three times and stored at −80 °C. Pellets were treated as previously described [7,30]. Samples were subjected to an LC MS/MS analysis as described below. Three biological replicates were used as treated (WT + Na$_2$S) and untreated (WT) samples. Sigma ratios (σ^R) were calculated for each protein using total area for cysteine peptides [30]. The fold change of S-sulfurated peptides (WT + Na$_2$S/WT) were normalized to the protein abundance from data acquired in the proteomic analysis described above. S-sulfurated peptides only detected in one condition (WT or WT + Na$_2$S) or proteins not identified in our no-enrichment proteomic analysis were assigned peaks areas equal to the lowest detected peptide or protein to eliminate division by zero during normalization [30].

2.4. LC-MS/MS Analysis of Proteome and S-Sulfurated Proteins

An LC-MS/MS analysis was carried out in the Laboratory of Biological Mass Spectrometry at Indiana University as previously described [30]. The resulting data were searched against the *E. faecalis TX4248* database (Uniprot UP000004846, 3273 entries) in Proteome Discoverer 2.1. Carbamidomethylation (CAM) of cysteine residues was set as a fixed modification. Protein N-terminal acetylation, oxidation of methionine, protein N-terminal methionine loss, protein N-terminal methionine loss and acetylation, and pyroglutamine formation were introduced as variable modifications. A total of three variable modifications were allowed. Trypsin digestion specificity with two missed cleavage was allowed. The mass tolerance for precursor and fragment ions was set to 10 ppm and 0.6 Da, respectively. The peptide peak area was quantified for MS1 ions and utilized to estimate fold-change in this label-free quantitation method.

2.5. Extraction and Measurement of Cellular Fatty Acids

Cell pellets from 14 mL cultures grown in biological triplicate as described above were resuspended in 1 mL methanolic NaOH [15% (w/v) NaOH in 50% (v/v) methanol] transferred to a glass, screw cap culture tube, vortexed for 5–10 s and saponified at 100 °C for 30 min. A total of 15 µg of pentadecanoic acid was added as an internal standard followed by fatty acid esterification, achieved by the addition of 2 mL of 3.25 N HCl in 46% (68%) (v/v) methanol at 80 °C for 10 min followed by extraction into 1.25 mL of 1:1 (v/v) methyl-*tert*-butyl ether in hexane for 10 min on a rotor (Barnstead Thermolyne Labquake Shaker, American Laboratory Trading, East Lyme, CT, USA). The aqueous phase was removed, and the organic phase was washed with 3 mL 1.2% (w/v) NaOH for 5 min on a rotor. The organic phase was promptly removed and stored until analysis. Samples were analyzed by GC-MS, by injecting 2 µL onto an SLB-5 MS 30 m × 0.25 mm × 0.25 um column. A sample run consisted of 35 °C (2 min) to 250 °C at 10 °C/min, then to 320 °C (3 min) at 20 °C/min. Fatty acids were identified based on the retention time of authentic standards. The MS was operated in single ion mode (SIM) using ions at 74 and 55 m/z. Chromatograms were extracted using these m/z and integrated, and peak areas were used to determine the relative abundance of each fatty acid. Fatty acids were designated in X:Y form, where X is the total number of carbon atoms, and Y is the number of double bonds, and each is presented as a fractional abundance of total fatty acids determined by the fraction of each fatty acid (peak area) to total fatty acids (sum of all peak areas).

2.6. Quantitation of Acetyl-CoA

Wild-type *E. faecalis* strain OG1RF was grown as described above in 100 mL cultures, and quantitation was performed using modifications of procedures described previously [31]. At an OD_{600} of 0.2, 2 mL of culture was centrifuged for 5 min, with the supernatant discarded and used to determine protein concentration. The remaining cell culture was quenched by the addition of a 3:2 (v/v) glycerol saline solution (−20 °C) to a ratio of 1:4 (v/v). Quenched cultures were placed at −20 °C for 5 min before centrifuging at 7100× g for 30 min at −11 °C. The supernatant was discarded, and the pellets were combined; washed with 2 mL of a 1:1 (v/v) glycerol saline solution (−20 °C); centrifuged for 20 min at −11 °C, with the supernatant discarded, and washed once more. Pellets were resuspended in 1 mL of 15% (v/v) methanol (cold) and transferred into a fresh 1.5 mL centrifuge tube and centrifuged at 10,000× g for 15 min at −11 °C, discarding the supernatant.

Cells were lysed by resuspending the pellet in 1.5 mL of 60% (v/v) cold methanol (−20 °C) and freeze-thawed in liquid nitrogen, followed by placement on ice. The process was repeated 5 times, and the cell debris was pelleted by centrifugation at a maximum speed for 15 min at −11 °C, and the supernatant was transferred to a new tube. The pellet was washed with 500 µL of 60% (v/v) methanol and centrifuged, and the supernatant was combined with that from the first centrifugation. The solutions were then dried down in a Speedvac concentrator and resuspended in 150 µL of LC-MS grade water and filtered through a 0.22 µm spin filter. A total of 10 µL was injected onto an Agilent AdvanceBio peptide C18 column (2.1 × 150 mm, 2.7 µm) equipped to an Aquity UPLC system coupled to a Waters G2S mass spectrometer. Acetyl-CoA was eluted using an acetonitrile-based gradient, slightly modified from that previously described (Solvent A: 0% (v/v) acetonitrile, 50 mM ammonium acetate; Solvent B: 100% (v/v) acetonitrile) at a flow rate of 250 µL/min [32]. A 15-min gradient was as follows: 0–1 min, 3% B; 1–7 min, 3–25% B; 7–8 min, 25–40% B; 8–11 min, 40% B; 11–15 min, 3% B. Quantitation was achieved via external calibration using the authentic acetyl-CoA standard (Sigma, St. Louis, MO, USA) and MassLynx software (version 4.2, Waters Corporation, Milford, MA, USA). The analysis was performed in biological triplicate.

2.7. Cloning and Purification of Recombinant Ef Pta

Ef Pta was cloned into the pHis parallel expression plasmid using the NcoI and SalI restriction sites, and the resulting plasmid was transformed into E. coli BL21 (DE3), cultured in LB medium at 37 °C until the OD_{600} reached 0.6–0.8, induced with 1 mM IPTG and expressed at 16–20 °C for 16 h. Cells were harvested by centrifugation and stored at −80 °C. The cell pellet was resuspended in a lysis buffer containing 25 mM Tris-HCl, 500 mM NaCl, 2 mM TCEP, 10% (v/v) glycerol and pH 8.0 and lysed by sonication. The cell lysate was clarified by centrifugation, and 70% (w/v) ammonium sulfate was added to salt out Ef Pta. The ammonium sulfate pellet was resuspended in the lysis buffer and was loaded on a HisTrap HP Ni-NTA column (Cytiva), which was pre-equilibrated with lysis buffer. The column was washed with lysis buffer followed by elution with an imidazole gradient from 0 to 500 mM. Fractions containing Ef Pta were combined, concentrated and further purified by size exclusion chromatography (Superdex G200 16/60 column, Cytiva) in a lysis buffer. Final fractions containing Pta with a purity of >95% estimated by SDS-PAGE were combined and stored with 10% (v/v) glycerol at −80 °C until use.

2.8. Enzyme Assays of Ef Pta Activity

Ef Pta is a reversible enzyme that can utilize either acetyl-CoA and inorganic phosphate or CoA and acetyl-phosphate as substrates, and both the forward and reverse reactions were assayed. Ef Pta was buffer-exchanged into fully degassed 25 mM Tris-HCl and 40 mM KCl at pH 8.0 in an anaerobic chamber. The acetyl-CoA-utilizing, CoA-forming reaction was measured using DTNB to derivatize the CoA thiol, and the TNB anion released was quantified by UV-Vis at 412 nm ($\varepsilon = 14{,}150$ M^{-1} cm^{-1}), as described previously [33]. The 150 µL reactions contained 50 nM Ef Pta, 5 mM KH_2PO_4, acetyl-CoA ranging from 10 µM to 5 mM and 500 µM DTNB, buffered by 25 mM Tris-HCl and 40 mM KCl at pH 8.0, at room temperature in an anaerobic chamber. The reactions were initiated with the addition of the enzyme and incubated for 2 min, at which time the absorption at 412 nm was measured. To measure the reverse reaction, the 150 µL reactions contained 50 nM Ef Pta, 5 mM acetylphosphate and CoA ranging from 10 µM to 5 mM, buffered by 25 mM Tris-HCl and 40 mM KCl at pH 8.0 at room temperature in an anaerobic chamber. The reactions were initiated by the addition of the enzyme and incubated for 30 s, and the production of acetyl-CoA was monitored via formation of the thioester bond at 233 nm ($\varepsilon = 4400$ M^{-1} cm^{-1}) [33,34].

To measure the production of acetyl-CoA, 50 µL reactions were prepared as described above. These reactions contained 20 or 150 µM of CoASSH from an in situ preparation [12] which contained Na_2S, CoA disulfide, CoA and CoASSH. This was compared to reactions containing 20 or 150 µM CoA in the absence or presence of Na_2S or CoA disulfide added at a concentration equal to that present in the in situ CoASSH preparation. The reactions were initiated with the addition of Ef Pta, incubated at room temperature for 30 s and quenched by addition of 150 µL 2 mM HPE-IAM in acetonitrile (1.5 mM final concentration). Samples were placed at −20 °C for 2 h to precipitate the protein and centrifuged at 4 °C for 20 min, and the supernatant was transferred to a clean 1.5 mL tube and dried down in a SpeedVac concentrator. Pellets were resuspended in 50 µL of HPLC grade water and then diluted at 1:20–1:100 in HPLC grade water and analyzed by LC-MS as described above. The concentration of acetyl-CoA was quantified by a series of authentic standards as described above.

2.9. Statistical Rationale and Bioinformatics Analysis

Proteins detected in fewer than two biological replicates were excluded from a statistical analysis of proteomic data, completed using an unpaired, two-tailed Student t-test with Welch's correction. Functional information for the selected proteins were gathered from the National Center for Biotechnology Information (NCBI; https://www.ncbi.nlm.nih.gov/, accessed on 3 September 2019), BioCyc (https://biocyc.org/web-services.shtml, accessed on 3 September 2019) and Kyoto Encyclopedia of Genes and Genomes (KEGG;

https://www.genome.jp/kegg/pathway.html, accessed on 3 September 2019) databases. Metabolism pathway information for the selected proteins was obtained from KEGG, and pathway analysis of *S*-sulfurated proteins was performed using the KEGG pathway mapper (https://www.genome.jp/kegg/mapper.html, accessed on 3 September 2019). A motif analysis of *S*-sulfuration sites was performed using pLogo (http://plogo.uconn.edu, accessed on 3 September 2019) [35]. For each modified cysteine, a 21-amino-acid sequence containing the *S*-sulfurated cysteine, with 10 amino acids flanking sequences on either side of the Cys, was selected. A background data set was constructed similarly using all cysteines identified in the reference genome for *E. faecalis* OG1RF (GenBank accession no. NZ_CP025020.1).

2.10. Cloning and Purification of Recombinant EfCoAPR

Gene expression and protein production were performed as previously described [12] with slight modifications. In brief, the *coaP* gene from *E. faecalis* strain OG1RF was fused with a hexahistidine tag and cloned into the pHIS parallel expression plasmid. The expression plasmid was transformed into *E. coli* BL21(DE3) and cultured in LB medium at 37 °C. *Ef*CoAPR expression was induced with 1 mM of IPTG for 16 h at 37 °C. After cell lysis by sonication, DNA removal, protein precipitation by ammonium sulfate and resuspension, His-tagged *Ef*CoAPR was purified by Ni-NTA affinity chromatography followed by size exclusion chromatography on a Superdex G200 HiLoad 16/600 (Cytiva, Marlborough, MA, USA) column using 20 mM MES at pH 6.0, 30 mM NaCl and 5% (v/v) glycerol buffer. Pure *Ef*CoAPR fractions were pooled, concentrated to $\approx$23 mg mL^{-1} using an Amicon Ultra 30 MWCO (Millipore, Burlington, MA, USA) by repeated concentration steps at 3500$\times$ *g* using an Eppendorf 5804R centrifuge and stored at -80 °C for further experiments.

2.11. X-ray Crystallography

Prior to crystallization experiments, *Ef*CoAPR was quickly thawed in a water bath at 42 °C and subjected to ultracentrifugation for 1 h at 217,200$\times$ *g* (Optima TL-100, TLA-100.3 fixed-angle rotor, Beckman Coulter). Initial crystallization screening was performed using a Mosquito LCP (SPT Labtech, Cambridge, UK) liquid dispenser robot and commercially available screens, e.g., JCSG +, BCS Screen, PACT Premier and Shot Gun, (Molecular Dimensions, Rotherham, UK) at protein concentrations ranging from 8–23 mg mL^{-1} using the vapor diffusion sitting-drop method. Poorly diffracting (8–10 Å) initial crystal hits from these screens were optimized using a cross-seeding approach as previously described [36] and the Seed Bead Steel Kit (Hampton Research, Aliso Viejo, CA, USA) following the manufacturer's instructions. Crystals appeared in several conditions, and a scale-up experiment was performed using a gradient of 18–22% (v/v) PEG 3350, 0.1 M Bis-Tris propane pH 6.4–6.6 and 0.2 M NaI or NaF. Native crystals were grown under 20% (v/v) PEG 3350, 0.1 M Bis-Tris propane buffer at pH 6.50 and 0.2 M sodium iodide; cryo-protected and sent to the European Synchrotron Radiation Facility (ESRF, Grenoble, France) [37] for data collection. Diffraction data were indexed, integrated and scaled within the autoPROC data processing pipeline [38,39], and data quality was assessed with the phenix.xtriage tool within the PHENIX suite of programs [39,40], with the structure solved by molecular replacement (MR) with PHASER [41] as implemented in PHENIX, using one chain (monomer) of the X-ray structure of CoADR-RHD from *Bacillus anthracis* (PDB 3ICS) [42] as the search model, devoid of any cofactors, solvent molecules and other ligands. Iterative model building and refinement were carried out in a cyclic manner with phenix.refine [43], BUSTER-TNT and COOT [44], until a complete model was built and refinement convergence achieved. The *Ef*CoAPR model was validated with MolProbity [45] within PHENIX with the atomic coordinates and structure factors deposited in the Protein Data Bank (http://wwpdb.org/, accessed on 3 September 2019) under accession code 8A56. Structural illustrations were rendered using PyMOL (Version 2.4.1, Schrödinger, LLC., New York, NY, USA) and COOT [43].

2.12. Molecular Dynamics (MD) Simulations

Simulations were carried out on *Ef*CoAPR with both cysteine residues unmodified and bound coenzyme A in its reduced state (CoASH) using GROMACS 2020.3 [46]. To build this system, we used atomic coordinates from the structure above (PDB 8A56) with all crystallographic water molecules in place and FAD coordinates as defined in the structure. Since only the PAP moiety of CoA could be resolved in the experimental electron density, we placed CoASH into the structure by superimposition with CoADR-RHD from *Bacillus anthracis* (PDB 3ICS) [42]. The atomic coordinates for the E474-Q479 loop from the B subunit were placed and refined using MODELLER [47]. The force field parameters were developed on the basis of the CHARMM General Force Field (CGenFF) [48]. The atom types and initial parameters were determined using the CGenFF webserver https://cgenff.paramchem.org, accessed on 3 September 2019) [48,49]. Parameters for FAD and CoASH were obtained from an electronic structure calculation using Gaussian03 at the HF/6–31G* level basis set, followed by a derivation of partial atomic charges using the RESP procedure [50]. The complex was placed into a truncated octahedral box of TIP3P water molecules, defining a distance of 15 Å between the border of the box and the closest atom of the solute. This gave us a total of 157,813 atoms in the system, with 46,933 water molecules and 1089 protein residues. The system was neutralized with Na^+ ions, and Na^+ and Cl^- ions were added to 0.15 M ionic strength.

Geometric optimization was performed with an energy minimization step of 5000 cycles with a 1000 kJ mol^{-1} nm^{-1} force constant applied over all atoms, excluding water molecules. Afterwards, the temperature was increased from 0 to 10 K using a Berendsen thermostat [51] with a coupling constant of 0.05 ps, in a 10 ps constant volume MD with a 0.1 fs time step, and a harmonic restraint potential of 1000 kJ mol^{-1} nm^{-1} applied over all protein residues and ligands. Thereafter, the temperature was increased from 10 to 300 K using a Berendsen thermostat (coupling constant of 0.05 ps), in a 200 ps constant volume MD with a 0.5 fs time step, applying a force constant of 1000 kJ mol^{-1} nm^{-1} to the protein backbone atoms and ligands. After the samples had been heated, the density was equilibrated with a 200 ps MD simulation at constant temperature (300 K) using V-rescale as a thermostat [52] and pressure with a time step of 1 ps (NTP ensemble), while applying a force constant of 1000 kJ mol^{-1} nm^{-1} to heavy atoms on the protomers and ligands. Additionally, another 10 ns MD of NTP ensemble was performed, with positional restraints on Cα atoms and the ligands. For production MD, 1400 ns simulations in the NTP ensemble were conducted, with a time step of 2 fs, under periodic boundary conditions [53] using the LINCS algorithm [54] to constrain all bonds. Long-range electrostatic interactions were handled with PME [55], setting a cutoff distance of 12 Å. All molecular visualizations and drawings were performed with the Visual Molecular Dynamics program [56].

3. Results

3.1. Global Proteomics Profiling of Wild-Type E. faecalis before and after Addition of Exogenous Na_2S

To elucidate the global response of the proteome to exogenous sulfide, we employed a label-free "bottom-up" proteomics analysis on soluble lysates to estimate the change in cellular abundance of specific proteins (Supplemental Table S1). In total, 1115 proteins were detected at least twice in four replicates, with 50 proteins observed only in the wild-type (WT) + Na_2S cells and 24 observed only in WT untreated cells (Figure 1A). Fifty-two proteins (4.9%) detectable in both WT and WT + Na_2S cells exhibited a significant change in cellular abundance, defined here as >2-fold change and $p < 0.001$, which includes the *cst*-like operon encoded enzyme CoAPR (Figure 1B). Strikingly, CoAPR is detected in untreated cells and is among the 25% least-abundant proteins that are detected; this suggests that the RSS-sensing transcriptional repressor of the *cst*-like operon CstR "senses" endogenous RSS prior to further induction by the exogenous sulfide (Figure 1C). The presence of CoAPR in unstressed WT cells is also consistent with the low endogenous level of coenzyme A persulfide (CoASSH) in this organism, as CoAPR specifically reduces CoASSH to the free thiol and H_2S [12]. After addition of Na_2S, CoAPR rises to the top 20% most abundant proteins detected consistent with the regulatory model of CstR (Figure 1D) [12,27].

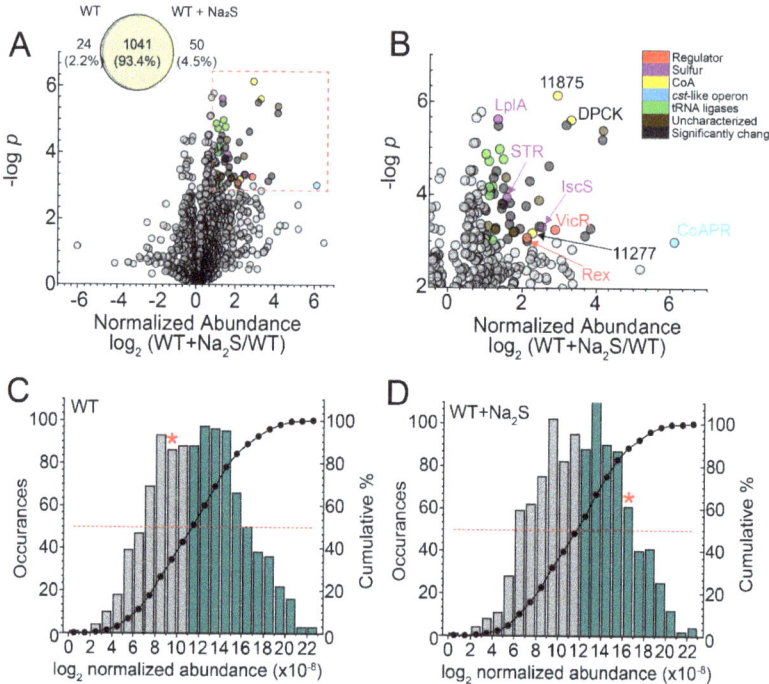

Figure 1. LC-MS/MS proteomics analysis of wild-type *E. faecalis*. Protein profiles of untreated (WT) vs. 0.2 mM Na_2S-treated (WT + Na_2S) *E. faecalis* cells from four biological replicates. (**A**) Venn diagram of proteins detected at least twice in four biological replicates, with volcano plot for proteins detected at least two times in four biological replicates. The significance threshold was set at $p < 0.001$ and fold-change in protein abundance at >2, as enclosed in the red dashed-line box. Circles corresponding to proteins within this significance threshold are shaded according to the annotated function in panel B. (**B**) Expanded view of proteins within a significance threshold, shaded according to the annotated function, with select proteins annotated with the protein name or locus tag (OG1RF_xxxxx). Histogram plot of the distribution of normalized abundance for all proteins detected in the (**C**) WT and (**D**) WT+ 0.2 mM Na_2S strains. The top-most 50% abundant proteins are indicated with a red dashed line, with the bars shaded blue. The red star (*) indicates the cellular abundance of CoAPR.

In addition to CoAPR, two transcriptional regulators, Rex (OG1RF_12010) and VicR (OG1RF_10965); several uncharacterized proteins and proteins involved in translation, including nine tRNA synthetases, were also increased in the proteome after addition of exogenous Na_2S (Figure 1B). Rex is NADH-regulated, contributes to $NAD^+/NADH$ homeostasis and impacts H_2O_2 detoxification in *E. faecalis* [57], while VicR is the soluble response regulator of the VicRK two-component membrane sensor kinase, the kinase activity of which is modulated by extracellular glutathione and dithiothreitol, a model reductant [58]. The concomitant increase in catalase (OG1RF_11314) and decrease the cellular abundance of FeoA, a known Rex target [57] (Supplemental Table S1), collectively suggests an overall change in the cellular redox potential with exogenous sulfide. Of additional interest is the increase in the cell abundance of dephospho-CoA kinase (DPCK) and two thioesterases (OG1RF_11875, OG1RF_11277) of unknown substrate specificity that catalyzed the hydrolysis of a thioester bond. DPCK catalyzed the final step in the de novo biosynthesis of CoA, which might suggest increased production of CoA under these conditions; this finding is consistent with the ≈1.5-fold increase in CoA 30 min post-addition of exogenous sulfide found in previous work [12]. In addition, an uncharacterized multidomain sulfurtransferase (STR, OG1RF_10483), lipoate-protein ligase (LplA, OG1RF_12105) and a candidate cysteine desulfurase (IscS, OG1RF_10258) involved in Fe-S cluster biogenesis were also significantly increased after addition of exogenous Na$_2$S. Two of these enzymes are known or projected to be involved in persulfide transfer (STR, IscS), while LplA lipoates enzymes that couple acyl-transfer from acetyl-CoA in large multienzyme dehydrogenases [59].

3.2. Proteome Persulfidation in E. faecalis

To explore H$_2$S/RSS signaling in *E. faecalis* further, we utilized our previously developed enrichment-reduction strategy [7,30] to profile proteome persulfidation in wild-type *E. faecalis* in the absence or presence of exogenous Na$_2$S. The extent to which a Cys residue is persulfidated after the addition of exogenous Na$_2$S vs. prior is reflected in the parameter σ^R. A σ^R value of 1.0 corresponds to peptides that are not persulfidated prior to the addition of Na$_2$S (24 proteins), and a σ^R value approaching 0 indicates peptides that are only persulfidated in the absence of exogenous sulfide (13 proteins). We identified 356 proteins (≈13% of the proteome) as persulfidated, and the majority of these proteins (90%) were persulfidated in both untreated and Na$_2$S-treated cells (Supplemental Figure S1A, Supplemental Table S2). This is consistent with previous studies of *S. aureus* [7] and *A. baumannii* [13] and suggests that the proteome acts as a reservoir of bioactive sulfane sulfur. These proteins map to many cellular processes, including fatty acid biosynthesis (FAS), amino acid biosynthesis, pyrimidine metabolism and central carbon metabolism. Efforts to identify a consensus sequence associated with sites of protein persulfidation in *E. faecalis* generally failed, even when we restricted our analysis to peptides with high σ^R (Supplemental Figure S2).

A consistent challenge in profiling proteome persulfidation, as well as many other cysteine thiol redox modifications [60], is the ability to distinguish persulfidated cysteines that are regulatory from those that are persulfidated collaterally on solvent-accessible or highly reactive cysteines. Since σ^R analysis alone does not consider changes in protein abundance, we measured the change in protein abundance using a label-free method (Figure 1, Supplemental Table S1) and used this change to normalize the change in persulfidation. We found that the vast majority of proteins with σ^R values greater than or less than one standard deviation from the mean (σ^R = 0.52) were found in the "wings" of the normalized abundance plot, a finding consistent with an identical analysis in *A. baumannii* (Supplemental Figure S1B) [13]. A better way to express these data is to compare the change in the persulfidation status of a particular peptide to its change in abundance in a log–log plot (Figure 2) [30]. Here, we predicted that a persulfidated peptide with a significant increase in persulfidation status coupled with relatively small change in protein abundance may be strong candidate regulatory protein targets (Figure 2).

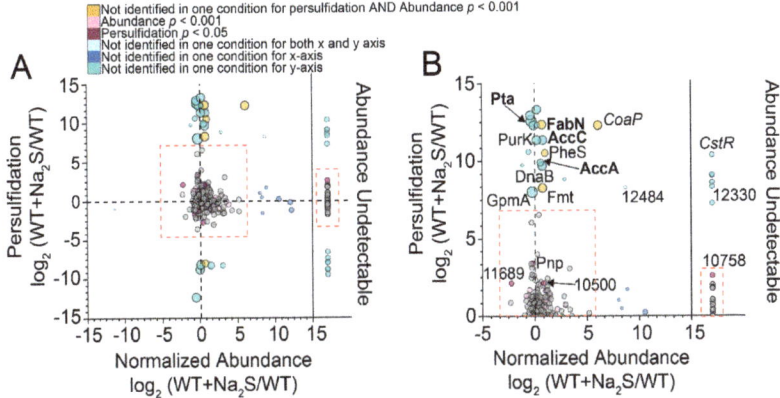

Figure 2. Changes in protein persulfidation relative to changes in protein abundance in *E. faecalis*

before and after the addition of exogenous sulfide. (**A**) Log–log plot of the change in protein persulfidation (WT + Na$_2$S/WT) vs. change in protein abundance (WT + Na$_2$S/WT). Each circle represents a single protein identified as persulfidated, colored according to the significance threshold in the legend. The red dashed boxes include proteins whose persulfidation status and/or normalized abundance was detectable in both WT and WT + Na$_2$S samples. Proteins outside these boxes were not detectable in one or more conditions and utilized a peak area one order of magnitude lower than the lowest detectable protein to calculate persulfidation or abundance changes. (**B**) Expanded view of proteins of which their persulfidation status increased after the addition of exogenous sulfide, with select proteins annotated with the protein name or locus tag (OG1RF_xxxxx).

An evaluation of protein thiols for which we have total persulfidation and abundance data, i.e., detectable and persulfidated in both conditions, revealed that a majority did not have a statistically significant change in persulfidation status or fractional abundance. This supports the idea that the proteome functions as a sink for sulfane sulfur that is not greatly impacted by the addition of a high dose of exogenous Na$_2$S to cells [7,13]. Those proteins that are more likely to represent regulatory targets via persulfidation are those that are only identified as persulfidated under conditions of Na$_2$S treatment, the majority of which may exhibit only small statistically significant changes in cell abundance (Figure 2B). A striking exception to this was CoAPR, which exhibited a large increase in protein abundance after the addition of Na$_2$S due to the transcriptional derepression by CstR [12] with only the cysteine derived from the C-terminal rhodanese domain (C508) identified as persulfidated in Na$_2$S-treated cells (Supplemental Table S2).

Other persulfidated proteins of note in this analysis included phosphotransacetylase (Pta), which catalyzed the reversible interconversion of acetyl-CoA and acetyl phosphate, and cysteines in enzymes involved in type II fatty acid biosynthesis (FAS), including AccA, AccC and FabN (Figure 2B; Supplemental Figure S3) [61,62]. AccA and AccC are part of a four-enzyme acetyl-CoA carboxylase (ACCase) complex, which defines the initial and committed step of FAS, carboxylating acetyl-CoA to make malonyl-CoA prior to linkage to the acyl-carrier protein (ACP) [62,63]. FabN is a bifunctional enzyme, possessing both 3-hydroxydecanoyl-ACP dehydratase activity, to create *trans*-2-decanoyl-ACP, and isomerase activity, converting *trans*-2-decenoyl-ACP to *cis*-3-decanoyl-ACP [64]. FabN is functionally analogous to, although structurally distinct from, FabA in *E. coli*, which defines a major point of regulation of the ratio of unsaturated to saturated fatty acids [61]. As such, *Ef* mutants lacking FabN exhibited unsaturated fatty acid auxotrophy, which could be partly rescued by supplementation by oleic acid (18:1) [65], revealing that *Ef* FabN is critically important in the biosynthesis of longer chain, unsaturated fatty acids [64]. Additionally, two other enzymes involved in FAS, including AccB (C119) of the ACCase complex and the primary β-ketoacyl-ACP synthase II, FabF (C262), were also persulfidated (Supplemental Figure S3, Supplemental Table S2). If persulfidation is regulatory for any of these enzymes, sulfide stress may impact the cellular concentrations of acyl-CoA species or the cellular composition of membrane-derived fatty acids.

3.3. Exogenous Na$_2$S Impacts Cellular Composition of Fatty Acids

To investigate the impact of exogenous sulfide on fatty acids and fatty acid biosynthesis, we extracted fatty acids from bacterial cultures before and after addition of Na$_2$S and quantified them as methyl esters by GC-MS [66]. This analysis revealed that 14:0, 16:0, 18:0 and 18:1 fatty acids dominated the profile, with a statistically significant increase in the relative abundance of 14:0 and 16:0 fatty acids following the addition of Na$_2$S (Figure 3A). We noted a corresponding decrease in the major unsaturated fatty acid species, 18:1 (*cis* and *trans* isomers were not resolved here), with little change in 16:1 species, and an accompanying decrease in the relative abundance of shorter chain saturated fatty acids ($\leq$12:0), the latter of which was anticipated as a result of their elongation to longer chain saturated fatty acids (Figure 3A,B). In addition, the ratio of total saturated to unsaturated fatty acids increased over time in cells treated with exogenous sulfide relative to untreated WT cells (Figure 3C). When we compared the relative abundance of each fatty acid between WT and

WT + Na$_2$S, we found that shorter chain fatty acids up to 14:0 followed the same trend, while longer fatty acids (>14:0) showed significant differences between the two conditions (Supplemental Figure S4). Together, these changes contribute to the observed difference in the ratio of total saturated to unsaturated fatty acids.

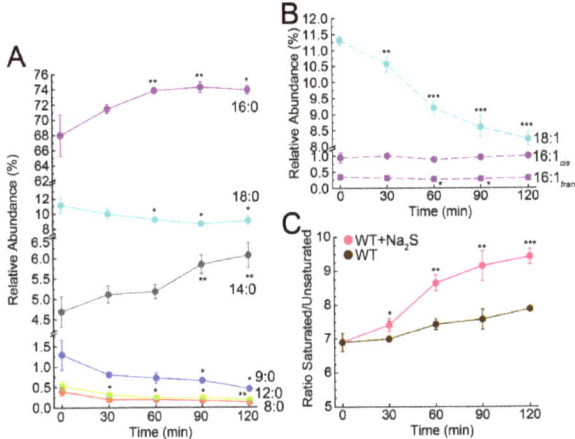

Figure 3. Fatty acid profiling in WT *E. faecalis*. Changes in the relative abundance for (**A**) saturated and (**B**) unsaturated fatty acids after the addition of exogenous Na$_2$S to cell cultures. (**C**) The ratio of total saturated to unsaturated fatty acids for Na$_2$S treated cells vs. untreated wild-type cells. Values represent the means ± S.D. derived from the results of biological triplicate experiments, with statistical significance established using a paired t-test relative to the endogenous, time 0 (*** $p \leq 0.001$, ** $p \leq 0.01$, * $p \leq 0.05$).

3.4. Exogenous Na$_2$S Impacts Acetyl-CoA via Enzyme Inhibition of Phosphotransacetylase (Pta) by CoASSH

Our fatty acid profiling results revealed a significant impact on the relative abundance of saturated vs. unsaturated fatty acids, consistent with regulatory inhibition of FabN activity (Figure 3 and Supplemental Figure S4). Persulfidation of three of the four subunits of ACCase motivated us to investigate a potential impact on acyl-CoA species under these conditions, since in *E. faecalis*, acetyl-CoA and malonyl-CoA are the predominant acyl-CoA species that are required for FAS (Supplemental Figure S3). Malonyl-CoA was found to be below our level of detection in both untreated and Na$_2$S-treated cells. In striking contrast, acetyl-CoA exhibited a nearly 20-fold increase 60 min post-addition of exogenous Na$_2$S (Figure 4A) in wild-type cells. This accumulation of acetyl-CoA was ≈12-fold higher than that quantitated from control WT cells grown for 60 min without addition of Na$_2$S (Figure 4A). This increase in acetyl-CoA may have originated from increased activity of acetyl-CoA producing enzymes, e.g., pyruvate dehydrogenase (PDH), acetate kinase (AckA) and Pta (Figure 4B), or decreased activity of the acetyl-CoA carboxylase (ACCase) complex [61,62].

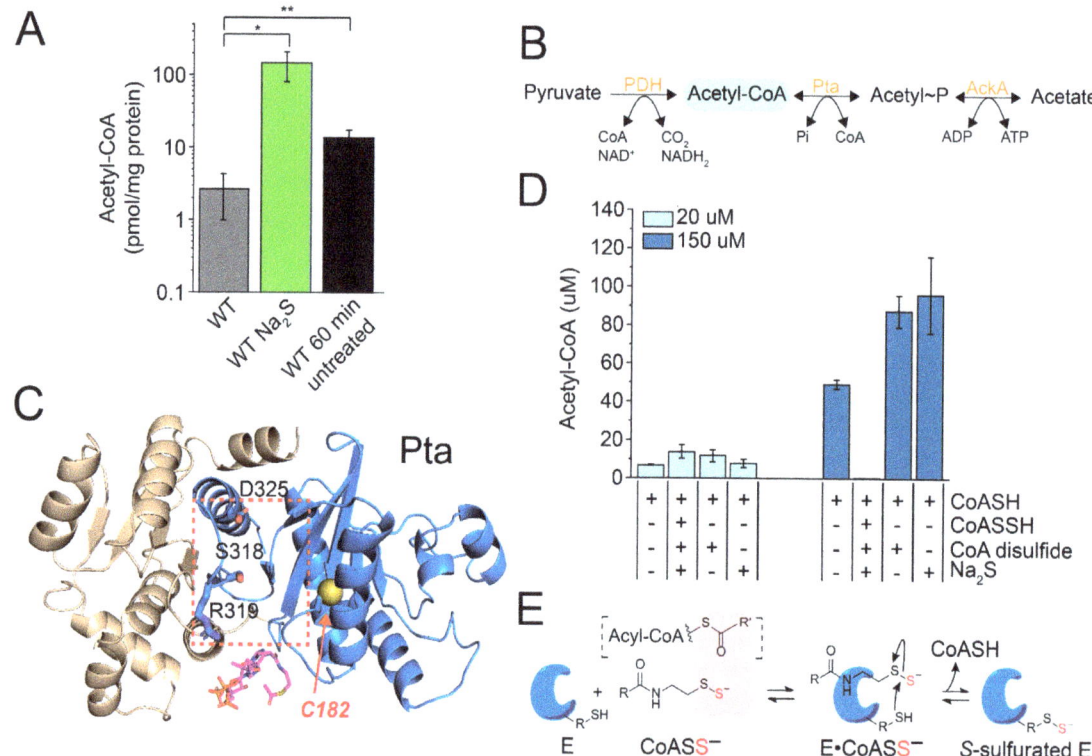

Figure 4. Acetyl-CoA accumulation via enzyme inhibition by CoASSH. (**A**) Quantitation of acetyl-CoA in WT cells treated with or without exogenous Na_2S. Values represent the means ± S.D. derived from results of $n = 5$ replicates, with statistical significance established using a paired t-test to wild-type untreated cells (** $p \leq 0.01$, * $p \leq 0.05$). (**B**) Metabolic pathways for the biosynthesis of acetyl-CoA in *E. faecalis*. (**C**) Ribbon representation of an AlphaFold2 [67,68] model of *Ef*Pta. The cleft between domain I (wheat) and domain II (blue) defines the active site (red box), where R319 provided electrostatic stabilization to the nucleotide end of bound CoASH (*magenta*, from PDB 6IOX), S318 hydrogen-bonds to the terminal thiol and D325 is the catalytic base [69]. C182, with the sulfur atom shown as a yellow sphere, is extensively persulfidated in cells. (**D**) Impact of CoASSH on the yield of acetyl-CoA by *Ef*Pta. (**E**) Protein *S*-sulfuration via CoASSH poisoning. Binding of CoASSH to an acyl-CoA or CoA-utilizing enzyme, E, which has a nearby Cys that participates in persulfide transfer from CoASSH results in the release of the free thiol and a *S*-sulfurated enzyme.

We chose *E. faecalis* Pta to investigate the extent to which the observed accumulation of acetyl-CoA could be traced to the combined activities of AckA and Pta, since Pta was identified as extensively persulfidated only under conditions of exogenous Na_2S treatment (Figure 2). The site of persulfidation in this enzyme, C182, is located on a loop in the CoA/acetyl-CoA binding pocket, as defined by a *Methanosarcina thermophila* Pta-CoA co-crystal structure [69]. Persulfidation at this location could have a regulatory impact on enzyme activity (Figure 4C). We purified *E. faecalis* Pta and characterized both the forward (acetyl-phosphate-forming) and reverse (acetyl-CoA-forming) reactions, which collectively showed that recombinant *Ef*Pta is a functional enzyme, with kinetic parameters comparable to those reported for other Pta enzymes in the literature (Supplemental Figure S5) [33,70,71].

We next investigated the extent to which *in situ*-prepared CoASSH could function as an inhibitor of Pta activity. The yield of acetyl-CoA was measured by HPLC from reactions containing Pta; acetyl-phosphate and either its natural substrate, CoASH, or a

CoASSH-containing mixture [12], which included equimolar CoASH and excess Na$_2$S and CoA disulfide. Control reactions were also performed, which included CoASH and either Na$_2$S or CoA disulfide at concentrations equivalent to those present in the in situ CoASSH mixture. At low concentrations of substrate (CoASH; 20 µM), the yield of acetyl-CoA was similar among reactions containing only CoA and CoASSH and in control reactions (Figure 4D). At high concentrations of the substrate (150 µM, above the K_m; see Supplemental Figure S5B), however, there was little detectable production of acetyl-CoA in the presence of the CoASSH mixture. This inhibition of activity was due to CoASSH specifically, since there was no negative impact on product formation from the control reactions containing excess Na$_2$S and CoA disulfide (Figure 4D). We did not investigate if Pta was persulfidated by CoASSH under these conditions, but it proved difficult to persulfidate Pta with various other sulfur donors, e.g., inorganic polysulfide, in vitro using standard methods (data not shown) [7]. These findings with Pta are consistent with a CoASSH "poisoning" model proposed previously (Figure 4E), where CoASSH functions as substrate mimic that forms long-lived complexes with CoA- and short-chain acyl-CoA-requiring enzymes [29,72]. If a nearby thiol is present, this may result in persulfide transfer and subsequent inhibition of enzyme activity.

3.5. Crystallographic Structure of Ligand-Bound EfCoAPR

In order to better understand the molecular basis of cellular resistance to CoASSH poisoning described above and likely mediated by CoAPR in *E. faecalis* (Figure 5A) [12], we determined the crystallographic structure of the enzyme as isolated from *E. coli* to a 2.05 Å resolution by molecular replacement using *Ba*CoADR-RHD [42] as the search model (Figure 5B; see Supplemental Table S3 for structure statistics). The asymmetric unit is composed of two molecules of *Ef*CoAPR in a tightly packed dimeric arrangement, consistent with a homodimer assembly state [42] and containing two FAD molecules and two molecules of 3′-phosphate-adenosine-5′-diphosphate (PAP) (Figure 5C), with the latter found in a region where CoA is expected to bind [42] (Supplemental Figure S6A). While inspection of the electron density revealed that the PAP moiety of CoA was well-ordered, the remainder of the CoA molecule could not be placed in our structure, which suggests considerable flexibility in the pantothenate portion of the ligand [42] (see below). The modelled PAP moiety was ~13.3 Å away from FAD riboflavin moiety, which was fully modelled and refined.

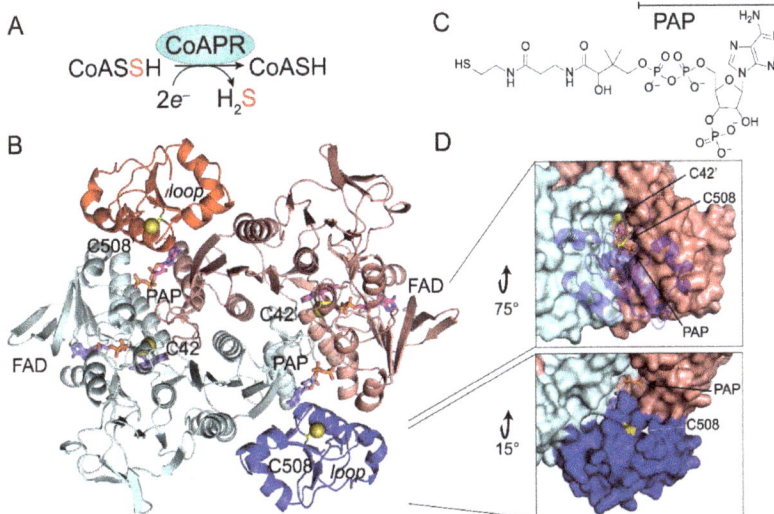

Figure 5. X-ray crystallographic analysis of *E. faecalis* CoAPR. (**A**) Reaction catalyzed by CoAPR; FAD

and pyridine nucleotide cofactors are not shown. (**B**) Ribbon diagram of the CoAPR homodimer, with one subunit shaded light blue (CDR domain)/blue (sulfurtransferase domain) and the other subunit shaded salmon (CDR domain)/red (sulfurtransferase domain). FAD, PAP and the two catalytically required Cys residues (C42, C508) are shown in stick. Loop, residues E474-Q479. (**C**) Chemical structure of coenzyme A with the PAP subdomain indicated. (**D**) Two views of the surface representation of the CoAPR dimer, illustrating the surface accessibility of the C508 thiol from the diphosphate moiety of PAP (lower panel) and looking through the cartoon representation of the sulfurtransferase domain to see the tunnel that extends along the protomer interface from the PAP to C42 and the flavin.

Each subunit is composed of two functional domains (Figure 5B). The N-terminal CoA disulfide reductase (CDR) domain consists of residues 1–446 and harbors the first catalytically active thiol, C42, while the C-terminal sulfurtransferase (rhodanese) domain is composed of residues 447–544 and contains the second catalytically required cysteine, C508 [12], which is persulfidated in cells (Figure 2). The dimer interface is extensive (3600 Å^2) and is largely stabilized by hydrophilic residues, contributed primarily by the CDR domains, with the FAD bound such that its ATP portion is close to the "bottom" of each protomer, with the isoalloxazine ring in van der Waals contact with the S$^\gamma$ of C42. The two sulfurtransferase domains of CoAPR are on the periphery of the dimer, effectively wedged between the two reductase domains. The 3′-phosphoadenosyl moiety of the PAP portion of the bound CoA forms an extensive part of this interface, deeply buried in the sulfurtransferase domain 10.7 Å from C508, wedged between the α1 helix of the opposite protomer, the terminal helix of the reductase domain of the same protomer and the core helix of the rhodanese domain (residues 512–525), which is immediately C-terminal to C508 (Figure 5B). C42 and C508′ make their closest approach from opposite protomers, but they are 26.6 Å apart.

The *Ef*CoAPR structure is similar to other FAD-dependent pyridine nucleotide-disulfide oxidoreductases, including those classified as CDRs, NADH (per)oxidases, NAD-dependent persulfide reductases (Npsr) [73,74] and *Bacillus anthracis* CoADR-RHD (*Ba*CoADR-RHD, 3ICS) [42]. In striking contrast to *Ef*CoAPR, the entire CoA molecule is visible in these three structures, with the CoA sulfur atom in close proximity to the flavin isoalloxazine ring of the opposite protomer [42,74,75]. The high structural similarity between *Ef*CoAPR and *Ba*CoADR-RHD models revealed nearly perfect superposition of the PAP moiety of CoA and FAD cofactors (Supplemental Figure S6A). The main structural differences between these models are found in two loop regions, in particular, the E474-Q479 loop in the rhodanese domain, which is disordered in *Ef*CoAPR but α-helical in *Ba*CDR-RHD (Figure 5B). This 474-Q479 loop appears to form a physical barrier that may gate direct access of C508 to the active site cavity. A tunnel ≈25 Å in length connects the aperture of the solvent-exposed catalytic C508 and the CoA cavity located in the rhodanese domain to the C42 and FAD binding groove, located in the CDR domain of the opposite protomer (Figure 5D and Supplemental Figure S6B). This tunnel may well be an essential feature of turnover, as it connects the FAD and CoA binding pockets to the solvent (see below).

3.6. Molecular Dynamics Simulations

To obtain additional insights into the dynamics of this complex [42], we carried out molecular dynamics simulations of our FAD- and CoASH-bound structure after building the remainder of CoASH into this model (Figure 6A). Two replica simulations of 1.4 μs each were performed, and in both runs, the pantothenate moiety of the CoA molecule corresponding to the same binding site (protomer B) left the vicinity of C42 (Figure 6A) and moved towards C508′ in the rhodanese domain of the other protomer (Figure 6B; Supplemental Video S1). In striking contrast, the pantothenate arm of the CoA bound to the adjacent protomer (protomer A) remained close to C42, routinely reaching distances below ≈3.5 Å (Supplementary Figure S7A). This suggests that each subunit might stabilize the CoA molecule in either an "extended" (Figure 6A) or "bent" (Figure 6B) conformation, a finding that might imply an "alternating active sites" model of catalysis, in which one subunit turns over while the other rests. The per-residue root mean-square fluctuation (RMSF) calculated over these simulations showed that the rhodanese domain presents distinct fluctuations between protomers (Supplemental Figure S7C), consistent with a concerted movement that may link CoASSH formation, folding of the E474-Q479 loop and significant dynamics associated with the rhodanese region (Supplemental Figure S7C). The relative position PAP moiety from CoA is stable along the MD trajectory, and only the pantothenate arm changes its position (Figure 6A,B and Supplemental Figure S8); furthermore, we found that the "arm" makes two slightly different approaches to C508 on opposite sides of the R513 side chain, with a minimum S-S distance of ≈6.5 Å (Figure 6C,D). The persulfidation of C508 may then bring these two reactive groups in sufficiently close proximity to perform the persulfide transfer.

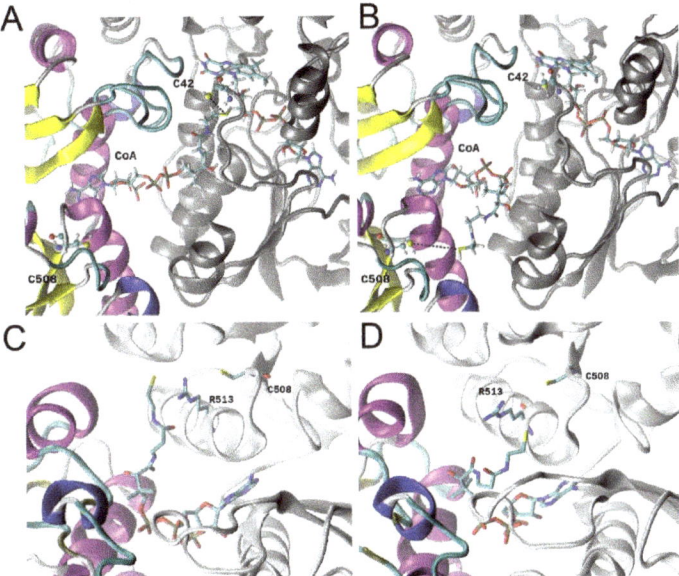

Figure 6. Representative snapshots of stable conformations of CoA relative to C508, obtained from 1.4 μs MD simulations. (**A**) Starting "extended" CoA conformation, protomer B; (**B**) representative "bent" CoA conformation, protomer B. The dimer backbone is depicted in the ribbon, with the CDR domain of one protomer colored based on a secondary structure and the rhodanese domain from the adjacent subunit shaded silver. All residues are depicted with sticks. The position of the pantothenate arm is slightly different in replica 1 (**C**) vs. replica 2 (**D**). approaching C508 from opposite sides of the R513 side chain (shown in sphere and stick).

These MD simulations provide significant support for the "swinging pantothenate arm" hypothesis [57], where the tightly bound CoA attacks a persulfide on C508, bringing CoASSH back to the reductase active site; the CoASSH is then attacked by the C42 with the release of the H_2S and formation of mixed disulfide, which is subsequently reduced by the flavin, which itself is reduced by a more weakly bound NAD(P)H [74]. Significant levels of C508 persulfidation in cells on par with those of candidate persulfidation targets Pta and FabN (Figure 2), coupled with no observable C42 persulfidation, are fully consistent with this mechanistic model. Whether or not the CoASH product is released was unclear from our structure and simulations. Given the extensive contacts in what might be a "closed" conformation (Figure 5B,D), the release of CoASH would seem to require access to a transiently "open" form that would disrupt the extensive interdomain interface into which PAP is wedged (Figure 5D). If CoASH is not released with each turnover, this would require high specificity in the initial persulfide transfer from CoASSH to the C-terminal sulfurtransferase domain; indeed, this domain possesses weak thiosulfate sulfurtransferase activity, suggesting that some other thiol persulfide, e.g., CoASSH, might be a better substrate for this persulfide transferase activity [12].

4. Discussion

The gastrointestinal tract is host to hundreds of microorganisms that have developed a symbiotic relationship with host epithelial cells in this niche based, in part, on the reduction of sulfur-containing molecules, e.g., sulfate, thiosulfate and tetrathionate, and the oxidation of H_2S. Perturbation of this symbiotic relationship results in gastrointestinal disease [20–22] due to increased H_2S or other sulfur species, e.g., tetrathionate, which provide a growth advantage to some pathogens in this niche [76]. *E. faecalis* encodes a CydAB, the alternate oxidase that is far less susceptible to H_2S-mediated inhibition [77–79], which may allow this organism to respire under normal and infection-relevant H_2S concentrations in the gut; indeed, the cell abundance of CydD, an assembly factor for CydAB biogenesis, increases under these conditions (Supplemental Table S1). In addition, *E. faecalis* CstR, which regulates the *cst*-like operon, may provide a growth advantage in this niche by lowering ambient persulfidation [28], but this is currently unknown. Here, we employed exogenous sulfide to investigate the proteomic response of *E. faecalis* to sulfide mis-regulation and profile protein persulfidation to determine potential targets of H_2S/RSS modification in this organism.

Our proteomic analysis revealed that ≈5% of the proteome that was detected under our conditions exhibited a significant change in normalized fractional abundance in response to exogenous sulfide. In fact, the *cst*-like operon-encoded protein CoAPR [12] was detectable in a soluble lysate in WT untreated cells, which may explain the significantly low endogenous concentrations of CoASSH compared to other low-molecular-weight persulfides (Figure 1). CoAPR then became one of the top 20% most abundant proteins detectable post-addition of Na_2S. This strongly suggests that *E. faecalis* protects the integrity of the CoA pool by preventing over-persulfidation of this important metabolite, with CoAPR being a significant component of this adaptive response. Consistent with this idea, we observed a significant increase in the cell abundance of DPCK, which is required for the biosynthesis of CoA, and two uncharacterized thioesterases, which may be deployed to hydrolyze an acyl-CoA substrate(s) to release CoA to meet cellular needs under these conditions (Figure 1B).

We found that ~13% of the proteome in *E. faecalis* harbored persulfidated cysteines, and the extent to which persulfidation changed relative to protein abundance was significant for only a handful of proteins (Figure 2). Proteins for which persulfidation status changed significantly relative to changes in protein abundance included CoAPR and its transcriptional regulator, CstR, as anticipated [12]. CstR is a di-thiol-containing transcriptional repressor, and our persulfidation profiling revealed that both cysteines, C31 and C62, in *E. faecalis* CstR were persulfidated in the cell, consistent with the capture of either a reaction intermediate or the product of the reaction of H_2S on a trisulfide bridge (C31-S-S-S-C62′), resulting in a persulfide adduct on each Cys residue [28]. Of the two cysteines in CoAPR, only the C-terminal rhodanese domain cysteine (C508) was persulfidated in vivo, consistent with a role in persulfide transfer in a "swinging pantothenate arm" reaction mechanism proposed by others [42,75] and for which we provided significant support from MD simulations (Figure 6). Indeed, the two active sites in CoAPR were separated by ≈27 Å across protomers (Figure 5B), and both are required by turnover and full product formation [12]; since the two active sites are spanned end-to-end by the CoA molecule, this solves the problem of getting these two active sites close enough to perform direct persulfide shuttling to create the anticipated mixed disulfide with C42 close to the flavin [12] (Figures 5 and 6). Additional work will be required to understand the specificity of persulfidation of C508, CoA product release (if any), the metabolic fate of the so-generated H_2S and the extent to which the rhodanese domains pack against the reductase dimer core in the absence of CoA, i.e., adopts an "open" conformation.

Several enzymes involved in the biosynthesis of fatty acids and acyl-CoA species exhibit significant changes in the abundance-normalized persulfidation status, including AccA, AccC, FabN and Pta (Figure 2). Persulfidation of these proteins may function as a regulatory switch via modification of a cysteine thiol, which impacts enzyme structure or turnover. Indeed, fatty acid profiling revealed significant changes in the relative abundance of fatty acids in response to exogenous sulfide, both in length and degree of saturation (Figure 3 and Supplemental Figure S4). These differences were largely derived from a significant increase in the most abundant fatty acid, 16:0, and a decrease in one longer (18:0) and three unsaturated (16:1$_{cis}$, 16:1$_{trans}$ and 18:1) fatty acids. Since the primary role of fatty acids is to form the phospholipid bilayer, these changes could induce significant alterations in the composition and physical properties of the cell membrane [80–82]. These changes in lipid composition may well be due to a negative regulatory effect of persulfidation of C21 in FabN, the deletion of which is known to impact the biosynthesis of unsaturated fatty acids [65]. Although there is no structure of *Ef* FabN, an AlphaFold2 model [67,68] revealed a "hot-dog" fold reminiscent of FabZ hexamers from *H. pylori* [83] and *P. aeruginosa* [84] and revealed that C21 is located in the α1-β loop, which is highly conserved in FabZs, close to the hot-dog (α3) helix, near the active site glutamate residue and the trimer interface, in this trimer of dimers architecture (Supplemental Figure S9A) [85]. Small displacements of the the α3 helix are known to impact enzyme specificity [85]; alternatively, persulfidation of C21 may lead to disassembly of the FabN hexamer to dimers and/or influence the way in which holo-ACP engages the hexamer [86].

The high levels of persulfidation of C50 in the biotin carboxylase (BC; AccC) subunit, which is conserved in the *E. coli* enzyme, may also be functionally important, since C50 forms a hydrogen bond at the interface with the biotin carboxylase carrier protein (BCCP; AccB) subunit of the heterooctameric *E. coli* BC$_4$•BCCP$_4$ biotin carboxylase complex [87,88]. Persulfidation, here, may destabilize the quaternary structure of the BC complex, thus inhibiting ACCase activity at this committed step of FAS. In addition, the AccA and AccD subunits form a heterotetrameric α$_2$β$_2$ carboxyltransferase enzyme [89], and C114, which is highly persulfidated in H$_2$S-treated cells, is located in the acetyl-CoA binding cleft, very close to the thiol/thioester end of the bound substrate (Supplemental Figure S9B). The extent to which these modifications are regulatory in vitro is not yet known, but the accumulation of cellular acetyl-CoA (Figure 4) and high cellular abundance of downstream FabH, which supplies acetoacetyl-CoA in the initiation of FAS (Supplemental Figure S3), may be reporting on reduced flux at early stages of FAS in Na$_2$S-stressed cells.

Membrane composition is known to impact antimicrobial activity [90] in bacteria, and in *E. faecalis*, the incorporation of exogenous fatty acids has been shown to provide protection from membrane damaging agents, including antibiotics [66,91]. The loss of FabN specifically leads to a relative increase in saturated fatty acids incorporated into phospholipids [65]. This is known to decrease membrane fluidity and results in an increase in the resistance to antibiotics including daptomycin [92]. In addition, FabN mutants also appear to elicit a decreased inflammatory response during infections, and these features may be broadly immunoprotective [65]. Protein lipidation, primarily palmitoylation, requires palmitic acid (16:0). Although its role in bacteria is not fully understood, some studies have suggested that bacterial palmitoylation is associated with infections, activates toxins and "hijacks" host enzymes to modify their proteins [93–96]. These data suggest that *E. faecalis* may be capable of leveraging infection-relevant H$_2$S/RSS to remodel the membrane in a way that is broadly protective against host stressors.

Finally, our finding of a significant accumulation of the major acyl-CoA species in *E. faecalis*, acetyl-CoA (Figure 4A), beyond FAS, may suggest that other enzymes that utilize or produce acetyl-CoA may well be subject to inhibition by CoASSH. Here, we demonstrated that CoASSH inhibits the acetyl-CoA-forming reaction by *E. faecalis* Pta, which suggests that the reverse reaction (acetyl-CoA utilizing) would also be inhibited (Figure 4D). These data with Pta, coupled with an analysis of AccAD carboxytransferase, are consistent with the hypothesis that CoASSH effectively poisons CoA- or acyl-CoA-requiring enzymes by binding as a substrate or product mimic, like that previously reported for human butyryl-CoA dehydrogenase [29]. CoASSH poisoning may result in persulfidation of a thiol in or near the active site, supported by the identification of several CoA and acyl-CoA requiring enzymes as extensively persulfidated in cells (Figure 4E), including Pta and AccAD (Supplemental Figure S9). This model requires that a cysteine residue be proximate to the persulfide "end" of a bound CoASSH and participate in sulfur transfer from CoASSH to generate CoA and a persulfidated enzyme. Although more support for this model is required, we suggest that an important metabolic impact in *E. faecalis* in response to exogenous sulfide is that of over-persulfidation of the CoA pool. In *E. faecalis*, CstR-regulated CoAPR (Figure 5) likely functions to maintain the integrity of the CoA pool, while in *S. aureus*, CstR-regulated enzymes collaborate in some way to minimize endogenous CoASSH to a level less than 1–2% of the total pool, depending on sulfur source. While, at first glance, this may seem like a modest impact (in *E. faecalis*, ambient levels of CoASSH are $\leq$10% that of *S. aureus*, at $\leq$0.1%) [12], if much of the CoA is bound to enzymes in cells, this would place a highly reactive hydropersulfide group within or in close physical proximity to the active sites of CoA- and short-chain acyl-CoA-requiring enzymes. The extent to which CoASSH poisoning in *E. faecalis* and other bacteria is operative remains to be determined.

5. Conclusions

In this work, we leveraged a global map of proteome persulfidation in *E. faecalis* to identify and discuss strong candidate regulatory persulfidation sites in enzymes associated with acyl-transfer reactions and fatty acid biosynthesis. H$_2$S/RSS mis-regulation induced significant perturbations in the fatty acid composition of the cell membrane and an increase of cellular acetyl-CoA, both consistent with a CoASSH poisoning model of primary acyl-CoA-dependent processes. The enzyme responsible for clearing toxic CoASSH in *E. faecalis* is CoA persulfide reductase (CoAPR), the structure and molecular dynamics analysis of which revealed a catalytic mechanism that is consistent with its persulfidation status in cells.

Supplementary Materials: The following are available online at https://www.mdpi.com/article/10.3390/antiox11081607/s1. Table S1: Excel file that lists all E. faecalis proteins detected in the label-free proteomics experiments; Table S2: Excel file that identifies the cysteine residues of all persulfidated (S-sulfurated) proteins in the proteome of E. faecalis; Table S3: Data collection, processing, refinement statistics and model quality parameters for the EfCoAPR CoA-bound structure; Video S1: Representation of the replica 1 MD simulation; Figure S1: Mapping proteome persulfidation in E. faecalis before and after the addition of exogenous sodium sulfide; Figure S2: Sequence motif analysis of S-sulfurated peptides; Figure S3: Fatty acid biosynthesis in E. faecalis; Figure S4: Relative abundance of fatty acids before and after the addition of Na2S; Figure S5: Enzymatic activity of E. faecalis Pta; Figure S6: Active site view and superposition of CoADR-RHD from B. anthracis and E. faecalis CoAPR; Figure S7: Distance between the sulfhydryl group of CoA and each of the two cysteine residues C42 and C508' and a stability analysis of the EfCoAPR dimer during these MD simulations; Figure S8: Relative position of PAP and pantothenate moieties from CoA; Figure S9: Models of major persulfidation targets in E. faecalis under conditions of sulfide stress. References [30,35,42,67,68,97–99] are cited in the supplementary materials.

Author Contributions: Investigation, B.J.C.W., S.S.C., K.A.E. and F.M.I.; formal analysis, B.J.C.W., S.S.C., K.A.E., J.C.T., F.M.I., J.A.B. and D.P.G.; funding acquisition, D.P.G. and J.A.B.; supervision, D.P.G. and J.A.B.; writing–original draft, B.J.C.W.; writing–review and editing, D.P.G. and J.A.B. All authors have read and agreed to the published version of the manuscript.

Funding: This work was supported by the U.S. National Institutes of Health (R35 GM118157 to D.P.G.) and FCT-Fundação para a Ciência e a Tecnologia, I.P. (MOSTMICRO-ITQB R&D Unit-UIDB/04612/2020, UIDP/04612/2020 and LS4FUTURE Associated Laboratory-LA/P/0087/2020). B.J.C.W. gratefully acknowledges receipt of a predoctoral fellowship from the Graduate Training Program in Quantitative and Chemical Biology (T32 GM131944) and the Kratz Fellowship from the Indiana University Department of Chemistry. S.S.C. and J.A.B. gratefully acknowledge FCT-Fundação para a Ciência e a Tecnologia, I.P. by the research fellowship 008/BI/2022 and by the framework of Article 23 of Decree-Law No.57/2017 of August 29, respectively.

Institutional Review Board Statement: Not applicable.

Informed Consent Statement: Not applicable.

Data Availability Statement: Crystallographic data have been deposited in the Protein Data Bank (http://www.wwpdb.org/), with the atomic coordinates and structure factors, under accession code 8A56. Models are available in ModelArchive (http://modelarchive.org/) with the accession codes ma-4xl3y (Pta), ma-eknu4 (FabN) and ma-df7nk (AccAD)$_2$.

Conflicts of Interest: The authors declare no conflict of interest.

Abbreviations

RSS, reactive sulfur species; H_2S, hydrogen sulfide; CoA, coenzyme A; CoASSH, CoA persulfide; LMW, low-molecular-weight; FA, fatty acid.

References

1. Shatalin, K.; Shatalina, E.; Mironov, A.; Nudler, E. H_2S: A universal defense against antibiotics in bacteria. *Science* **2011**, *334*, 986–990. [CrossRef] [PubMed]
2. Toliver-Kinsky, T.; Cui, W.; Toro, G.; Lee, S.J.; Shatalin, K.; Nudler, E.; Szabo, C. H_2S, a Bacterial Defense Mechanism against the Host Immune Response. *Infect. Immun.* **2019**, *87*, e00272-18. [CrossRef] [PubMed]
3. Mironov, A.; Seregina, T.; Nagornykh, M.; Luhachack, L.G.; Korolkova, N.; Lopes, L.E.; Kotova, V.; Zavilgelsky, G.; Shakulov, R.; Shatalin, K.; et al. Mechanism of H_2S-mediated protection against oxidative stress in *Escherichia coli*. *Proc. Natl. Acad. Sci. USA* **2017**, *114*, 6022–6027. [CrossRef] [PubMed]
4. Luhachack, L.; Rasouly, A.; Shamovsky, I.; Nudler, E. Transcription factor YcjW controls the emergency H_2S production in *E. coli*. *Nat. Commun.* **2019**, *10*, 2868. [CrossRef]
5. Saini, A.; Chinta, K.C.; Reddy, V.P.; Glasgow, J.N.; Stein, A.; Lamprecht, D.A.; Rahman, M.A.; Mackenzie, J.S.; Truebody, B.E.; Adamson, J.H.; et al. Hydrogen sulfide stimulates *Mycobacterium tuberculosis* respiration, growth and pathogenesis. *Nat. Commun.* **2020**, *11*, 557. [CrossRef]
6. Shukla, P.; Khodade, V.S.; SharathChandra, M.; Chauhan, S.; Mishra, S.; Siddaramappa, S.; Pradeep, B.E.; Singh, A.; Chakrapani, H. "On demand" redox buffering by H_2S contributes to antibiotic resistance revealed by a bacteria-specific H_2S donor. *Chem. Sci.* **2017**, *8*, 4967–4972. [CrossRef]
7. Peng, H.; Zhang, Y.; Palmer, L.D.; Kehl-Fie, T.E.; Skaar, E.P.; Trinidad, J.C.; Giedroc, D.P. Hydrogen Sulfide and Reactive Sulfur Species Impact Proteome S-Sulfhydration and Global Virulence Regulation in *Staphylococcus aureus*. *ACS Infect. Dis.* **2017**, *3*, 744–755. [CrossRef]
8. Ida, T.; Sawa, T.; Ihara, H.; Tsuchiya, Y.; Watanabe, Y.; Kumagai, Y.; Suematsu, M.; Motohashi, H.; Fujii, S.; Matsunaga, T.; et al. Reactive cysteine persulfides and S-polythiolation regulate oxidative stress and redox signaling. *Proc. Natl. Acad. Sci. USA* **2014**, *111*, 7606–7611. [CrossRef]
9. Cuevasanta, E.; Zeida, A.; Carballal, S.; Wedmann, R.; Morzan, U.N.; Trujillo, M.; Radi, R.; Estrin, D.A.; Filipovic, M.R.; Alvarez, B. Insights into the mechanism of the reaction between hydrogen sulfide and peroxynitrite. *Free Radic. Biol. Med.* **2015**, *80*, 93–100. [CrossRef]
10. Ono, K.; Kitamura, Y.; Zhang, T.; Tsutsuki, H.; Rahman, A.; Ihara, T.; Akaike, T.; Sawa, T. Cysteine Hydropersulfide Inactivates beta-Lactam Antibiotics with Formation of Ring-Opened Carbothioic S-Acids in Bacteria. *ACS Chem. Biol.* **2021**, *16*, 731–739. [CrossRef]
11. Everett, S.A.; Wardman, P. Perthiols as antioxidants: Radical-scavenging and prooxidative mechanisms. *Methods Enzymol.* **1995**, *251*, 55–69. [PubMed]
12. Shen, J.; Walsh, B.J.C.; Flores-Mireles, A.L.; Peng, H.; Zhang, Y.; Zhang, Y.; Trinidad, J.C.; Hultgren, S.J.; Giedroc, D.P. Hydrogen Sulfide Sensing through Reactive Sulfur Species (RSS) and Nitroxyl (HNO) in *Enterococcus faecalis*. *ACS Chem. Biol.* **2018**, *13*, 1610–1620. [CrossRef]
13. Walsh, B.J.C.; Wang, J.; Edmonds, K.A.; Palmer, L.D.; Zhang, Y.; Trinidad, J.C.; Skaar, E.P.; Giedroc, D.P. The Response of *Acinetobacter baumannii* to Hydrogen Sulfide Reveals Two Independent Persulfide-Sensing Systems and a Connection to Biofilm Regulation. *mBio* **2020**, *11*, e01254-20. [CrossRef]
14. Peng, H.; Shen, J.; Edmonds, K.A.; Luebke, J.L.; Hickey, A.K.; Palmer, L.D.; Chang, F.J.; Bruce, K.A.; Kehl-Fie, T.E.; Skaar, E.P.; et al. Sulfide homeostasis and nitroxyl intersect via formation of reactive sulfur species in *Staphylococcus aureus*. *mSphere* **2017**, *2*, e00082-17. [CrossRef] [PubMed]
15. Truong, D.H.; Eghbal, M.A.; Hindmarsh, W.; Roth, S.H.; O'Brien, P.J. Molecular mechanisms of hydrogen sulfide toxicity. *Drug Metab. Rev.* **2006**, *38*, 733–744. [CrossRef] [PubMed]

16. Peng, H.; Zhang, Y.; Trinidad, J.C.; Giedroc, D.P. Thioredoxin Profiling of Multiple Thioredoxin-Like Proteins in *Staphylococcus aureus*. *Front. Microbiol.* **2018**, *9*, 2385. [CrossRef]
17. Motta, J.P.; Flannigan, K.L.; Agbor, T.A.; Beatty, J.K.; Blackler, R.W.; Workentine, M.L.; Da Silva, G.J.; Wang, R.; Buret, A.G.; Wallace, J.L. Hydrogen sulfide protects from colitis and restores intestinal microbiota biofilm and mucus production. *Inflamm. Bowel Dis.* **2015**, *21*, 1006–1017. [CrossRef]
18. Wallace, J.L.; Motta, J.P.; Buret, A.G. Hydrogen sulfide: An agent of stability at the microbiome-mucosa interface. *Am. J. Physiol.-Gastrointest. Liver Physiol.* **2018**, *314*, G143–G149. [CrossRef]
19. Guo, C.; Liang, F.; Shah Masood, W.; Yan, X. Hydrogen sulfide protected gastric epithelial cell from ischemia/reperfusion injury by Keap1 S-sulfhydration, MAPK dependent anti-apoptosis and NF-kappaB dependent anti-inflammation pathway. *Eur. J. Pharmacol.* **2014**, *725*, 70–78. [CrossRef]
20. Pitcher, M.C.; Cummings, J.H. Hydrogen sulphide: A bacterial toxin in ulcerative colitis? *Gut* **1996**, *39*, 1–4. [CrossRef]
21. Attene-Ramos, M.S.; Wagner, E.D.; Plewa, M.J.; Gaskins, H.R. Evidence that hydrogen sulfide is a genotoxic agent. *Mol. Cancer Res.* **2006**, *4*, 9–14. [CrossRef] [PubMed]
22. Xu, G.Y.; Winston, J.H.; Shenoy, M.; Zhou, S.; Chen, J.D.; Pasricha, P.J. The endogenous hydrogen sulfide producing enzyme cystathionine-beta synthase contributes to visceral hypersensitivity in a rat model of irritable bowel syndrome. *Mol. Pain* **2009**, *5*, 44. [CrossRef] [PubMed]
23. Barton, L.L.; Ritz, N.L.; Fauque, G.D.; Lin, H.C. Sulfur Cycling and the Intestinal Microbiome. *Dig. Dis. Sci.* **2017**, *62*, 2241–2257. [CrossRef] [PubMed]
24. Stacy, A.; Andrade-Oliveira, V.; McCulloch, J.A.; Hild, B.; Oh, J.H.; Perez-Chaparro, P.J.; Sim, C.K.; Lim, A.I.; Link, V.M.; Enamorado, M.; et al. Infection trains the host for microbiota-enhanced resistance to pathogens. *Cell* **2021**, *184*, 615–627. [CrossRef] [PubMed]
25. Walsh, B.J.C.; Giedroc, D.P. H$_2$S and reactive sulfur signaling at the host-bacterial pathogen interface. *J. Biol. Chem.* **2020**, *295*, 13150–13168. [CrossRef]
26. Grossoehme, N.; Kehl-Fie, T.E.; Ma, Z.; Adams, K.W.; Cowart, D.M.; Scott, R.A.; Skaar, E.P.; Giedroc, D.P. Control of Copper Resistance and Inorganic Sulfur Metabolism by Paralogous Regulators in *Staphylococcus aureus*. *J. Biol. Chem.* **2011**, *286*, 13522–13531. [CrossRef]
27. Luebke, J.L.; Shen, J.; Bruce, K.E.; Kehl-Fie, T.E.; Peng, H.; Skaar, E.P.; Giedroc, D.P. The CsoR-like sulfurtransferase repressor (CstR) is a persulfide sensor in *Staphylococcus aureus*. *Mol. Microbiol.* **2014**, *94*, 1343–1360. [CrossRef]
28. Fakhoury, J.N.; Zhang, Y.; Edmonds, K.A.; Bringas, M.; Luebke, J.L.; Gonzalez-Gutierrez, G.; Capdevila, D.A.; Giedroc, D.P. Functional asymmetry and chemical reactivity of CsoR family persulfide sensors. *Nucleic. Acids Res.* **2021**, *49*, 12556–12576. [CrossRef]
29. Landry, A.P.; Moon, S.; Kim, H.; Yadav, P.K.; Guha, A.; Cho, U.S.; Banerjee, R. A Catalytic Trisulfide in Human Sulfide Quinone Oxidoreductase Catalyzes Coenzyme A Persulfide Synthesis and Inhibits Butyrate Oxidation. *Cell Chem. Biol.* **2019**, *26*, 1515–1525.e4. [CrossRef]
30. Walsh, B.J.C.; Giedroc, D.P. Proteomics Profiling of S-sulfurated Proteins in *Acinetobacter baumannii*. *Bio. Protoc.* **2021**, *11*, e4000. [CrossRef]
31. Smart, K.F.; Aggio, R.B.; Van Houtte, J.R.; Villas-Boas, S.G. Analytical platform for metabolome analysis of microbial cells using methyl chloroformate derivatization followed by gas chromatography-mass spectrometry. *Nat. Prot.* **2010**, *5*, 1709–1729. [CrossRef] [PubMed]
32. Neubauer, S.; Chu, D.B.; Marx, H.; Sauer, M.; Hann, S.; Koellensperger, G. LC-MS/MS-based analysis of coenzyme A and short-chain acyl-coenzyme A thioesters. *Anal. Bioanal. Chem.* **2015**, *407*, 6681–6688. [CrossRef] [PubMed]
33. Campos-Bermudez, V.A.; Bologna, F.P.; Andreo, C.S.; Drincovich, M.F. Functional dissection of Escherichia coli phosphotransacetylase structural domains and analysis of key compounds involved in activity regulation. *FEBS J.* **2010**, *277*, 1957–1966. [CrossRef] [PubMed]
34. Decker, K. Acetyl-Coenzyme A UV-Spectrophotometric Assay. In *Methods of Enzymatic Analysis (Second English Edition)*; Elsevier Inc.: Amsterdam, The Netherlands; Verlag Chemie GmbH: Weinheim, Germany, 1974; Volume 4, pp. 1988–2044.
35. O'Shea, J.P.; Chou, M.F.; Quader, S.A.; Ryan, J.K.; Church, G.M.; Schwartz, D. pLogo: A probabilistic approach to visualizing sequence motifs. *Nat. Methods* **2013**, *10*, 1211–1212. [CrossRef]
36. D'Arcy, A.; Villard, F.; Marsh, M. An automated microseed matrix-screening method for protein crystallization. *Acta Crystallogr. Sect. D Biol. Crystallogr.* **2007**, *63*, 550–554. [CrossRef]
37. Theveneau, P.; Baker, R.; Barrett, R.; Beteva, A.; Bowler, M.W.; Carpentier, P.; Caserotto, H.; de Sanctis, D.; Dobias, F.; Flot, D.; et al. The Upgrade Programme for the Structural Biology beam lines at the European Synchrotron Radiation Facility—High throughput sample evaluation and automation. *J. Phys. Conf. Ser.* **2013**, *425*, 012001. [CrossRef]
38. Vonrhein, C.; Flensburg, C.; Keller, P.; Sharff, A.; Smart, O.; Paciorek, W.; Womack, T.; Bricogne, G. Data processing and analysis with the autoPROC toolbox. *Acta Crystallogr. D Biol. Crystallogr.* **2011**, *67*, 293–302. [CrossRef]
39. Winn, M.D.; Ballard, C.C.; Cowtan, K.D.; Dodson, E.J.; Emsley, P.; Evans, P.R.; Keegan, R.M.; Krissinel, E.B.; Leslie, A.G.; McCoy, A.; et al. Overview of the CCP4 suite and current developments. *Acta Crystallogr. Sect. D Biol. Crystallogr.* **2011**, *67*, 235–242. [CrossRef]

40. Adams, P.D.; Afonine, P.V.; Bunkoczi, G.; Chen, V.B.; Davis, I.W.; Echols, N.; Headd, J.J.; Hung, L.W.; Kapral, G.J.; Grosse-Kunstleve, R.W.; et al. PHENIX: A comprehensive Python-based system for macromolecular structure solution. *Acta Crystallogr. Sect. D Biol. Crystallogr.* **2010**, *66*, 213–221. [CrossRef]
41. McCoy, A.J.; Grosse-Kunstleve, R.W.; Adams, P.D.; Winn, M.D.; Storoni, L.C.; Read, R.J. Phaser crystallographic software. *J. Appl. Crystallogr.* **2007**, *40*, 658–674. [CrossRef]
42. Wallen, J.R.; Mallett, T.C.; Boles, W.; Parsonage, D.; Furdui, C.M.; Karplus, P.A.; Claiborne, A. Crystal structure and catalytic properties of Bacillus anthracis CoADR-RHD: Implications for flavin-linked sulfur trafficking. *Biochemistry* **2009**, *48*, 9650–9667. [CrossRef] [PubMed]
43. Afonine, P.V.; Grosse-Kunstleve, R.W.; Echols, N.; Headd, J.J.; Moriarty, N.W.; Mustyakimov, M.; Terwilliger, T.C.; Urzhumtsev, A.; Zwart, P.H.; Adams, P.D. Towards automated crystallographic structure refinement with phenix.refine. *Acta Crystallogr. Sect. D Biol. Crystallogr.* **2012**, *68*, 352–367. [CrossRef] [PubMed]
44. Emsley, P.; Cowtan, K. Coot: Model-building tools for molecular graphics. *Acta Crystallogr. Sect. D Biol. Crystallogr.* **2004**, *60*, 2126–2132. [CrossRef] [PubMed]
45. Chen, V.B.; Arendall, W.B., 3rd; Headd, J.J.; Keedy, D.A.; Immormino, R.M.; Kapral, G.J.; Murray, L.W.; Richardson, J.S.; Richardson, D.C. MolProbity: All-atom structure validation for macromolecular crystallography. *Acta Crystallogr. Sect. D Biol. Crystallogr.* **2010**, *66*, 12–21. [CrossRef]
46. Abraham, M.J.; Murtola, T.; Schulz, R.; Pall, S.; Smith, J.C.; Hess, B.; Lindahl, E. GROMACS: High performance molecular simulations through multi-level parallelism from laptops to supercomputers. *SoftwareX* **2015**, *1–2*, 19–25. [CrossRef]
47. Webb, B.; Sali, A. Comparative Protein Structure Modeling Using MODELLER. *Curr. Protoc. Protein Sci.* **2016**, *86*, 2.9.1–2.9.37. [CrossRef]
48. Vanommeslaeghe, K.; Hatcher, E.; Acharya, C.; Kundu, S.; Zhong, S.; Shim, J.; Darian, E.; Guvench, O.; Lopes, P.; Vorobyov, I.; et al. CHARMM general force field: A force field for drug-like molecules compatible with the CHARMM all-atom additive biological force fields. *J. Comput. Chem.* **2010**, *31*, 671–690. [CrossRef]
49. Vanommeslaeghe, K.; Raman, E.P.; MacKerell, A.D., Jr. Automation of the CHARMM General Force Field (CGenFF) II: Assignment of bonded parameters and partial atomic charges. *J. Chem. Inf. Model.* **2012**, *52*, 3155–3168. [CrossRef]
50. Bayly, C.I.; Cieplak, P.; Cornell, W.; Kollman, P.A. A well-behaved electrostatic potential based method using charge restraints for deriving atomic charges: The RESP model. *J. Phys. Chem.* **1993**, *97*, 10269–10280. [CrossRef]
51. Berendsen, H.J.C.; Postma, J.P.M.; Van Gunsteren, W.F.; Dinola, A.; Haak, J.R. Molecular Dynamics with Coupling to an External Bath. *J. Chem. Phys.* **1984**, *81*, 3684–3690. [CrossRef]
52. Bussi, G.; Donadio, D.; Parrinello, M. Canonical Sampling through Velocity Rescaling. *J. Chem. Phys.* **2007**, *126*, 014101. [CrossRef] [PubMed]
53. Essmann, U.; Perera, L.; Berkowitz, M.L.; Darden, T.; Lee, H.; Pedersen, L.G. A Smooth Particle Mesh Ewald Method. *J. Chem. Phys.* **1995**, *103*, 8577–8593. [CrossRef]
54. Hess, B.; Bekker, H.; Berendsen, H.J.C.; Fraaije, J.G.E.M. LINCS: A Linear Constraint Solver for Molecular Simulations. *J. Comput. Chem.* **1997**, *18*, 1463–1472. [CrossRef]
55. Darden, T.; York, D.; Pedersen, L.G. Particle Mesh Ewald: An N·log(N) Method for Ewald Sums in Large Systems. *J. Chem. Phys.* **1993**, *98*, 10089–10092. [CrossRef]
56. Humphrey, W.; Dalke, A.; Schulten, K. VMD: Visual Molecular Dynamics. *J. Mol. Graph.* **1996**, *14*, 33–38, 27–38. [CrossRef]
57. Vesic, D.; Kristich, C.J. A Rex family transcriptional repressor influences H_2O_2 accumulation by *Enterococcus faecalis*. *J. Bacteriol.* **2013**, *195*, 1815–1824. [CrossRef]
58. Ma, P.; Yuille, H.M.; Blessie, V.; Gohring, N.; Igloi, Z.; Nishiguchi, K.; Nakayama, J.; Henderson, P.J.; Phillips-Jones, M.K. Expression, purification and activities of the entire family of intact membrane sensor kinases from *Enterococcus faecalis*. *Mol. Membr. Biol.* **2008**, *25*, 449–473. [CrossRef]
59. Cronan, J.E.; Zhao, X.; Jiang, Y. Function, attachment and synthesis of lipoic acid in Escherichia coli. *Adv. Microb. Physiol.* **2005**, *50*, 103–146.
60. Yang, J.; Carroll, K.S.; Liebler, D.C. The Expanding Landscape of the Thiol Redox Proteome. *Mol. Cell. Proteom.* **2016**, *15*, 1–11. [CrossRef]
61. Zhang, Y.M.; Rock, C.O. Membrane lipid homeostasis in bacteria. *Nat. Rev. Microbiol.* **2008**, *6*, 222–233. [CrossRef]
62. Beld, J.; Lee, D.J.; Burkart, M.D. Fatty acid biosynthesis revisited: Structure elucidation and metabolic engineering. *Mol. Biosyst.* **2015**, *11*, 38–59. [CrossRef] [PubMed]
63. Cronan, J.E., Jr.; Waldrop, G.L. Multi-subunit acetyl-CoA carboxylases. *Prog. Lipid Res.* **2002**, *41*, 407–435. [CrossRef]
64. Wang, H.; Cronan, J.E. Functional replacement of the FabA and FabB proteins of *Escherichia coli* fatty acid synthesis by *Enterococcus faecalis* FabZ and FabF homologues. *J. Biol. Chem.* **2004**, *279*, 34489–34495. [CrossRef] [PubMed]
65. Diederich, A.K.; Duda, K.A.; Romero-Saavedra, F.; Engel, R.; Holst, O.; Huebner, J. Deletion of *fabN* in *Enterococcus faecalis* results in unsaturated fatty acid auxotrophy and decreased release of inflammatory cytokines. *Innate Immun.* **2016**, *22*, 284–293. [CrossRef]
66. Saito, H.E.; Harp, J.R.; Fozo, E.M. Incorporation of exogenous fatty acids protects *Enterococcus faecalis* from membrane-damaging agents. *Appl. Environ. Microbiol.* **2014**, *80*, 6527–6538. [CrossRef]

67. Jumper, J.; Evans, R.; Pritzel, A.; Green, T.; Figurnov, M.; Ronneberger, O.; Tunyasuvunakool, K.; Bates, R.; Zidek, A.; Potapenko, A.; et al. Highly accurate protein structure prediction with AlphaFold. *Nature* **2021**, *596*, 583–589. [CrossRef]
68. Mirdita, M.; Ovchinnikov, S.; Steinegger, M. ColabFold—Making protein folding accessible to all. *bioRxiv* **2021**. [CrossRef]
69. Lawrence, S.H.; Luther, K.B.; Schindelin, H.; Ferry, J.G. Structural and functional studies suggest a catalytic mechanism for the phosphotransacetylase from *Methanosarcina thermophila*. *J. Bacteriol.* **2006**, *188*, 1143–1154. [CrossRef]
70. Brinsmade, S.R.; Escalante-Semerena, J.C. In vivo and in vitro analyses of single-amino acid variants of the *Salmonella enterica* phosphotransacetylase enzyme provide insights into the function of its N-terminal domain. *J. Biol. Chem.* **2007**, *282*, 12629–12640. [CrossRef]
71. Xu, Q.S.; Jancarik, J.; Lou, Y.; Kuznetsova, K.; Yakunin, A.F.; Yokota, H.; Adams, P.; Kim, R.; Kim, S.H. Crystal structures of a phosphotransacetylase from *Bacillus subtilis* and its complex with acetyl phosphate. *J. Struct. Funct. Genom.* **2005**, *6*, 269–279. [CrossRef]
72. Williamson, G.; Engel, P.C.; Mizzer, J.P.; Thorpe, C.; Massey, V. Evidence that the greening ligand in native butyryl-CoA dehydrogenase is a CoA persulfide. *J. Biol. Chem.* **1982**, *257*, 4314–4320. [CrossRef]
73. Lee, K.H.; Humbarger, S.; Bahnvadia, R.; Sazinsky, M.H.; Crane, E.J., 3rd. Characterization of the mechanism of the NADH-dependent polysulfide reductase (Npsr) from *Shewanella loihica* PV-4: Formation of a productive NADH-enzyme complex and its role in the general mechanism of NADH and FAD-dependent enzymes. *Biochim. Biophys. Acta* **2014**, *1844*, 1708–1717. [CrossRef]
74. Shabdar, S.; Anaclet, B.; Castineiras, A.G.; Desir, N.; Choe, N.; Crane, E.J., 3rd; Sazinsky, M.H. Structural and Kinetic Characterization of Hyperthermophilic NADH-Dependent Persulfide Reductase from *Archaeoglobus fulgidus*. *Archaea* **2021**, *2021*, 8817136. [CrossRef] [PubMed]
75. Warner, M.D.; Lukose, V.; Lee, K.H.; Lopez, K.; Sazinsky, M.H.; Crane, E.J., 3rd. Characterization of an NADH-dependent persulfide reductase from *Shewanella loihica* PV-4: Implications for the mechanism of sulfur respiration via FAD-dependent enzymes. *Biochemistry* **2011**, *50*, 194–206. [CrossRef] [PubMed]
76. Winter, S.E.; Thiennimitr, P.; Winter, M.G.; Butler, B.P.; Huseby, D.L.; Crawford, R.W.; Russell, J.M.; Bevins, C.L.; Adams, L.G.; Tsolis, R.M.; et al. Gut inflammation provides a respiratory electron acceptor for *Salmonella*. *Nature* **2010**, *467*, 426–429. [CrossRef]
77. Korshunov, S.; Imlay, K.R.; Imlay, J.A. The cytochrome bd oxidase of *Escherichia coli* prevents respiratory inhibition by endogenous and exogenous hydrogen sulfide. *Mol. Microbiol.* **2016**, *101*, 62–77. [CrossRef]
78. Jones-Carson, J.; Husain, M.; Liu, L.; Orlicky, D.J.; Vazquez-Torres, A. Cytochrome *bd*-Dependent Bioenergetics and Antinitrosative Defenses in *Salmonella* Pathogenesis. *MBio* **2016**, *7*, e02052-16. [CrossRef]
79. Forte, E.; Borisov, V.B.; Falabella, M.; Colaco, H.G.; Tinajero-Trejo, M.; Poole, R.K.; Vicente, J.B.; Sarti, P.; Giuffre, A. The Terminal Oxidase Cytochrome bd Promotes Sulfide-resistant Bacterial Respiration and Growth. *Sci. Rep.* **2016**, *6*, 23788. [CrossRef]
80. Spector, A.A.; Yorek, M.A. Membrane lipid composition and cellular function. *J. Lipid Res.* **1985**, *26*, 1015–1035. [CrossRef]
81. Leekumjorn, S.; Cho, H.J.; Wu, Y.; Wright, N.T.; Sum, A.K.; Chan, C. The role of fatty acid unsaturation in minimizing biophysical changes on the structure and local effects of bilayer membranes. *Biochim. Biophys. Acta* **2009**, *1788*, 1508–1516. [CrossRef]
82. Brenner, R.R. Effect of unsaturated acids on membrane structure and enzyme kinetics. *Prog. Lipid Res.* **1984**, *23*, 69–96. [CrossRef]
83. Shen, S.; Hang, X.; Zhuang, J.; Zhang, L.; Bi, H.; Zhang, L. A back-door Phenylalanine coordinates the stepwise hexameric loading of acyl carrier protein by the fatty acid biosynthesis enzyme beta-hydroxyacyl-acyl carrier protein dehydratase (FabZ). *Int. J. Biol. Macromol.* **2019**, *128*, 5–11. [CrossRef] [PubMed]
84. Kimber, M.S.; Martin, F.; Lu, Y.; Houston, S.; Vedadi, M.; Dharamsi, A.; Fiebig, K.M.; Schmid, M.; Rock, C.O. The structure of (3R)-hydroxyacyl-acyl carrier protein dehydratase (FabZ) from *Pseudomonas aeruginosa*. *J. Biol. Chem.* **2004**, *279*, 52593–52602. [CrossRef] [PubMed]
85. Lu, Y.J.; White, S.W.; Rock, C.O. Domain swapping between *Enterococcus faecalis* FabN and FabZ proteins localizes the structural determinants for isomerase activity. *J. Biol. Chem.* **2005**, *280*, 30342–30348. [CrossRef] [PubMed]
86. Zhang, L.; Xiao, J.; Xu, J.; Fu, T.; Cao, Z.; Zhu, L.; Chen, H.Z.; Shen, X.; Jiang, H.; Zhang, L. Crystal structure of FabZ-ACP complex reveals a dynamic seesaw-like catalytic mechanism of dehydratase in fatty acid biosynthesis. *Cell Res.* **2016**, *26*, 1330–1344. [CrossRef] [PubMed]
87. Broussard, T.C.; Kobe, M.J.; Pakhomova, S.; Neau, D.B.; Price, A.E.; Champion, T.S.; Waldrop, G.L. The three-dimensional structure of the biotin carboxylase-biotin carboxyl carrier protein complex of *E. coli* acetyl-CoA carboxylase. *Structure* **2013**, *21*, 650–657. [CrossRef]
88. Broussard, T.C.; Price, A.E.; Laborde, S.M.; Waldrop, G.L. Complex formation and regulation of *Escherichia coli* acetyl-CoA carboxylase. *Biochemistry* **2013**, *52*, 3346–3357. [CrossRef]
89. Bilder, P.; Lightle, S.; Bainbridge, G.; Ohren, J.; Finzel, B.; Sun, F.; Holley, S.; Al-Kassim, L.; Spessard, C.; Melnick, M.; et al. The structure of the carboxyltransferase component of acetyl-coA carboxylase reveals a zinc-binding motif unique to the bacterial enzyme. *Biochemistry* **2006**, *45*, 1712–1722. [CrossRef]
90. Lee, T.H.; Hofferek, V.; Separovic, F.; Reid, G.E.; Aguilar, M.I. The role of bacterial lipid diversity and membrane properties in modulating antimicrobial peptide activity and drug resistance. *Curr. Opin. Chem. Biol.* **2019**, *52*, 85–92. [CrossRef]
91. Harp, J.R.; Saito, H.E.; Bourdon, A.K.; Reyes, J.; Arias, C.A.; Campagna, S.R.; Fozo, E.M. Exogenous Fatty Acids Protect *Enterococcus faecalis* from Daptomycin-Induced Membrane Stress Independently of the Response Regulator LiaR. *Appl. Environ. Microbiol.* **2016**, *82*, 4410–4420. [CrossRef]

92. Rashid, R.; Cazenave-Gassiot, A.; Gao, I.H.; Nair, Z.J.; Kumar, J.K.; Gao, L.; Kline, K.A.; Wenk, M.R. Comprehensive analysis of phospholipids and glycolipids in the opportunistic pathogen *Enterococcus faecalis*. *PLoS ONE* **2017**, *12*, e0175886. [CrossRef] [PubMed]
93. Sobocinska, J.; Roszczenko-Jasinska, P.; Ciesielska, A.; Kwiatkowska, K. Protein Palmitoylation and Its Role in Bacterial and Viral Infections. *Front. Immunol.* **2017**, *8*, 2003. [CrossRef] [PubMed]
94. Bray, B.A.; Sutcliffe, I.C.; Harrington, D.J. Impact of lgt mutation on lipoprotein biosynthesis and in vitro phenotypes of Streptococcus agalactiae. *Microbiology* **2009**, *155*, 1451–1458. [CrossRef] [PubMed]
95. Hicks, S.W.; Charron, G.; Hang, H.C.; Galan, J.E. Subcellular targeting of *Salmonella* virulence proteins by host-mediated S-palmitoylation. *Cell Host Microbe* **2011**, *10*, 9–20. [CrossRef]
96. Spera, J.M.; Guaimas, F.; Corvi, M.M.; Ugalde, J.E. Brucella Hijacks Host-Mediated Palmitoylation To Stabilize and Localize PrpA to the Plasma Membrane. *Infect. Immun.* **2018**, *86*, e00402-18. [CrossRef]
97. Karplus, P.A.; Diederichs, K. Linking crystallographic model and data quality. *Science* **2012**, *336*, 1030–1033.
98. Word, J.M.; Lovell, S.C.; LaBean, T.H.; Taylor, H.C.; Zalis, M.E.; Presley, B.K.; Richardson, J.S.; Richardson, D.C. Visualizing and quantifying molecular goodness-of-fit: Small-probe contact dots with explicit hydrogen atoms. *J. Mol. Biol.* **1999**, *285*, 1711–1733.
99. Zhang, Y.M.; White, S.W.; Rock, C.O. Inhibiting bacterial fatty acid synthesis. *J. Biol. Chem.* **2006**, *281*, 17541–17544.

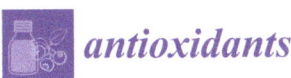

Review

Protective Roles of Hydrogen Sulfide in Alzheimer's Disease and Traumatic Brain Injury

Bindu D. Paul [1,2,3,4,*] and Andrew A. Pieper [5,6,7,8,9,10,11]

1. Department of Pharmacology and Molecular Sciences, Johns Hopkins University School of Medicine, Baltimore, MD 21205, USA
2. The Solomon H. Snyder Department of Neuroscience, Johns Hopkins University School of Medicine, Baltimore, MD 21205, USA
3. Department of Psychiatry and Behavioral Sciences, Johns Hopkins University School of Medicine, Baltimore, MD 21205, USA
4. Lieber Institute for Brain Development, Baltimore, MD 21205, USA
5. Brain Health Medicines Center, Harrington Discovery Institute, University Hospitals Cleveland Medical Center, Cleveland, OH 44106, USA; andrew.pieper@harringtondiscovery.org
6. Department of Psychiatry, Case Western Reserve University, Cleveland, OH 44106, USA
7. Geriatric Psychiatry, GRECC, Louis Stokes Cleveland VA Medical Center, Cleveland, OH 44106, USA
8. Institute for Transformative Molecular Medicine, School of Medicine, Case Western Reserve University, Cleveland, OH 44106, USA
9. Department of Pathology, Case Western Reserve University, School of Medicine, Cleveland, OH 44106, USA
10. Department of Neuroscience, Case Western Reserve University, School of Medicine, Cleveland, OH 44106, USA
11. Translational Therapeutics Core, Cleveland Alzheimer's Disease Research Center, Cleveland, OH 44106, USA
* Correspondence: bpaul8@jhmi.edu

Abstract: The gaseous signaling molecule hydrogen sulfide (H_2S) critically modulates a plethora of physiological processes across evolutionary boundaries. These include responses to stress and other neuromodulatory effects that are typically dysregulated in aging, disease, and injury. H_2S has a particularly prominent role in modulating neuronal health and survival under both normal and pathologic conditions. Although toxic and even fatal at very high concentrations, emerging evidence has also revealed a pronounced neuroprotective role for lower doses of endogenously generated or exogenously administered H_2S. Unlike traditional neurotransmitters, H_2S is a gas and, therefore, is unable to be stored in vesicles for targeted delivery. Instead, it exerts its physiologic effects through the persulfidation/sulfhydration of target proteins on reactive cysteine residues. Here, we review the latest discoveries on the neuroprotective roles of H_2S in Alzheimer's disease (AD) and traumatic brain injury, which is one the greatest risk factors for AD.

Keywords: transsulfuration; cysteine; hydrogen sulfide; Alzheimer's disease; Huntington's disease; traumatic brain injury; mitochondria; neuroprotection; learning and memory; dementia

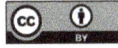

1. Introduction

The mere mention of hydrogen sulfide (H_2S) conjures up images of rotten eggs and sewers. H_2S is a colorless, but not odorless, gas with the smell of rotten eggs and potent toxicity at high concentrations. In 1713, the Italian physician Bernardino Ramazzini first described H_2S toxicity when he reported eye inflammation in workers who cleaned "privies and cesspits" (Ramazzini B. De Morbis Artificum Diatriba. Mutinae (Modena). Antonii Capponi, 1700 [1]). It was later discovered that H_2S can be produced by both bacteria and eukaryotes and that the transsulfuration pathway mediates the interconversion of homocysteine and cysteine via the intermediate cystathionine [2,3]. This was followed by further biochemical characterization of the mammalian enzymes involved in H_2S synthesis by several independent research groups [4–7].

Traditionally studied in readily accessible peripheral organs such as the liver, investigation of H_2S in the brain gained momentum when Warenycia and colleagues observed that the inhalation of H_2S by rats increased brain sulfides in direct proportion to the dose of gas inhaled and also mortality [8]. These investigators further revealed the presence of endogenous sulfides in normal brains without the inhalation of H_2S, suggesting for the first time a normal physiologic role for H_2S in the brain. Additionally, around that same time, elevated sulfide levels were observed in the brain of two fatal cases of H_2S poisoning, further generating recognition and interest in the role of H_2S in the brain [9]. Taken together, the detection of sulfides in the brain spurred detailed studies that ultimately forged a new field of research into this ancient signaling molecule [10].

Initial studies on H_2S predominantly revolved around its toxic effects in mammals [11–13], most notably with respect to mitochondrial bioenergetics [14,15]. Indeed, at high concentrations, H_2S inhibits cytochrome c oxidase and uncouples oxidative phosphorylation, which decreases adenosine triphosphate (ATP) production [16,17]. At lower concentrations, however, H_2S exerts stimulatory and protective effects on mitochondria [18–20]. For example, H_2S stimulates mitochondrial bioenergetics in multiple ways, including enhancing mitochondrial biogenesis and promoting mitophagy of damaged mitochondria [18]. Depending on the method and condition used, H_2S levels can range anywhere from nanomolar levels to micromolar levels, with physiologic levels of H_2S in the nanomolar range (reviewed in [21]). There is a dire need for specific and sensitive probes that can be utilized to detect and measure H_2S in vivo. Diminished H_2S production has been observed in several neurodegenerative diseases, including Huntington's disease (HD), Parkinson's disease (PD), and Alzheimer's disease (AD). On the other hand, elevated H_2S is also deleterious. For instance, the triplicated gene for cystathionine β-synthase (CBS) on chromosome 21 in Down syndrome increases H_2S levels throughout the body, which suppresses complex IV of the mitochondrial electron transport chain [22–24]. This article focuses on the neuroprotective roles of H_2S in vivo in the brain and its protective efficacy in both AD and traumatic brain injury (TBI), one of the leading risks factors for AD [25].

2. Biosynthesis of H_2S in the Brain

H_2S is generated in vivo in the brain by three enzymes: cystathionine γ-lyase (CSE), CBS, and 3-mercaptopyruvate sulfur transferase (3-MST) through a coordinated and highly regulated process known as the transsulfuration pathway [7,26–29] (Figure 1). Notably, the expression of the biosynthetic enzymes for H_2S is spatially compartmentalized. Specifically, CSE is exclusively localized to neurons, CBS is expressed in Bergmann glia and astrocytes [30,31], and 3-MST has also been localized to neurons [32]. All three enzymes utilize cysteine directly or indirectly to produce H_2S. 3-MST acts on 3-mercaptopyruvate (3-MP) produced by cysteine aminotransferase (CAT) to produce H_2S. In the absence of CAT, 3-MST cannot produce H_2S unless 3-MP is present. Apart from these pathways, H_2S can also be generated from the acid labile pool, iron–sulfur protein clusters, and the sulfane sulfur pool in the presence of endogenous reductants [33,34]. Higher levels of bound sulfur are found in the brain, with free H_2S being maintained at low levels under basal conditions. H_2S is also released from bound sulfur in homogenates of neurons and astrocytes under alkaline conditions, akin to what occurs in vivo when high extracellular concentrations of K^+ ions are released by neuronal excitation [34]. The significance of the spatial compartmentalization of CSE, 3-MST, and CBS in the brain is not clear, and these enzymes may have cell-type-specific roles that are yet to be identified. It is increasingly evident that astrocytes have important signaling roles, ranging from immune signaling, synaptic plasticity, and metabolic functions to providing a support system for neurons [35–37]. The role of CBS in these processes is yet to be elucidated. Additionally, of the three H_2S-generating enzymes, CSE is highly inducible, whereas CBS is constitutively expressed [27]. CBS can be regulated at the post-translational level by S-adenosyl methionine (SAM), an allosteric modulator [38]. Levels of SAM are decreased in the cerebrospinal fluid and brain tissue of AD patients, which could lead to a decrease in H_2S levels [39,40].

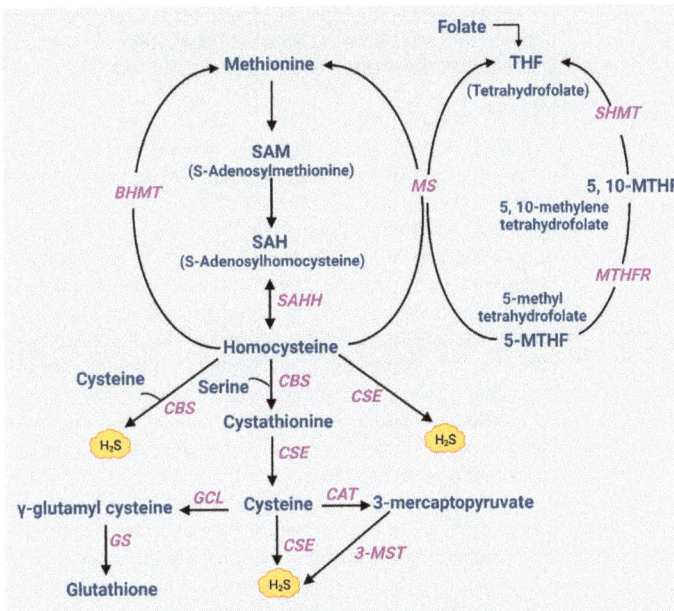

Figure 1. The transsulfuration and transmethylation pathways. Transsulfuration involves transfer of sulfur from homocysteine to cysteine. Homocysteine is generated from dietary methionine via S-adenosylmethionine (SAM) and S-adenosylhomocysteine (SAH). SAH is converted to homocysteine by S-adenosylhomocysteine hydrolase (SAHH). Homocysteine is then used either for generation of H_2S via the transsulfuration pathway or moved into the transmethylation pathway to generate methionine. With respect to the transsulfuration pathway, cystathionine β-synthase (CBS) converts homocysteine to H_2S or condenses homocysteine with serine to form cystathionine, which is then converted to cysteine by cystathionine γ-lyase (CSE). Cysteine is directly utilized by CSE to form H_2S or alternatively converted to 3-mercaptopyruvate by cysteine aminotyransferase (CAT). 3-mercaptopyruvate sulfurtransferase (3-MST) then converts 3-MST to H_2S. Cysteine can also be utilized to produce glutathione (GSH) by the sequential actions of glutamyl cysteine ligase (GCL) and GSH synthase (GS). The other pathway for homocysteine involves the regeneration of methionine via the transmethylation pathway. Methylation of homocysteine may occur either through a folate-independent or dependent pathway. In the folate-dependent pathway shown here, the vitamin B_{12}-dependent enzyme methionine synthase (MS) converts homocysteine to methionine and tetrahydrofolate (THF), utilizing 5-methyltetrahydrofolate (5-MTHF) as the methyl donor. Next, serine hydroxymethyltransferase (SHMT) converts THF to 5,10-methylenetetrahydrofolate (5,10-MTHF), utilizing serine and vitamin B_6. 5,10-MTHF is reduced to 5-MTHF by 5,10-methylenetetrahydrofolate reductase (MTHFR), remethylating another molecule of homocysteine in the process [29].

3. H_2S Signaling in Cognitive Functions

One of the earliest studies on the neuromodulator action of H_2S in the central nervous system, conducted by Kimura and associates in 1996, showed that H_2S acted on N-methyl D-aspartate (NMDA) receptors to modulate long-term potentiation and neurotransmission [10]. The same group also reported that H_2S diminished oxidative stress in neurons [41], which was later attributed to the restoration of glutathione (GSH) levels and the stabilization of the mitochondria [42]. Oxidative stress plays a central role in pathogenesis of several neurodegenerative diseases, and thus restoring dysregulated H_2S metabolism in these conditions was proposed to be beneficial [43]. However, it is important to note that H_2S exhibits a bell-shaped dose response curve, with lower concentrations being generally beneficial and higher doses being toxic. The importance of this equilibrium is underscored by the tight regulation of endogenous H$_2$S synthesis. Here, we review the current understanding of the role of H$_2$S in two major forms of neuropsychiatric disease characterized by cognitive impairment: AD and TBI.

3.1. Alzheimer's Disease

Alzheimer's disease (AD), a multifactorial neurodegenerative condition characterized by the progressive loss of cognitive function and memory, is the leading worldwide cause of dementia [44,45]. Indeed, approximately 6.5 million Americans aged 65 and older are living with Alzheimer's dementia today [46]. The neuropathological hallmarks of Alzheimer's disease classically include the deposition of neurofibrillary tangles and paired helical fragments comprising the microtubule associated protein tau as well as the accumulation of plaques composed of Aβ peptides [47,48]. However, several lines of evidence also reveal that cognitively normal individuals often have deposits of amyloid plaques, and efforts to treat AD through addressing these two major forms of pathology have not yet succeeded [49,50]. The utility and safety of amyloid-based approaches has also recently been called into question by the Alves et al., whose meta-analysis of the published literature has shown that these therapeutic approaches may compromise long-term brain health by accelerating brain atrophy [51].

Notably, several studies have shown that the suboptimal or excessive levels of metabolites or cofactors of the transsulfuration pathway are also linked to dementia and cognitive deficits, pointing towards another possible therapeutic target for AD (Figure 1). For example, as described below, hyperhomocysteinemia has been linked to dementia.

3.1.1. Hyperhomocysteinemia and Its Causes

Homocysteine is formed from S-adenosyl homocysteine by S-adenosylhomocysteine hydrolase (SAHH), and hyperhomocysteinemia has been established as an independent risk factor for dementia and cardiovascular diseases. Homocysteine is utilized as a substrate for both CSE and CBS to produce H$_2$S. While CBS utilizes a combination of cysteine and homocysteine to produce H$_2$S, CSE utilizes homocysteine alone to generate the gasotransmitter [52,53]. A subset of patients displaying homocysteinemia exhibited diminished CBS activity and substantial cardiovascular disability [54]. Thus, both elevated homocysteine levels and decreased H$_2$S levels mediated vascular complications observed in subjects with impaired CBS activity [55]. Several studies have also shown that levels of homocysteine correlated with the severity of AD [56,57], and increased serum homocysteine was generally observed by the time people reached their nineties [58–61]. Elevated homocysteine levels additionally occur in TBI, one of the greatest risk factors for AD. Homocysteine can elicit toxicity in multiple ways, including the aberrant processing of the amyloid precursor protein (APP), overactivation of the NMDA receptor, DNA damage, and oxidative stress [29].

As described above, homocysteine resides at the intersection of the transsulfuration and transmethylation pathways, where it is either converted to cysteine via cystathionine or remethylated to methionine (Figure 1). Hyperhomocysteinemia may arise due to several reasons, including decreased expression or activity of the enzymes methylenetetrahydrofolate reductase (MTHFR), methionine synthase (MS), CBS, or CSE. MTHFR acts on 5,10-methylenetetrahydrofolate to produce 5-methyltetrahydrofolate, the methyl donor for remethylation of homocysteine to form methionine by MS. Notably, mutations in the *MTHFR* gene, which decrease the activity of the protein, have been linked to AD [62]. Along similar lines, mutations in the *CTH* gene are also associated with AD [63,64]. Decreased levels of folate, vitamin B$_{12}$ (a cofactor for MS), or S-adenosyl methionine (SAM) also lead to hyperhomocysteinemia. SAM is a methyl donor generated from S-adenosylhomocysteine (SAH), which also serves as a cofactor for CBS activity [38]. SAM levels are decreased in AD, which may compromise the levels of cystathionine formed from homocysteine by CBS as well as H$_2$S production because CBS utilizes homocysteine along with cysteine to produce H$_2$S [39,40,53]. The administration of SAM to the APP/Presenilin-1 (PS1) mouse model of AD and to cultured astrocytes conferred cellular protection and stimulated the transsulfuration pathway [65]. Similarly, in both an Aβ intrahippocampal injection rat model and cultured SH-SY5Y cells, SAM enhanced GSH levels and prevented inflammatory changes and oxidative stress [66].

3.1.2. Cysteine and GSH Metabolism

GSH, a tripeptide of glycine, glutamate, and cysteine, is one of the most abundant antioxidants in cells and tissues [67]. Among its many roles, GSH serves as a cofactor for several enzymes, modulates redox balance in cells, and provides a reservoir for glutamatergic neurotransmission [68]. The availability of cysteine is the rate limiting step for the synthesis of GSH, and, therefore, any alterations in cysteine may compromise GSH metabolism and elevate oxidative stress [69]. Aging, the biggest risk factor for developing AD, has also been associated with declining cysteine levels, and, as such, it has been designated as a "cysteine deficiency syndrome" [70]. Dysregulated cysteine metabolism has been observed in AD as well [71,72]. Cysteine levels are also regulated by the activity of its transporters, which exhibit suboptimal activity in several models of AD. Furthermore, soluble Aβ oligomers inhibit both basal and insulin-like growth factor-1 (IGF-1)-stimulated cysteine uptake through the neuronal cysteine transporter, the excitatory amino acid transporter 3 (EAAT3/EAAC1) [73]. Another study reported an increase in detergent-insoluble EAAC1 in the hippocampus of AD patients compared to normal subjects [74].

Along with declining cysteine levels, GSH is also significantly diminished in mouse models of AD prior to amyloid-β deposition, with the magnitude of the decrease in GSH correlating exponentially with the magnitude of increased intraneuronal Aβ accumulation [75]. Decreased GSH and antioxidant enzymes have also been linked to disease progression in AD [76]. While one meta-analysis of studies of postmortem tissues from subjects with mild cognitive impairment (MCI) and AD did not detect significant changes in GSH [77], it is important to note that the postmortem preservation of metabolites is notoriously variable. By contrast, recent magnetic resonance spectroscopy (MRS) studies have revealed significant depletion of brain GSH in MCI and AD, including the highly affected hippocampal brain region [78–81]. GSH depletion may also compromise the activity of GSH-requiring enzymes, such as glyoxalase 1 and 2 (GLO1 and 2), which are dysregulated in AD [82]. GLO1 and GLO2 are a part of the glyoxalase system that prevents glycation reactions mediated by alpha-ketoaldehydes such as methylglyoxal and glyoxal [83].

3.1.3. H_2S and AD

Although disrupted H_2S balance in AD was reported several decades ago, the molecular mechanisms are only beginning to be understood [29]. Diminished brain H_2S levels in AD were first observed in 2002 and correlated to decreased CBS activity [84]. Decreased H_2S was also observed in the plasma of AD patients and correlated with severity of disease [85]. The same study also observed an increase in homocysteine levels. Diminished H_2S that correlated with brain energy levels in the APP/PS1 mouse model of AD was additionally demonstrated using a fluorescent probe that simultaneously measured ATP [86]. In addition, decreased CSE levels have been observed in different models of AD, as described below [72,87].

Initial studies investigating the neuroprotective role of H_2S in AD involved the administration of H_2S donors, which exerted protective effects in several AD models. In a rat model involving the hippocampal injection of Aβ1-40, for example, the fast release H_2S donor sodium hydrosulfide (NaHS) prevented neuroinflammation by suppressing the increase in cytokines, such as Tumor necrosis factor alpha (TNF-α), interleukin 1-beta (IL-1β), IL-6, and pro-inflammatory cyclooxygenase-2 (COX-2) [88]. NaHS also prevented amyloid-β-induced toxicity in microglial cultures, reduced inflammation, preserved mitochondrial function [89], and prevented Aβ-induced toxicity in PC12 cells [90,91]. Furthermore, NaHS prevented spatial memory impairment and neuroinflammation in an amyloid-based rat model of AD [92]. A separate study utilizing NaHS and Tabiano's spa-water (rich in sulfur compounds) ameliorated behavioral deficits in three experimental models of AD [93]. H_2S donors were also tested in a *C. elegans* model of AD and shown to reduce Aβ aggregation, increase levels of acetylcholine, and reduce oxidative stress [94]. Another study reported that dietary methionine restriction in APP/PS1 mice ameliorated neurodegeneration, improved cognition, and increased H_2S production [95]. Several studies have also reported on the beneficial effects of natural products or plant-based foods that are rich sources of H_2S, including garlic [96]. In 2007, for example, it was demonstrated that the garlic-derived compounds diallyl sulfide (DAS), diallyl disulfide (DADS), and diallyl trisulfide (DATS) all release H_2S, with diallyl trisulfide (DATS) showing the greatest activity [97,98]. S-allylcysteine (SAC), another garlic compound, also increases H_2S by increasing expression of CSE [99,100]. After these findings, garlic extracts and their endogenous sulfur containing compounds were tested and found to be efficacious in models of AD [101–106]. A summary of beneficial effects of H_2S in models of AD is shown below in Table 1.

Table 1. Neuroprotective effects of hydrogen sulfide.

H_2S Donor/ Boosting Agent	System	Effect	Ref.
NaHS	β (Aβ 25-35)-treated PC12 cells	Prevented β (Aβ 25-35)-induced cytotoxicity and apoptosis by reducing the loss of MMP and attenuating the increase in intracellular ROS.	[90]
NaHS	PC12 cells	Decreased beta secretase-1 (BACE-1) levels and Aβ1-42 release. Increased phosphorylation of Akt.	[91]
NaHS	Aβ1-40-induced toxicity in BV-2 microglial cells	Attenuated Aβ1-40-induced lactate dehydrogenase (LDH) release and expression of growth arrest DNA damage (GADD 153). Inhibited release of nitric oxide, induction of inducible nitric oxide synthase (iNOS), and expression of tumor necrosis factor α (TNF-α) and cyclooxygenase 2 (COX-2).	[89]
NaHS	Rat Amyloid β (Aβ 1-40)-injection model	Ameliorated learning and memory deficits. Suppressed Aβ(1-40)-induced apoptosis in the hippocampal CA1 region. Diminished hippocampal inflammation, astrogliosis, and microgliosis.	[92]
NaHS	APP/PS1 mouse model of AD	Improved spatial memory. Decreased expression of BACE1, PS1, and amyloidogenic C99 fragment. Increased expression of ADAM17 and nonamyloidogenic C83 fragment.	[107]
NaHS	APP/PS1 mouse model of AD	Increased hippocampal H_2S levels, intracellular ATP, and mitochondrial COX IV activity. Improved hippocampus-dependent contextual fear memory and novel object recognition. Decreased Aβ accumulation in mitochondria.	[108]
NaHS	APP/PS1 mouse model of AD	Inhibited γ-secretase activity and decreases mitochondrial Aβ production in neurons.	[109]
NaHS	Rat amyloid β (Aβ 25-35)-injection model	Prevented neuronal loss, apoptosis, and activation of pro-caspase-3. Decreased expression of phosphodiesterase 5 (PDE-5) in the hippocampus. Upregulated expression of peroxisome proliferator-activated receptor (PPAR)-α and PPAR-γ. Prevented Aβ 25-35-decrease in IκB-α degradation and increase in nuclear factor-κB (NF-κB) p65 phosphorylation levels.	[110]

Table 1. Cont.

H$_2$S Donor/ Boosting Agent	System	Effect	Ref.
NaHS	Primary hippocampal neuronal culture from C57/BL6 mice at P0-P1	Reduced Aβ-induced apoptosis. Decreased release of cytochrome C into the cytosol and caspase-3 activity. Decreased translocation of the phosphatase and tensin homologs deleted on chromosome 10 (PTEN) from the cytosol to the mitochondria. Increased p-AKT/AKT levels in PI3K-dependent manner.	[111]
NaHS	APP/PS1 mouse model of AD	Mitigated cognitive deficits. Decreased the number of senile plaques, Aβ1-40 and Aβ1-42 levels, neuronal loss, beta-amyloid precursor (APP), and BACE1. Increased CBS and 3MST. Augmented antioxidant effects through induction of nuclear factor erythroid-2-related factor 2 (Nrf2), heme oxygenase-1(HO-1), and glutathione S-transferase (GST).	[112]
Memit (Derived from memantine by replacing the free amine group with an isothiocyanate moiety)	Aβ oligomers-induced damage in human neurons and rat	Decreased Aβ(1-42)-induced aggregation and Aβ oligomer-induced damage in human neurons and rat microglial cells. Increased neuroprotective autophagy.	[113]
H$_2$S releasing peptide conjugates	C. elegans	Reduced Aβ1–42 amyloid deposits and ROS. Increased acetylcholine levels.	[94]
Sulfanagen	APP/PS1 mouse model of AD	Stimulated 3-MST and prevented neuropathology.	[114]
Methionine restriction	APP/PS1 mouse model of AD	Decreased Aβ accumulation. Improved cognitive function. Restored synapse ultrastructure. Alleviated mitochondrial dysfunction by enhancing mitochondrial biogenesis in male mice. Balanced the redox status and activated cystathionine-β-synthase (CBS)/ H$_2$S pathway.	[95]
Naringin	Rat Amyloid β (Aβ)-injection model	Improved spatial memory. Increased H$_2$S production.	[115]
NaHS	LPS-induced AD-like cognitive deficits in Wistar albino rats	Reduced inflammation. Decreased oxidative stress, apoptosis, and histopathological alterations.	[116]
NaHS in combination with the NMDA-receptor antagonist, MK801	Homocysteine (intracerebral injection)-induced AD-like neurodegeneration	Ameliorated BBB disruption, impaired cerebral blood flow (CBF), and diminished synaptic function.	[117]
NaHS	Mouse primary hippocampal neurons (E16–18), 3xTg-AD mouse model of AD	Reduced neuronal death in Aβ1-42 treated primary hippocampal neuronal culture and increased neurite length. Increased plasma H$_2$S and decreased anxiety-like behavior and cognitive deficits in 3xTg-AD mice. Reduced amyloid deposits and hyperphosphorylation of Tau. Decreased inflammatory responses, oxidative stress, and gliosis in 3×Tg-AD mice.	[118]
NaHS, sulfurous water	3xTg-AD mouse model of AD	Prevented learning and memory deficits. Reduced size of amyloid β plaques. Decreased activity of c-jun N-terminal kinases, extracellular signal-regulated kinases, and p38.	[119]
NaHS, Tabiano's spa-water	Rat Aβ1–40 injection model of AD, Streptozotocin-induced AD, 3xTg-AD mouse model of AD	Improved learning and memory deficits in all three models. Decreased amyloid deposits in the rat models of AD. The spa-water decreased oxidative and nitrosative stress, MAPK activation, inflammation, and apoptosis in 3xTg-AD mice.	[93]
Na-GYY4137	3xTg-AD mouse model of AD	Improved motor and cognitive function in 3xTg-AD mice. Increased overall sulfhydration. Inhibited Tau phosphorylation by sulfhydrating glycogen synthase kinase (GSK3β) and inhibiting its activity.	[72]

Persulfidation, AD, and Aging

One of the modes by which H_2S signals is through post-translational modification, termed sulfhydration or persulfidation, which both refer to the same chemical reaction in which the thiol group of cysteine is converted to an –SSH or persulfide group [52,120,121]. Here, H_2S cannot directly modify an –SH group, and the main mechanisms by which persulfides are generated are by reactions of H_2S with oxidized cysteines or disulfides or by reactions of cysteine residues with sulfide radicals, polysulfides, and other persulfides [121,122]. Persulfidation is a reversible modification regulated by the endogenous thioredoxin/thioredoxin reductase system [123–125]. Notably, persulfidation and H_2S signaling are compromised in several age-related neurodegenerative diseases, including AD, HD, PD, and spinocerebellar ataxia (SCA) [126–129].

Although there are numerous studies on the beneficial effects of H_2S in AD, analysis of persulfidation (the major mode by which the gaseous molecule signals) in AD is scarce. More recently, the status of persulfidation has been studied directly in AD (Figure 2). For example, overall persulfidation is decreased in mouse models of AD as well as postmortem samples from human AD subjects [72]. Notably, persulfidation of Glycogen synthase kinase-3β (GSK-3β), the major kinase that phosphorylates Tau, is decreased in AD. Administration of Na-GYY4137 to the 3xTg-AD model of AD rectified the persulfidation deficits and prevented motor and cognitive decline [29,72]. Suboptimal persulfidation was also observed in the APP/PS1 mouse model of AD, where decreased expression of CSE was observed, in addition to the human hippocampal and cortex samples [87]. This study also demonstrated a role for the autophagy-related activating factor 6 (ATF6) in expression of CSE. Stereotaxic injection of lentiviral particles encoding CTH into the ventricular system of the brain rescued spatial memory deficits in *Atf6* CKO/APP/PS1 mice. The transport of ATF6 from the endoplasmic reticulum to the Golgi apparatus under ER stress is mediated by the Soluble NSF attachment protein (αSNAP)/ SNAP receptor (SNARE) pathway. Persulfidation of αSNAP is also decreased in ATF6 knockout mice, which may indicate a role in AD.

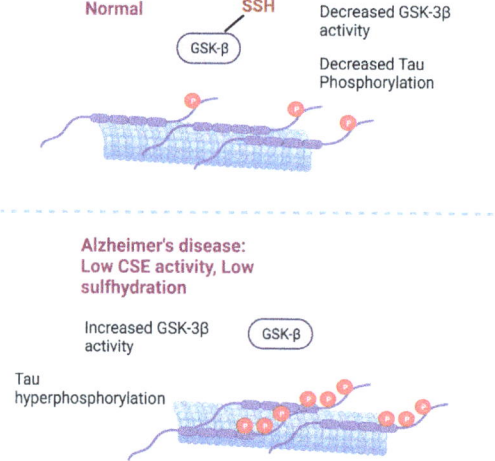

Figure 2. Disruption of H_2S signaling in Alzheimer's disease (AD). During normal conditions, glycogen synthase kinase-3β (GSK-3β) is sulfhydrated, which inhibits its catalytic activity and prevents hyper-phosphorylation of Tau (Top panel). In AD, decreased CSE activity leads to lower sulfhydration of GSK-3β, which leads to elevated phosphorylation of Tau.

Lastly, aging is the biggest risk factor for developing AD, and diminished persulfidation is also ubiquitously observed across evolutionary boundaries during aging. Importantly, several of the proteins whose persulfidation levels are altered may modulate AD pathology and disease progression [122,130]. A systematic analysis of these targets is warranted to elucidate the links between persulfidation and AD. For instance, MTHFR, a key enzyme regulating intracellular homocysteine metabolism, is normally persulfidated, and decreased persulfidation of MTHFR promotes hyperhomocysteinemia, a risk factor for AD [131].

3.2. Traumatic Brain Injury

TBI and H_2S

Traumatic brain injury (TBI) is one of the most prevalent forms of neurodegenerative disease, and typically entails chronic and progressive neuropsychiatric impairment even after a single injury. This pathologic process is poorly understood, and, to date, there are no protective treatments for patients. It is well-established that there is considerable overlap in pathology between TBI and AD [25], and H_2S is involved in various biological functions after TBI, including the response to oxidative stress in the brain. Due to the brain's voracious need for the constant generation of ATP, which generates free radicals as a by-product, and the brain's abundance of metal ions and phospholipids that generate additional oxidative products, the brain, even under normal circumstances, is constantly exposed to high levels of oxidative stress. This vulnerability is further exacerbated by TBI because of an increased energy requirement for self-repair processes after injury that ultimately leads to an inability to maintain mitochondrial membrane potential, resulting in complete energy failure and cell death. Early results in cellular models indicated protective efficacy of H_2S in this scenario. For example, H_2S generated by mitochondrial 3-MST directly reduced the generation of ROS and protected PC12 cells from apoptosis after severe oxidative stress [132]. In cultured neurons, H_2S promoted the neuronal production of GSH and the scavenging of oxygen free radicals, hydrogen peroxide, and lipid peroxides [42,133]. Thus, whether changes in brain H_2S might be involved in the pathophysiology of TBI, and whether supplemental H_2S might be neuroprotective in TBI, became an active area of investigation.

There is now substantial evidence in animal models that TBI decreases brain levels of H_2S and that exogenous supplementation of H_2S protects the brain after injury. In 2013, Zhang et al. observed that subjecting mice to the weight drop model of TBI acutely decreased levels of hippocampal and cortical CBS mRNA and protein, and this correlated with decreased levels of H_2S [134]. They additionally demonstrated that pretreatment with the H_2S donor NaHS partially reduced lesion volume after injury [134]. That same year, Jiang et al. showed the protective efficacy of NaHS in an additional model of TBI induced by controlled cortical impact (CCI) in rats [135]. Specifically, CCI acutely decreased brain H_2S, and the preservation of brain H_2S with NaHS treatment beginning before injury blocked brain edema, blood–brain barrier (BBB) impairment, and the acquisition of motor deficits. They also reported that NaHS-treated rats showed reduced TBI lesion volume and were protected from TBI-induced decreases in brain superoxide dismutase and choline acetyltransferase activity, as well as TBI-induced increases in the oxidative products 8-iso-prostaglandin F2 alpha and malondialdehyde, up to 72 h after injury [135].

These results were further bolstered when Zhang et al. extended their work in the weight drop model of TBI the following year, showing that NaHS pretreatment prevented cerebral edema and cognitive impairment in the Morris water maze after TBI, as well as cleavage of caspase-3, decreased Bcl-2, and elevated neuronal apoptosis [136]. Preserved cognition in the Morris water maze by NaHS pretreatment in rats exposed to CCI was also independently established by the Hajisoltani laboratory [137], and Xu et al. additionally demonstrated that NaHS-mediated modulation of the PI3K/Akt/mTOR signaling pathway after TBI in mice was associated with BBB protection, the inhibition of neuronal apoptosis, remyelination of axons, and preservation of mitochondrial function [138]. Evidence for protective efficacy of H$_2$S in the CCI model of TBI was also demonstrated by Campolo et al., who showed that the administration of 2-(6-methoxynapthalen-2-yl)-propionic acid 4-thiocarbamoyl-phenyl ester (ATB-346), a H$_2$S-releasing derivative of naproxen, attenuated TBI-induced brain edema, neuronal cell death, and motor impairment, while naproxen (which does not release H$_2$S) had no protective efficacy [139]. ATB-346 was also associated with significantly decreased expression of inducible nitric oxide synthase (iNOS), cyclooxygenase 2 (COX-2), tumor necrosis factor alpha (TNFα), and interleukin 1-beta (IL-1β), as well as normalized levels of glial-derived neurotrophic factor (GDNF) and nerve growth factor (NGF), and increased levels of vascular endothelial growth factor (VEGF), after TBI [139]. While all of these changes would be considered likely beneficial to brain health in the setting of TBI, it is unclear whether any of these occur as a direct result of H$_2$S action or if this simply reflects the profile of a healthier brain by virtue of other upstream effects of H$_2$S. Interestingly, Zhang et al. have shown that increased expression of 3-MST in neurons occurs predominantly in those neurons that survive after TBI [140], implicating a regulated and direct protective role of endogenous H$_2$S after TBI. More recently, H$_2$S-mediated protection in TBI in rats has been linked to the modulation of glutamate-mediated oxidative stress via the p53/glutaminase2 pathway [141]. In addition, the Centurion laboratory recently reported that subchronic treatment with NaHS protected rats from hemodynamic and sympathetic nervous system impairments after TBI and also restored CSE and CBS expression in the brain [142]. It has also been demonstrated that subchronic NaHS after TBI in rats prevents hypertension, vascular impairment, and oxidative stress [143]. In conclusion, there are a myriad of central and peripheral beneficial effects of H$_2$S on TBI outcomes, although the precise mechanisms by which these protective effects occur are currently unknown (Figure 3).

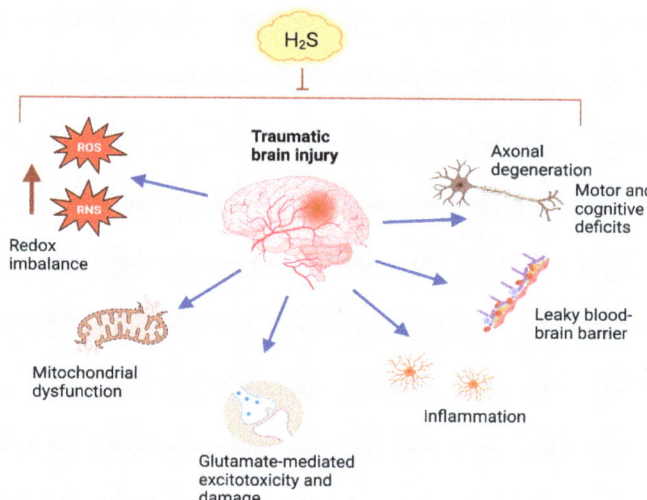

Figure 3. Neuroprotective effects of H$_2$S in traumatic brain injury (TBI). TBI impacts several physiological processes that lead to motor and cognitive deficits. TBI causes increases in reactive oxygen and nitrogen species (ROS and RNS), leading to oxidative and nitrosative stress and mitochondrial dysfunction. TBI also elicits glutamate-induced neurotoxicity and inflammation and causes a leaky blood–brain barrier. All of these processes influence each other and ultimately culminate in neurodegeneration.

4. Dysregulation of Iron Homeostasis in AD, TBI and Intersection with H$_2$S Signaling

Iron is a transition metal with important roles in the brain, ranging from being a component of iron–sulfur cluster proteins and heme proteins to participating in DNA synthesis and neurotransmitter metabolism. However, the dysregulation of iron homeostasis can be deleterious, as ferrous iron (Fe^{2+}) reacts with H_2O_2 and produces $^{\bullet}OH$ and HO_2 to oxidize lipids, proteins, and DNA [43]. Additionally, superoxide radicals ($O_2^{\bullet-}$) produced by mitochondria during respiration reduce Fe^{3+} to Fe^{2+} by the Haber–Weiss reaction [144]. The accumulation of iron in the brain is a common feature of aging, several neurodegenerative diseases, and TBI and is known to drive neuronal loss [145–149]. Specifically, disrupted iron metabolism and its aberrant redox cycling trigger ferroptosis, an iron-dependent cell death pathway that elicits lipid peroxidation and damage to cellular components in several neurodegenerative diseases, including AD [150–153]. Ferroptosis was described over a decade ago as a distinct form of cell death linked to aging, neurodegeneration, immune system dysfunction, and cancer [151,154]. It is well-established that ferroptosis is intimately linked to depletion of cysteine, a component of GSH in cells, and several studies have shown that cysteine/cystine deprivation can elicit this form of cell death. As cysteine serves as the substrate for generation of H_2S, the involvement of this gasotransmitter in ferroptosis has been explored. To date, H_2S donors have been shown to alleviate damage caused by ferroptosis in various contexts by activating cytoprotective signaling pathways [155–157]. The effect of H_2S on ferroptosis in the brain in the context of injury and neurodegeneration is yet to be systematically studied and could inform the development of novel therapeutics.

5. Therapeutic Opportunities

Although significant advances in the elucidation of signaling mediated by H_2S have been made, clinical translation has yet to follow. While there is abundant evidence of the neuroprotective efficacy of H_2S donors in rodents, *Drosophila*, and worm models, examples of translation to human disease are scarce. However, some H_2S-donating hybrid drugs have made it into clinical trials, including a phase 2B study that demonstrated a reduction in gastrointestinal toxicity of the hybrid H_2S-releasing analgesic/anti-inflammatory drug ATB-346, as compared to the non-steroidal anti-inflammatory drug (NSAID) naproxen that produces a similar inhibition of the inflammatory cyclooxygenase-2 (COX2) molecule. [158]. The safety and side-effects of these compounds are still being evaluated. Harnessing H_2S donors can prove challenging, as the timing and dose of the donors likely requires optimization. For example, numerous reports have demonstrated a biphasic dose–response curve for H_2S, with higher doses being toxic. An alternate approach involves the use of natural H_2S donors such as garlic extracts, which are rich in sulfur compounds that release H_2S and may be beneficial in cardiovascular disorders [97,98]. The use of such donors might also be considered in ameliorating symptoms of AD, TBI, and other neurodegenerative disorders involving diminished H_2S signaling. The opposite may be true of diseases involving elevated H_2S, such as Down syndrome, in which the trisomy of chromosome 21 leads to excess H_2S production due to an extra copy of CBS [23,24]. Thus, depending on the paucity or excess of H_2S, appropriate treatment strategies will need to be developed.

6. Conclusions

AD is a complex, multifactorial disease, with most cases arising sporadically. The susceptibility factors for developing AD are several, with aging and TBI being major risk factors. There are several commonalities between AD and TBI, including dysregulated gasotransmitter signaling. Accumulating evidence shows that deficiencies in the gaseous signaling molecule H_2S can drive pathology in AD and TBI and that the augmentation of H_2S levels affords therapeutic benefits in these conditions. Stimulating H_2S production or restoring the homeostasis of the various metabolites of the transsulfuration and transmethylation pathway that contribute to cysteine, GSH, or H_2S production may be beneficial for these or other related forms of neurodegenerative disease. H_2S is a gaseous molecule and cannot be stored in vesicles, unlike conventional neurotransmitters, but elicits effects through sulfhydration, which can be used as a marker for its action. Accurate measurement of the various forms and metabolites H_2S would further deepen our knowledge pertaining to the physiological relevance of this gaseous messenger molecule.

Author Contributions: Conceptualization, B.D.P. and A.A.P., writing—original draft preparation, B.D.P. and A.A.P.; writing—review and editing, B.D.P. and A.A.P. All authors have read and agreed to the published version of the manuscript.

Funding: B.D.P. and A.A.P. are supported by the American Heart Association and Paul Allen Foundation grant 19PABH134580006. B.D.P. is also supported by NIH NIDA, grants P50 DA044123, NIH NIA 1R21AG073684-01, and R01AG071512, and funding from the Solve-ME foundation and the Catalyst Award from Johns Hopkins University. A.A.P. is supported as the Case Western Reserve University Rebecca E. Barchas, MD, Professor in Translational Psychiatry and the University Hospitals Morley-Mather Chair in Neuropsychiatry. A.A.P. also acknowledges support from The Valour Foundation, Brockman Foundation, Department of Veterans Affairs Merit Award I01BX005976, NIH/NIGMS RM1 GM142002, NIH/NIA RO1AG066707, NIH/NIA 1 U01 AG073323, and NIH/NIA 1 P30 AGO62428-01 (Translational Therapeutics Core of the Cleveland Alzheimer's Disease Research Center), Elizabeth Ring Mather & William Gwinn Mather Fund, S. Livingston Samuel Mather Trust, G.R. Lincoln Family Foundation, Wick Foundation, Leonard Krieger Fund of the Cleveland Foundation, Maxine and Lester Stoller Parkinson's Research Fund, and the Louis Stokes VA Medical Center resources and facilities.

Acknowledgments: We acknowledge BioRender for the use of icons in figures.

Conflicts of Interest: The authors declare no conflict of interest.

Abbreviations

3-MST	3-mercaptopyruvate sulfurtransferase
AD	Alzheimer's disease
APP	Amyloid precursor protein
ATB346	2-(6-methoxynapthalen-2-yl)-propionic acid 4-thiocarbamoyl-phenyl ester
ATF6	Activating factor 6
BBB	Blood–brain barrier
CAT	Cysteine aminotransferase
CBF	Cerebral blood flow
CBS	Cystathionine β-synthase
CSE	Cystathionine γ-lyase
CCI	Controlled cortical impact
COX-2	Cyclo-oxygenase-2
DADS	Diallyl disulfide
DATS	Diallyl trisulfide
EAAT3/EAAC1	Excitatory amino acid transporter 3
GDNF	Glial-derived neurotrophic factor
GLO-1,2	Glyoxalase 1,2
GSH	Glutathione
GSK-3β	Glycogen synthase kinase-3β
HD	Huntington's disease
iNOS	Inducible nitric oxide synthase
MCI	Mild cognitive impairment
MRS	Magnetic resonance spectroscopy
MTHFR	Methylenetetrahydrofolate reductase
NGF	Nerve growth factor
Nrf2	Nuclear factor erythroid-2-related factor 2
PD	Parkinson's disease
PDE5	Phosphodiesterase 5
PS1	Presenilin-1
ROS	Reactive Oxygen Species
RNS	Reactive Nitrogen Species
SAC	S-allyl cysteine
SAHH	S-adenosylhomocysteine hydrolase

SAM	S-adenosyl methionine
SCA	Spinocerebellar ataxia
α-SNAP	α-soluble NSF attachment protein
SNARE	Soluble NSF attachment protein receptor
TNF-α	Tumor necrosis factor alpha
VEGF	Vascular endothelial growth factor

References

1. Ramazzini, B. De Morbis Artificum Diatriba. Mutinae (Modena). Antonii Capponi. In *Google Scholar*; 1700. Available online: https://www.ncbi.nlm.nih.gov/pmc/articles/PMC1446785/ (accessed on 1 April 2023).
2. du Vigneaud, V.; Loring, G.S.; Craft, H.A. The oxidation of the sulfur of homocystine, methionine, and S-methylcysteine in the animal body. *J. Biol. Chem.* **1934**, *105*, 481–488. [CrossRef]
3. Binkley, F.; Du Vigneato, V. The formation of cysteine from homocysteine and serine by liver tissue of rats. *J. Biol. Chem.* **1942**, *144*, 507–511. [CrossRef]
4. Hanson, H.; Eisfeld, G. Intermediary sulfur metabolism. III. Formation of hydrogen sulfide from cystine and cysteine by the liver. *Z. Gesamte Inn. Med.* **1952**, *7*, 801–810. [PubMed]
5. Chatagner, F.; Sauret-Ignazi, G. Role of transamination and pyridoxal phosphate in the enzymatic formation of hydrogen sulfide from cysteine by the rat liver under anaerobiosis. *Bull. Soc. Chim. Biol.* **1956**, *38*, 415–428.
6. Ubuka, T.; Yuasa, S.; Ishimoto, Y.; Shimomura, M. Desulfuration of l-cysteine through transamination and transsulfuration in rat liver. *Physiol. Chem. Phys.* **1977**, *9*, 241–246.
7. Stipanuk, M.H.; Beck, P.W. Characterization of the enzymic capacity for cysteine desulphhydration in liver and kidney of the rat. *Biochem. J.* **1982**, *206*, 267–277. [CrossRef]
8. Warenycia, M.W.; Goodwin, L.R.; Benishin, C.G.; Reiffenstein, R.J.; Francom, D.M.; Taylor, J.D.; Dieken, F.P. Acute hydrogen sulfide poisoning. Demonstration of selective uptake of sulfide by the brainstem by measurement of brain sulfide levels. *Biochem. Pharmacol.* **1989**, *38*, 973–981. [CrossRef]
9. Goodwin, L.R.; Francom, D.; Dieken, F.P.; Taylor, J.D.; Warenycia, M.W.; Reiffenstein, R.J.; Dowling, G. Determination of sulfide in brain tissue by gas dialysis/ion chromatography: Postmortem studies and two case reports. *J. Anal. Toxicol.* **1989**, *13*, 105–109. [CrossRef]
10. Abe, K.; Kimura, H. The possible role of hydrogen sulfide as an endogenous neuromodulator. *J. Neurosci.* **1996**, *16*, 1066–1071. [CrossRef]
11. Wang, R. Physiological implications of hydrogen sulfide: A whiff exploration that blossomed. *Physiol. Rev.* **2012**, *92*, 791–896. [CrossRef] [PubMed]
12. Haouzi, P.; Sonobe, T.; Judenherc-Haouzi, A. Hydrogen sulfide intoxication induced brain injury and methylene blue. *Neurobiol. Dis.* **2020**, *133*, 104474. [CrossRef]
13. Reiffenstein, R.J.; Hulbert, W.C.; Roth, S.H. Toxicology of hydrogen sulfide. *Annu. Rev. Pharmacol. Toxicol.* **1992**, *32*, 109–134. [CrossRef]
14. Nicholls, P.; Kim, J.K. Sulphide as an inhibitor and electron donor for the cytochrome c oxidase system. *Can. J. Biochem.* **1982**, *60*, 613–623. [CrossRef] [PubMed]
15. Blackstone, E.; Morrison, M.; Roth, M.B. H2S induces a suspended animation-like state in mice. *Science* **2005**, *308*, 518. [CrossRef]
16. Nicholls, P.; Marshall, D.C.; Cooper, C.E.; Wilson, M.T. Sulfide inhibition of and metabolism by cytochrome c oxidase. *Biochem. Soc. Trans.* **2013**, *41*, 1312–1316. [CrossRef] [PubMed]
17. Collman, J.P.; Ghosh, S.; Dey, A.; Decreau, R.A. Using a functional enzyme model to understand the chemistry behind hydrogen sulfide induced hibernation. *Proc. Natl. Acad. Sci. USA* **2009**, *106*, 22090–22095. [CrossRef]
18. Paul, B.D.; Snyder, S.H.; Kashfi, K. Effects of hydrogen sulfide on mitochondrial function and cellular bioenergetics. *Redox Biol.* **2021**, *38*, 101772. [CrossRef] [PubMed]
19. Modis, K.; Bos, E.M.; Calzia, E.; van Goor, H.; Coletta, C.; Papapetropoulos, A.; Hellmich, M.R.; Radermacher, P.; Bouillaud, F.; Szabo, C. Regulation of mitochondrial bioenergetic function by hydrogen sulfide. Part II. Pathophysiological and therapeutic aspects. *Br. J. Pharmacol.* **2014**, *171*, 2123–2146. [CrossRef]
20. Szabo, C.; Ransy, C.; Modis, K.; Andriamihaja, M.; Murghes, B.; Coletta, C.; Olah, G.; Yanagi, K.; Bouillaud, F. Regulation of mitochondrial bioenergetic function by hydrogen sulfide. Part I. Biochemical and physiological mechanisms. *Br. J. Pharmacol.* **2014**, *171*, 2099–2122. [CrossRef]
21. Cirino, G.; Szabo, C.; Papapetropoulos, A. Physiological roles of hydrogen sulfide in mammalian cells, tissues, and organs. *Physiol. Rev.* **2023**, *103*, 31–276. [CrossRef] [PubMed]
22. Panagaki, T.; Randi, E.B.; Augsburger, F.; Szabo, C. Overproduction of H(2)S, generated by CBS, inhibits mitochondrial Complex IV and suppresses oxidative phosphorylation in Down syndrome. *Proc. Natl. Acad. Sci. USA* **2019**, *116*, 18769–18771. [CrossRef] [PubMed]
23. Ichinohe, A.; Kanaumi, T.; Takashima, S.; Enokido, Y.; Nagai, Y.; Kimura, H. Cystathionine beta-synthase is enriched in the brains of Down's patients. *Biochem. Biophys. Res. Commun.* **2005**, *338*, 1547–1550. [CrossRef]

24. Szabo, C. The re-emerging pathophysiological role of the cystathionine-beta-synthase—Hydrogen sulfide system in Down syndrome. *FEBS J.* **2020**, *287*, 3150–3160. [CrossRef]
25. Barker, S.; Paul, B.D.; Pieper, A.A. Increased risk of aging-related neurodegenerative disease after traumatic brain injury. *biomedicines* **2023**, *11*, 1154. [CrossRef]
26. Paul, B.D.; Snyder, S.H. Modes of physiologic H2S signaling in the brain and peripheral tissues. *Antioxid. Redox Signal.* **2015**, *22*, 411–423. [CrossRef]
27. Sbodio, J.I.; Snyder, S.H.; Paul, B.D. Regulators of the transsulfuration pathway. *Br. J. Pharmacol.* **2019**, *176*, 583–593. [CrossRef]
28. Paul, B.D.; Snyder, S.H. Gasotransmitter hydrogen sulfide signaling in neuronal health and disease. *Biochem. Pharmacol.* **2018**, *149*, 101–109. [CrossRef]
29. Paul, B.D. Neuroprotective Roles of the Reverse Transsulfuration Pathway in Alzheimer's Disease. *Front Aging Neurosci* **2021**, *13*, 659402. [CrossRef]
30. Morikawa, T.; Kajimura, M.; Nakamura, T.; Hishiki, T.; Nakanishi, T.; Yukutake, Y.; Nagahata, Y.; Ishikawa, M.; Hattori, K.; Takenouchi, T.; et al. Hypoxic regulation of the cerebral microcirculation is mediated by a carbon monoxide-sensitive hydrogen sulfide pathway. *Proc. Natl. Acad. Sci. USA* **2012**, *109*, 1293–1298. [CrossRef] [PubMed]
31. Enokido, Y.; Suzuki, E.; Iwasawa, K.; Namekata, K.; Okazawa, H.; Kimura, H. Cystathionine beta-synthase, a key enzyme for homocysteine metabolism, is preferentially expressed in the radial glia/astrocyte lineage of developing mouse CNS. *FASEB J.* **2005**, *19*, 1854–1856. [CrossRef] [PubMed]
32. Shibuya, N.; Tanaka, M.; Yoshida, M.; Ogasawara, Y.; Togawa, T.; Ishii, K.; Kimura, H. 3-Mercaptopyruvate sulfurtransferase produces hydrogen sulfide and bound sulfane sulfur in the brain. *Antioxid. Redox Signal.* **2009**, *11*, 703–714. [CrossRef] [PubMed]
33. Shen, X.; Peter, E.A.; Bir, S.; Wang, R.; Kevil, C.G. Analytical measurement of discrete hydrogen sulfide pools in biological specimens. *Free Radic. Biol. Med.* **2012**, *52*, 2276–2283. [CrossRef] [PubMed]
34. Ishigami, M.; Hiraki, K.; Umemura, K.; Ogasawara, Y.; Ishii, K.; Kimura, H. A source of hydrogen sulfide and a mechanism of its release in the brain. *Antioxid. Redox Signal.* **2009**, *11*, 205–214. [CrossRef]
35. Khaspekov, L.G.; Frumkina, L.E. Molecular Mechanisms of Astrocyte Involvement in Synaptogenesis and Brain Synaptic Plasticity. *Biochemistry* **2023**, *88*, 502–514. [CrossRef]
36. Farizatto, K.L.G.; Baldwin, K.T. Astrocyte-synapse interactions during brain development. *Curr. Opin. Neurobiol.* **2023**, *80*, 102704. [CrossRef]
37. Jorgacevski, J.; Potokar, M. Immune Functions of Astrocytes in Viral Neuroinfections. *Int. J. Mol. Sci.* **2023**, *24*, 3514. [CrossRef]
38. Finkelstein, J.D.; Kyle, W.E.; Martin, J.L.; Pick, A.M. Activation of cystathionine synthase by adenosylmethionine and adenosylethionine. *Biochem. Biophys. Res. Commun.* **1975**, *66*, 81–87. [CrossRef]
39. Morrison, L.D.; Smith, D.D.; Kish, S.J. Brain S-adenosylmethionine levels are severely decreased in Alzheimer's disease. *J. Neurochem.* **1996**, *67*, 1328–1331. [CrossRef]
40. Linnebank, M.; Popp, J.; Smulders, Y.; Smith, D.; Semmler, A.; Farkas, M.; Kulic, L.; Cvetanovska, G.; Blom, H.; Stoffel-Wagner, B.; et al. S-adenosylmethionine is decreased in the cerebrospinal fluid of patients with Alzheimer's disease. *Neurodegener. Dis.* **2010**, *7*, 373–378. [CrossRef]
41. Kimura, H.; Shibuya, N.; Kimura, Y. Hydrogen sulfide is a signaling molecule and a cytoprotectant. *Antioxid. Redox Signal.* **2012**, *17*, 45–57. [CrossRef]
42. Kimura, Y.; Goto, Y.; Kimura, H. Hydrogen sulfide increases glutathione production and suppresses oxidative stress in mitochondria. *Antioxid. Redox Signal.* **2010**, *12*, 1–13. [CrossRef] [PubMed]
43. Sbodio, J.I.; Snyder, S.H.; Paul, B.D. Redox Mechanisms in Neurodegeneration: From Disease Outcomes to Therapeutic Opportunities. *Antioxid. Redox Signal.* **2019**, *30*, 1450–1499. [CrossRef]
44. Masters, C.L.; Bateman, R.; Blennow, K.; Rowe, C.C.; Sperling, R.A.; Cummings, J.L. Alzheimer's disease. *Nat. Rev. Dis. Primers* **2015**, *1*, 15056. [CrossRef] [PubMed]
45. Lane, C.A.; Hardy, J.; Schott, J.M. Alzheimer's disease. *Eur. J. Neurol.* **2018**, *25*, 59–70. [CrossRef] [PubMed]
46. 2022 Alzheimer's disease facts and figures. *Alzheimers Dement.* **2022**, *18*, 700–789. [CrossRef]
47. Braak, H.; Braak, E. Staging of Alzheimer's disease-related neurofibrillary changes. *Neurobiol. Aging* **1995**, *16*, 271–278, discussion 278–284. [CrossRef]
48. Braak, H.; Braak, E. Neuropathological stageing of Alzheimer-related changes. *Acta Neuropathol.* **1991**, *82*, 239–259. [CrossRef]
49. Snitz, B.E.; Weissfeld, L.A.; Lopez, O.L.; Kuller, L.H.; Saxton, J.; Singhabahu, D.M.; Klunk, W.E.; Mathis, C.A.; Price, J.C.; Ives, D.G.; et al. Cognitive trajectories associated with beta-amyloid deposition in the oldest-old without dementia. *Neurology* **2013**, *80*, 1378–1384. [CrossRef]
50. Rentz, D.M.; Locascio, J.J.; Becker, J.A.; Moran, E.K.; Eng, E.; Buckner, R.L.; Sperling, R.A.; Johnson, K.A. Cognition, reserve, and amyloid deposition in normal aging. *Ann. Neurol.* **2010**, *67*, 353–364. [CrossRef]
51. Alves, F.; Kallinowski, P.; Ayton, S. Accelerated Brain Volume Loss Caused by Anti-beta-Amyloid Drugs: A Systematic Review and Meta-analysis. *Neurology* **2023**. [CrossRef]
52. Paul, B.D.; Snyder, S.H. H(2)S signalling through protein sulfhydration and beyond. *Nat. Rev. Mol. Cell Biol.* **2012**, *13*, 499–507. [CrossRef]
53. Chen, X.; Jhee, K.H.; Kruger, W.D. Production of the neuromodulator H2S by cystathionine beta-synthase via the condensation of cysteine and homocysteine. *J. Biol. Chem.* **2004**, *279*, 52082–52086. [CrossRef]

54. Beard, R.S., Jr.; Bearden, S.E. Vascular complications of cystathionine beta-synthase deficiency: Future directions for homocysteine-to-hydrogen sulfide research. *Am. J. Physiol. Heart Circ. Physiol.* **2011**, *300*, H13–H26. [CrossRef]
55. Sen, U.; Mishra, P.K.; Tyagi, N.; Tyagi, S.C. Homocysteine to hydrogen sulfide or hypertension. *Cell Biochem. Biophys.* **2010**, *57*, 49–58. [CrossRef]
56. Kitzlerova, E.; Fisar, Z.; Jirak, R.; Zverova, M.; Hroudova, J.; Benakova, H.; Raboch, J. Plasma homocysteine in Alzheimer's disease with or without co-morbid depressive symptoms. *Neuro Endocrinol. Lett.* **2014**, *35*, 42–49.
57. Farina, N.; Jerneren, F.; Turner, C.; Hart, K.; Tabet, N. Homocysteine concentrations in the cognitive progression of Alzheimer's disease. *Exp. Gerontol.* **2017**, *99*, 146–150. [CrossRef] [PubMed]
58. McCaddon, A.; Davies, G.; Hudson, P.; Tandy, S.; Cattell, H. Total serum homocysteine in senile dementia of Alzheimer type. *Int. J. Geriatr. Psychiatry* **1998**, *13*, 235–239. [CrossRef]
59. Smith, A.D.; Refsum, H.; Bottiglieri, T.; Fenech, M.; Hooshmand, B.; McCaddon, A.; Miller, J.W.; Rosenberg, I.H.; Obeid, R. Homocysteine and Dementia: An International Consensus Statement. *J. Alzheimers Dis.* **2018**, *62*, 561–570. [CrossRef]
60. Clarke, R.; Smith, A.D.; Jobst, K.A.; Refsum, H.; Sutton, L.; Ueland, P.M. Folate, vitamin B12, and serum total homocysteine levels in confirmed Alzheimer disease. *Arch. Neurol.* **1998**, *55*, 1449–1455. [CrossRef] [PubMed]
61. Zhang, L.; Xie, X.; Sun, Y.; Zhou, F. Blood and CSF Homocysteine Levels in Alzheimer's Disease: A Meta-Analysis and Meta-Regression of Case-Control Studies. *Neuropsychiatr. Dis. Treat.* **2022**, *18*, 2391–2403. [CrossRef] [PubMed]
62. Castro, R.; Rivera, I.; Ravasco, P.; Jakobs, C.; Blom, H.J.; Camilo, M.E.; de Almeida, I.T. 5,10-Methylenetetrahydrofolate reductase 677C–>T and 1298A–>C mutations are genetic determinants of elevated homocysteine. *QJM* **2003**, *96*, 297–303. [CrossRef] [PubMed]
63. Wang, J.; Hegele, R.A. Genomic basis of cystathioninuria (MIM 219500) revealed by multiple mutations in cystathionine gamma-lyase (CTH). *Hum. Genet.* **2003**, *112*, 404–408. [CrossRef]
64. Wang, J.; Huff, A.M.; Spence, J.D.; Hegele, R.A. Single nucleotide polymorphism in CTH associated with variation in plasma homocysteine concentration. *Clin. Genet.* **2004**, *65*, 483–486. [CrossRef]
65. Wan, X.; Ma, B.; Wang, X.; Guo, C.; Sun, J.; Cui, J.; Li, L. S-Adenosylmethionine Alleviates Amyloid-beta-Induced Neural Injury by Enhancing Trans-Sulfuration Pathway Activity in Astrocytes. *J. Alzheimers Dis.* **2020**, *76*, 981–995. [CrossRef]
66. Li, Q.; Cui, J.; Fang, C.; Liu, M.; Min, G.; Li, L. S-Adenosylmethionine Attenuates Oxidative Stress and Neuroinflammation Induced by Amyloid-beta Through Modulation of Glutathione Metabolism. *J. Alzheimers Dis.* **2017**, *58*, 549–558. [CrossRef]
67. Forman, H.J.; Zhang, H.; Rinna, A. Glutathione: Overview of its protective roles, measurement, and biosynthesis. *Mol. Aspects Med.* **2009**, *30*, 1–12. [CrossRef]
68. Sedlak, T.W.; Paul, B.D.; Parker, G.M.; Hester, L.D.; Snowman, A.M.; Taniguchi, Y.; Kamiya, A.; Snyder, S.H.; Sawa, A. The glutathione cycle shapes synaptic glutamate activity. *Proc. Natl. Acad. Sci. USA* **2019**, *116*, 2701–2706. [CrossRef]
69. Griffith, O.W. Biologic and pharmacologic regulation of mammalian glutathione synthesis. *Free. Radic. Biol. Med.* **1999**, *27*, 922–935. [CrossRef] [PubMed]
70. Droge, W. Oxidative stress and ageing: Is ageing a cysteine deficiency syndrome? *Philos. Trans. R. Soc. Lond. B Biol. Sci.* **2005**, *360*, 2355–2372. [CrossRef]
71. Han, H.; Wang, F.; Chen, J.; Li, X.; Fu, G.; Zhou, J.; Zhou, D.; Wu, W.; Chen, H. Changes in Biothiol Levels Are Closely Associated with Alzheimer's Disease. *J. Alzheimers Dis.* **2021**, *82*, 527–540. [CrossRef] [PubMed]
72. Giovinazzo, D.; Bursac, B.; Sbodio, J.I.; Nalluru, S.; Vignane, T.; Snowman, A.M.; Albacarys, L.M.; Sedlak, T.W.; Torregrossa, R.; Whiteman, M.; et al. Hydrogen sulfide is neuroprotective in Alzheimer's disease by sulfhydrating GSK3beta and inhibiting Tau hyperphosphorylation. *Proc. Natl. Acad. Sci. USA* **2021**, *118*, e2017225118. [CrossRef] [PubMed]
73. Hodgson, N.; Trivedi, M.; Muratore, C.; Li, S.; Deth, R. Soluble oligomers of amyloid-beta cause changes in redox state, DNA methylation, and gene transcription by inhibiting EAAT3 mediated cysteine uptake. *J. Alzheimers Dis.* **2013**, *36*, 197–209. [CrossRef]
74. Duerson, K.; Woltjer, R.L.; Mookherjee, P.; Leverenz, J.B.; Montine, T.J.; Bird, T.D.; Pow, D.V.; Rauen, T.; Cook, D.G. Detergent-insoluble EAAC1/EAAT3 aberrantly accumulates in hippocampal neurons of Alzheimer's disease patients. *Brain Pathol.* **2009**, *19*, 267–278. [CrossRef]
75. Pontrello, C.G.; McWhirt, J.M.; Glabe, C.G.; Brewer, G.J. Age-Related Oxidative Redox and Metabolic Changes Precede Intraneuronal Amyloid-beta Accumulation and Plaque Deposition in a Transgenic Alzheimer's Disease Mouse Model. *J. Alzheimers Dis.* **2022**, *90*, 1501–1521. [CrossRef]
76. Ansari, M.A.; Scheff, S.W. Oxidative stress in the progression of Alzheimer disease in the frontal cortex. *J. Neuropathol. Exp. Neurol.* **2010**, *69*, 155–167. [CrossRef]
77. Zabel, M.; Nackenoff, A.; Kirsch, W.M.; Harrison, F.E.; Perry, G.; Schrag, M. Markers of oxidative damage to lipids, nucleic acids and proteins and antioxidant enzymes activities in Alzheimer's disease brain: A meta-analysis in human pathological specimens. *Free. Radic. Biol. Med.* **2018**, *115*, 351–360. [CrossRef] [PubMed]
78. Mandal, P.K.; Saharan, S.; Tripathi, M.; Murari, G. Brain glutathione levels–a novel biomarker for mild cognitive impairment and Alzheimer's disease. *Biol. Psychiatry* **2015**, *78*, 702–710. [CrossRef] [PubMed]
79. Shukla, D.; Mandal, P.K.; Mishra, R.; Punjabi, K.; Dwivedi, D.; Tripathi, M.; Badhautia, V. Hippocampal Glutathione Depletion and pH Increment in Alzheimer's Disease: An in vivo MRS Study. *J. Alzheimers Dis.* **2021**, *84*, 1139–1152. [CrossRef]

80. Chen, J.J.; Thiyagarajah, M.; Song, J.; Chen, C.; Herrmann, N.; Gallagher, D.; Rapoport, M.J.; Black, S.E.; Ramirez, J.; Andreazza, A.C.; et al. Altered central and blood glutathione in Alzheimer's disease and mild cognitive impairment: A meta-analysis. *Alzheimers Res. Ther.* **2022**, *14*, 23. [CrossRef]
81. Dwivedi, D.; Megha, K.; Mishra, R.; Mandal, P.K. Glutathione in Brain: Overview of Its Conformations, Functions, Biochemical Characteristics, Quantitation and Potential Therapeutic Role in Brain Disorders. *Neurochem. Res.* **2020**, *45*, 1461–1480. [CrossRef]
82. Navarro, J.F.; Croteau, D.L.; Jurek, A.; Andrusivova, Z.; Yang, B.; Wang, Y.; Ogedegbe, B.; Riaz, T.; Stoen, M.; Desler, C.; et al. Spatial Transcriptomics Reveals Genes Associated with Dysregulated Mitochondrial Functions and Stress Signaling in Alzheimer Disease. *iScience* **2020**, *23*, 101556. [CrossRef]
83. Thornalley, P.J. Glyoxalase I–structure, function and a critical role in the enzymatic defence against glycation. *Biochem. Soc. Trans.* **2003**, *31*, 1343–1348. [CrossRef]
84. Eto, K.; Asada, T.; Arima, K.; Makifuchi, T.; Kimura, H. Brain hydrogen sulfide is severely decreased in Alzheimer's disease. *Biochem. Biophys. Res. Commun.* **2002**, *293*, 1485–1488. [CrossRef] [PubMed]
85. Liu, X.Q.; Liu, X.Q.; Jiang, P.; Huang, H.; Yan, Y. Plasma levels of endogenous hydrogen sulfide and homocysteine in patients with Alzheimer's disease and vascular dementia and the significance thereof. *Zhonghua Yi Xue Za Zhi* **2008**, *88*, 2246–2249.
86. Sun, P.; Chen, H.C.; Lu, S.; Hai, J.; Guo, W.; Jing, Y.H.; Wang, B. Simultaneous Sensing of H(2)S and ATP with a Two-Photon Fluorescent Probe in Alzheimer's Disease: Toward Understanding Why H(2)S Regulates Glutamate-Induced ATP Dysregulation. *Anal. Chem.* **2022**, *94*, 11573–11581. [CrossRef] [PubMed]
87. Zhang, J.Y.; Ma, S.; Liu, X.; Du, Y.; Zhu, X.; Liu, Y.; Wu, X. Activating transcription factor 6 regulates cystathionine to increase autophagy and restore memory in Alzheimer's disease model mice. *Biochem. Biophys. Res. Commun.* **2022**, *615*, 109–115. [CrossRef] [PubMed]
88. Fan, H.; Guo, Y.; Liang, X.; Yuan, Y.; Qi, X.; Wang, M.; Ma, J.; Zhou, H. Hydrogen sulfide protects against amyloid beta-peptide induced neuronal injury via attenuating inflammatory responses in a rat model. *J. Biomed. Res.* **2013**, *27*, 296–304. [CrossRef] [PubMed]
89. Liu, Y.Y.; Bian, J.S. Hydrogen sulfide protects amyloid-beta induced cell toxicity in microglia. *J. Alzheimers Dis.* **2010**, *22*, 1189–1200. [CrossRef] [PubMed]
90. Tang, X.Q.; Yang, C.T.; Chen, J.; Yin, W.L.; Tian, S.W.; Hu, B.; Feng, J.Q.; Li, Y.J. Effect of hydrogen sulphide on beta-amyloid-induced damage in PC12 cells. *Clin. Exp. Pharmacol. Physiol.* **2008**, *35*, 180–186. [CrossRef]
91. Zhang, H.; Gao, Y.; Zhao, F.; Dai, Z.; Meng, T.; Tu, S.; Yan, Y. Hydrogen sulfide reduces mRNA and protein levels of beta-site amyloid precursor protein cleaving enzyme 1 in PC12 cells. *Neurochem. Int.* **2011**, *58*, 169–175. [CrossRef]
92. Xuan, A.; Long, D.; Li, J.; Ji, W.; Zhang, M.; Hong, L.; Liu, J. Hydrogen sulfide attenuates spatial memory impairment and hippocampal neuroinflammation in beta-amyloid rat model of Alzheimer's disease. *J. Neuroinflammation* **2012**, *9*, 202. [CrossRef]
93. Giuliani, D.; Ottani, A.; Zaffe, D.; Galantucci, M.; Strinati, F.; Lodi, R.; Guarini, S. Hydrogen sulfide slows down progression of experimental Alzheimer's disease by targeting multiple pathophysiological mechanisms. *Neurobiol. Learn. Mem.* **2013**, *104*, 82–91. [CrossRef]
94. Ali, R.; Hameed, R.; Chauhan, D.; Sen, S.; Wahajuddin, M.; Nazir, A.; Verma, S. Multiple Actions of H(2)S-Releasing Peptides in Human beta-Amyloid Expressing C. elegans. *ACS Chem. Neurosci.* **2022**, *13*, 3378–3388. [CrossRef]
95. Xi, Y.; Zhang, Y.; Zhou, Y.; Liu, Q.; Chen, X.; Liu, X.; Grune, T.; Shi, L.; Hou, M.; Liu, Z. Effects of methionine intake on cognitive function in mild cognitive impairment patients and APP/PS1 Alzheimer's Disease model mice: Role of the cystathionine-beta-synthase/H(2)S pathway. *Redox Biol.* **2023**, *59*, 102595. [CrossRef]
96. Rose, P.; Moore, P.K.; Zhu, Y.Z. Garlic and Gaseous Mediators. *Trends Pharmacol. Sci.* **2018**, *39*, 624–634. [CrossRef] [PubMed]
97. Benavides, G.A.; Squadrito, G.L.; Mills, R.W.; Patel, H.D.; Isbell, T.S.; Patel, R.P.; Darley-Usmar, V.M.; Doeller, J.E.; Kraus, D.W. Hydrogen sulfide mediates the vasoactivity of garlic. *Proc. Natl. Acad. Sci. USA* **2007**, *104*, 17977–17982. [CrossRef]
98. Liang, D.; Wu, H.; Wong, M.W.; Huang, D. Diallyl Trisulfide Is a Fast H2S Donor, but Diallyl Disulfide Is a Slow One: The Reaction Pathways and Intermediates of Glutathione with Polysulfides. *Org. Lett.* **2015**, *17*, 4196–4199. [CrossRef]
99. Chuah, S.C.; Moore, P.K.; Zhu, Y.Z. S-allylcysteine mediates cardioprotection in an acute myocardial infarction rat model via a hydrogen sulfide-mediated pathway. *Am. J. Physiol. Heart Circ. Physiol.* **2007**, *293*, H2693–H2701. [CrossRef] [PubMed]
100. Ghazimoradi, M.M.; Ghoushi, E.; Ghobadi Pour, M.; Karimi Ahmadabadi, H.; Rafieian-Kopaei, M. A review on garlic as a supplement for Alzheimer's disease: A mechanistic insight into its direct and indirect effects. *Curr. Pharm. Des.* **2023**, *29*, 519–526. [CrossRef]
101. Ray, B.; Chauhan, N.B.; Lahiri, D.K. The "aged garlic extract:" (AGE) and one of its active ingredients S-allyl-L-cysteine (SAC) as potential preventive and therapeutic agents for Alzheimer's disease (AD). *Curr. Med. Chem.* **2011**, *18*, 3306–3313. [CrossRef] [PubMed]
102. Chauhan, N.B. Effect of aged garlic extract on APP processing and tau phosphorylation in Alzheimer's transgenic model Tg2576. *J. Ethnopharmacol.* **2006**, *108*, 385–394. [CrossRef] [PubMed]
103. Tedeschi, P.; Nigro, M.; Travagli, A.; Catani, M.; Cavazzini, A.; Merighi, S.; Gessi, S. Therapeutic Potential of Allicin and Aged Garlic Extract in Alzheimer's Disease. *Int. J. Mol. Sci.* **2022**, *23*, 6950. [CrossRef] [PubMed]
104. Griffin, B.; Selassie, M.; Gwebu, E.T. Effect of Aged Garlic Extract on the Cytotoxicity of Alzheimer beta-Amyloid Peptide in Neuronal PC12 Cells. *Nutr. Neurosci.* **2000**, *3*, 139–142. [CrossRef]

105. Gupta, V.B.; Indi, S.S.; Rao, K.S. Garlic extract exhibits antiamyloidogenic activity on amyloid-beta fibrillogenesis: Relevance to Alzheimer's disease. *Phytother. Res.* **2009**, *23*, 111–115. [CrossRef]
106. Luo, J.F.; Dong, Y.; Chen, J.Y.; Lu, J.H. The effect and underlying mechanisms of garlic extract against cognitive impairment and Alzheimer's disease: A systematic review and meta-analysis of experimental animal studies. *J. Ethnopharmacol.* **2021**, *280*, 114423. [CrossRef]
107. He, X.L.; Yan, N.; Zhang, H.; Qi, Y.W.; Zhu, L.J.; Liu, M.J.; Yan, Y. Hydrogen sulfide improves spatial memory impairment and decreases production of Abeta in APP/PS1 transgenic mice. *Neurochem. Int.* **2014**, *67*, 1–8. [CrossRef]
108. Yang, Y.J.; Zhao, Y.; Yu, B.; Xu, G.G.; Wang, W.; Zhan, J.Q.; Tang, Z.Y.; Wang, T.; Wei, B. GluN2B-containing NMDA receptors contribute to the beneficial effects of hydrogen sulfide on cognitive and synaptic plasticity deficits in APP/PS1 transgenic mice. *Neuroscience* **2016**, *335*, 170–183. [CrossRef]
109. Zhao, F.L.; Qiao, P.F.; Yan, N.; Gao, D.; Liu, M.J.; Yan, Y. Hydrogen Sulfide Selectively Inhibits gamma-Secretase Activity and Decreases Mitochondrial Abeta Production in Neurons from APP/PS1 Transgenic Mice. *Neurochem. Res.* **2016**, *41*, 1145–1159. [CrossRef]
110. Li, X.H.; Deng, Y.Y.; Li, F.; Shi, J.S.; Gong, Q.H. Neuroprotective effects of sodium hydrosulfide against beta-amyloid-induced neurotoxicity. *Int. J. Mol. Med.* **2016**, *38*, 1152–1160. [CrossRef]
111. Cui, W.; Zhang, Y.; Yang, C.; Sun, Y.; Zhang, M.; Wang, S. Hydrogen sulfide prevents Abeta-induced neuronal apoptosis by attenuating mitochondrial translocation of PTEN. *Neuroscience* **2016**, *325*, 165–174. [CrossRef]
112. Liu, Y.; Deng, Y.; Liu, H.; Yin, C.; Li, X.; Gong, Q. Hydrogen sulfide ameliorates learning memory impairment in APP/PS1 transgenic mice: A novel mechanism mediated by the activation of Nrf2. *Pharmacol. Biochem. Behav.* **2016**, *150–151*, 207–216. [CrossRef] [PubMed]
113. Sestito, S.; Daniele, S.; Pietrobono, D.; Citi, V.; Bellusci, L.; Chiellini, G.; Calderone, V.; Martini, C.; Rapposelli, S. Memantine prodrug as a new agent for Alzheimer's Disease. *Sci. Rep.* **2019**, *9*, 4612. [CrossRef] [PubMed]
114. Rao, S.P.; Xie, W.; Christopher Kwon, Y.I.; Juckel, N.; Xie, J.; Dronamraju, V.R.; Vince, R.; Lee, M.K.; More, S.S. Sulfanegen stimulates 3-mercaptopyruvate sulfurtransferase activity and ameliorates Alzheimer's disease pathology and oxidative stress in vivo. *Redox Biol.* **2022**, *57*, 102484. [CrossRef] [PubMed]
115. Salehpour, M.; Ashabi, G.; Kashef, M.; Marashi, E.S.; Ghasemi, T. Aerobic Training with Naringin Supplementation Improved Spatial Cognition via H(2)S Signaling Pathway in Alzheimer's Disease Model Rats. *Exp. Aging Res.* **2022**, 1–14. [CrossRef]
116. Aboulhoda, B.E.; Rashed, L.A.; Ahmed, H.; Obaya, E.M.M.; Ibrahim, W.; Alkafass, M.A.L.; Abd El-Aal, S.A.; ShamsEldeen, A.M. Hydrogen sulfide and mesenchymal stem cells-extracted microvesicles attenuate LPS-induced Alzheimer's disease. *J. Cell. Physiol.* **2021**, *236*, 5994–6010. [CrossRef] [PubMed]
117. Kamat, P.K.; Kyles, P.; Kalani, A.; Tyagi, N. Hydrogen Sulfide Ameliorates Homocysteine-Induced Alzheimer's Disease-Like Pathology, Blood-Brain Barrier Disruption, and Synaptic Disorder. *Mol. Neurobiol.* **2016**, *53*, 2451–2467. [CrossRef] [PubMed]
118. Huang, H.J.; Chen, S.L.; Hsieh-Li, H.M. Administration of NaHS Attenuates Footshock-Induced Pathologies and Emotional and Cognitive Dysfunction in Triple Transgenic Alzheimer's Mice. *Front. Behav. Neurosci.* **2015**, *9*, 312. [CrossRef]
119. Vandini, E.; Ottani, A.; Zaffe, D.; Calevro, A.; Canalini, F.; Cavallini, G.M.; Rossi, R.; Guarini, S.; Giuliani, D. Mechanisms of Hydrogen Sulfide against the Progression of Severe Alzheimer's Disease in Transgenic Mice at Different Ages. *Pharmacology* **2019**, *103*, 50–60. [CrossRef]
120. Mustafa, A.K.; Gadalla, M.M.; Sen, N.; Kim, S.; Mu, W.; Gazi, S.K.; Barrow, R.K.; Yang, G.; Wang, R.; Snyder, S.H. H2S signals through protein S-sulfhydration. *Sci. Signal.* **2009**, *2*, ra72. [CrossRef]
121. Paul, B.D.; Snyder, S.H. H2S: A Novel Gasotransmitter that Signals by Sulfhydration. *Trends Biochem. Sci.* **2015**, *40*, 687–700. [CrossRef]
122. Petrovic, D.; Kouroussis, E.; Vignane, T.; Filipovic, M.R. The Role of Protein Persulfidation in Brain Aging and Neurodegeneration. *Front. Aging Neurosci.* **2021**, *13*, 674135. [CrossRef] [PubMed]
123. Doka, E.; Pader, I.; Biro, A.; Johansson, K.; Cheng, Q.; Ballago, K.; Prigge, J.R.; Pastor-Flores, D.; Dick, T.P.; Schmidt, E.E.; et al. A novel persulfide detection method reveals protein persulfide- and polysulfide-reducing functions of thioredoxin and glutathione systems. *Sci. Adv.* **2016**, *2*, e1500968. [CrossRef]
124. Krishnan, N.; Fu, C.; Pappin, D.J.; Tonks, N.K. H2S-Induced sulfhydration of the phosphatase PTP1B and its role in the endoplasmic reticulum stress response. *Sci. Signal.* **2011**, *4*, ra86. [CrossRef]
125. Wedmann, R.; Onderka, C.; Wei, S.; Szijarto, I.A.; Miljkovic, J.L.; Mitrovic, A.; Lange, M.; Savitsky, S.; Yadav, P.K.; Torregrossa, R.; et al. Improved tag-switch method reveals that thioredoxin acts as depersulfidase and controls the intracellular levels of protein persulfidation. *Chem. Sci.* **2016**, *7*, 3414–3426. [CrossRef]
126. Vandiver, M.S.; Paul, B.D.; Xu, R.; Karuppagounder, S.; Rao, F.; Snowman, A.M.; Ko, H.S.; Lee, Y.I.; Dawson, V.L.; Dawson, T.M.; et al. Sulfhydration mediates neuroprotective actions of parkin. *Nat. Commun.* **2013**, *4*, 1626. [CrossRef]
127. Paul, B.D.; Sbodio, J.I.; Snyder, S.H. Mutant Huntingtin Derails Cysteine Metabolism in Huntington's Disease at Both Transcriptional and Post-Translational Levels. *Antioxidants* **2022**, *11*, 1470. [CrossRef] [PubMed]
128. Sbodio, J.I.; Snyder, S.H.; Paul, B.D. Golgi stress response reprograms cysteine metabolism to confer cytoprotection in Huntington's disease. *Proc. Natl. Acad. Sci. USA* **2018**, *115*, 780–785. [CrossRef]

129. Snijder, P.M.; Baratashvili, M.; Grzeschik, N.A.; Leuvenink, H.G.D.; Kuijpers, L.; Huitema, S.; Schaap, O.; Giepmans, B.N.G.; Kuipers, J.; Miljkovic, J.L.; et al. Overexpression of Cystathionine gamma-Lyase Suppresses Detrimental Effects of Spinocerebellar Ataxia Type 3. *Mol. Med.* **2016**, *21*, 758–768. [CrossRef] [PubMed]
130. Zivanovic, J.; Kouroussis, E.; Kohl, J.B.; Adhikari, B.; Bursac, B.; Schott-Roux, S.; Petrovic, D.; Miljkovic, J.L.; Thomas-Lopez, D.; Jung, Y.; et al. Selective Persulfide Detection Reveals Evolutionarily Conserved Antiaging Effects of S-Sulfhydration. *Cell Metab.* **2019**, *30*, 1152–1170.e1113. [CrossRef]
131. Ji, D.; Luo, C.; Liu, J.; Cao, Y.; Wu, J.; Yan, W.; Xue, K.; Chai, J.; Zhu, X.; Wu, Y.; et al. Insufficient S-Sulfhydration of Methylenetetrahydrofolate Reductase Contributes to the Progress of Hyperhomocysteinemia. *Antioxid. Redox Signal.* **2022**, *36*, 1–14. [CrossRef]
132. Yin, W.L.; He, J.Q.; Hu, B.; Jiang, Z.S.; Tang, X.Q. Hydrogen sulfide inhibits MPP$^+$-induced apoptosis in PC12 cells. *Life Sci.* **2009**, *85*, 269–275. [CrossRef]
133. Kimura, Y.; Kimura, H. Hydrogen sulfide protects neurons from oxidative stress. *FASEB J.* **2004**, *18*, 1165–1167. [CrossRef] [PubMed]
134. Zhang, M.; Shan, H.; Wang, T.; Liu, W.; Wang, Y.; Wang, L.; Zhang, L.; Chang, P.; Dong, W.; Chen, X.; et al. Dynamic change of hydrogen sulfide after traumatic brain injury and its effect in mice. *Neurochem. Res.* **2013**, *38*, 714–725. [CrossRef] [PubMed]
135. Jiang, X.; Huang, Y.; Lin, W.; Gao, D.; Fei, Z. Protective effects of hydrogen sulfide in a rat model of traumatic brain injury via activation of mitochondrial adenosine triphosphate-sensitive potassium channels and reduction of oxidative stress. *J. Surg. Res.* **2013**, *184*, e27–e35. [CrossRef] [PubMed]
136. Zhang, M.; Shan, H.; Chang, P.; Wang, T.; Dong, W.; Chen, X.; Tao, L. Hydrogen sulfide offers neuroprotection on traumatic brain injury in parallel with reduced apoptosis and autophagy in mice. *PLoS ONE* **2014**, *9*, e87241. [CrossRef]
137. Karimi, S.A.; Hosseinmardi, N.; Janahmadi, M.; Sayyah, M.; Hajisoltani, R. The protective effect of hydrogen sulfide (H(2)S) on traumatic brain injury (TBI) induced memory deficits in rats. *Brain Res. Bull.* **2017**, *134*, 177–182. [CrossRef]
138. Xu, K.; Wu, F.; Xu, K.; Li, Z.; Wei, X.; Lu, Q.; Jiang, T.; Wu, F.; Xu, X.; Xiao, J.; et al. NaHS restores mitochondrial function and inhibits autophagy by activating the PI3K/Akt/mTOR signalling pathway to improve functional recovery after traumatic brain injury. *Chem. Biol. Interact.* **2018**, *286*, 96–105. [CrossRef]
139. Campolo, M.; Esposito, E.; Ahmad, A.; Di Paola, R.; Paterniti, I.; Cordaro, M.; Bruschetta, G.; Wallace, J.L.; Cuzzocrea, S. Hydrogen sulfide-releasing cyclooxygenase inhibitor ATB-346 enhances motor function and reduces cortical lesion volume following traumatic brain injury in mice. *J. Neuroinflamm.* **2014**, *11*, 196. [CrossRef]
140. Zhang, M.; Shan, H.; Chang, P.; Ma, L.; Chu, Y.; Shen, X.; Wu, Q.; Wang, Z.; Luo, C.; Wang, T.; et al. Upregulation of 3-MST Relates to Neuronal Autophagy After Traumatic Brain Injury in Mice. *Cell. Mol. Neurobiol.* **2017**, *37*, 291–302. [CrossRef]
141. Sun, J.; Li, X.; Gu, X.; Du, H.; Zhang, G.; Wu, J.; Wang, F. Neuroprotective effect of hydrogen sulfide against glutamate-induced oxidative stress is mediated via the p53/glutaminase 2 pathway after traumatic brain injury. *Aging* **2021**, *13*, 7180–7189. [CrossRef]
142. Huerta de la Cruz, S.; Rocha, L.; Santiago-Castaneda, C.; Sanchez-Lopez, A.; Pinedo-Rodriguez, A.D.; Medina-Terol, G.J.; Centurion, D. Hydrogen Sulfide Subchronic Treatment Improves Hypertension Induced by Traumatic Brain Injury in Rats through Vasopressor Sympathetic Outflow Inhibition. *J. Neurotrauma* **2022**, *39*, 181–195. [CrossRef]
143. Lopez-Preza, F.I.; Huerta de la Cruz, S.; Santiago-Castaneda, C.; Silva-Velasco, D.L.; Beltran-Ornelas, J.H.; Tapia-Martinez, J.; Sanchez-Lopez, A.; Rocha, L.; Centurion, D. Hydrogen sulfide prevents the vascular dysfunction induced by severe traumatic brain injury in rats by reducing reactive oxygen species and modulating eNOS and H(2)S-synthesizing enzyme expression. *Life Sci.* **2023**, *312*, 121218. [CrossRef]
144. Kehrer, J.P. The Haber-Weiss reaction and mechanisms of toxicity. *Toxicology* **2000**, *149*, 43–50. [CrossRef]
145. Lin, Q.; Shahid, S.; Hone-Blanchet, A.; Huang, S.; Wu, J.; Bisht, A.; Loring, D.; Goldstein, F.; Levey, A.; Crosson, B.; et al. Magnetic resonance evidence of increased iron content in subcortical brain regions in asymptomatic Alzheimer's disease. *Hum. Brain Mapp.* **2023**. [CrossRef] [PubMed]
146. Kenkhuis, B.; Bush, A.I.; Ayton, S. How iron can drive neurodegeneration. *Trends Neurosci.* **2023**, *46*, 333–335. [CrossRef]
147. Mahoney-Sanchez, L.; Bouchaoui, H.; Ayton, S.; Devos, D.; Duce, J.A.; Devedjian, J.C. Ferroptosis and its potential role in the physiopathology of Parkinson's Disease. *Prog. Neurobiol.* **2021**, *196*, 101890. [CrossRef]
148. Robicsek, S.A.; Bhattacharya, A.; Rabai, F.; Shukla, K.; Dore, S. Blood-Related Toxicity after Traumatic Brain Injury: Potential Targets for Neuroprotection. *Mol. Neurobiol.* **2020**, *57*, 159–178. [CrossRef]
149. Nisenbaum, E.J.; Novikov, D.S.; Lui, Y.W. The presence and role of iron in mild traumatic brain injury: An imaging perspective. *J. Neurotrauma* **2014**, *31*, 301–307. [CrossRef] [PubMed]
150. Braughler, J.M.; Duncan, L.A.; Chase, R.L. The involvement of iron in lipid peroxidation. Importance of ferric to ferrous ratios in initiation. *J. Biol. Chem.* **1986**, *261*, 10282–10289. [CrossRef] [PubMed]
151. Dixon, S.J.; Lemberg, K.M.; Lamprecht, M.R.; Skouta, R.; Zaitsev, E.M.; Gleason, C.E.; Patel, D.N.; Bauer, A.J.; Cantley, A.M.; Yang, W.S.; et al. Ferroptosis: An iron-dependent form of nonapoptotic cell death. *Cell* **2012**, *149*, 1060–1072. [CrossRef]
152. Ashraf, A.; Jeandriens, J.; Parkes, H.G.; So, P.W. Iron dyshomeostasis, lipid peroxidation and perturbed expression of cystine/glutamate antiporter in Alzheimer's disease: Evidence of ferroptosis. *Redox Biol.* **2020**, *32*, 101494. [CrossRef] [PubMed]
153. Wu, Y.; Torabi, S.F.; Lake, R.J.; Hong, S.; Yu, Z.; Wu, P.; Yang, Z.; Nelson, K.; Guo, W.; Pawel, G.T.; et al. Simultaneous Fe^{2+}/Fe^{3+} imaging shows Fe^{3+} over Fe^{2+} enrichment in Alzheimer's disease mouse brain. *Sci. Adv.* **2023**, *9*, eade7622. [CrossRef] [PubMed]

154. Stockwell, B.R. Ferroptosis turns 10: Emerging mechanisms, physiological functions, and therapeutic applications. *Cell* **2022**, *185*, 2401–2421. [CrossRef]
155. Wang, Y.; Ying, X.; Wang, Y.; Zou, Z.; Yuan, A.; Xiao, Z.; Geng, N.; Qiao, Z.; Li, W.; Lu, X.; et al. Hydrogen sulfide alleviates mitochondrial damage and ferroptosis by regulating OPA3-NFS1 axis in doxorubicin-induced cardiotoxicity. *Cell. Signal.* **2023**, *107*, 110655. [CrossRef]
156. Yu, Y.; Li, X.; Wu, X.; Li, X.; Wei, J.; Chen, X.; Sun, Z.; Zhang, Q. Sodium hydrosulfide inhibits hemin-induced ferroptosis and lipid peroxidation in BV2 cells via the CBS/H(2)S system. *Cell. Signal.* **2023**, *104*, 110594. [CrossRef] [PubMed]
157. Yu, M.; Wang, W.; Dang, J.; Liu, B.; Xu, J.; Li, J.; Liu, Y.; He, L.; Ying, Y.; Cai, J.; et al. Hydrogen sulfide protects retinal pigment epithelium cells against ferroptosis through the AMPK- and p62-dependent non-canonical NRF2-KEAP1 pathway. *Exp. Cell Res.* **2023**, *422*, 113436. [CrossRef]
158. Wallace, J.L.; Nagy, P.; Feener, T.D.; Allain, T.; Ditroi, T.; Vaughan, D.J.; Muscara, M.N.; de Nucci, G.; Buret, A.G. A proof-of-concept, Phase 2 clinical trial of the gastrointestinal safety of a hydrogen sulfide-releasing anti-inflammatory drug. *Br. J. Pharmacol.* **2020**, *177*, 769–777. [CrossRef]

Disclaimer/Publisher's Note: The statements, opinions and data contained in all publications are solely those of the individual author(s) and contributor(s) and not of MDPI and/or the editor(s). MDPI and/or the editor(s) disclaim responsibility for any injury to people or property resulting from any ideas, methods, instructions or products referred to in the content.

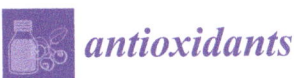

Review

H₂S Donors with Cytoprotective Effects in Models of MI/R Injury and Chemotherapy-Induced Cardiotoxicity

Qiwei Hu and John C. Lukesh III *

Department of Chemistry, Wake Forest University, Wake Downtown Campus, 455 Vine Street, Winston-Salem, NC 27101, USA
* Correspondence: lukeshjc@wfu.edu

Abstract: Hydrogen sulfide (H_2S) is an endogenous signaling molecule that greatly influences several important (patho)physiological processes related to cardiovascular health and disease, including vasodilation, angiogenesis, inflammation, and cellular redox homeostasis. Consequently, H_2S supplementation is an emerging area of interest, especially for the treatment of cardiovascular-related diseases. To fully unlock the medicinal properties of hydrogen sulfide, however, the development and refinement of H_2S releasing compounds (or donors) are required to augment its bioavailability and to better mimic its natural enzymatic production. Categorizing donors by the biological stimulus that triggers their H_2S release, this review highlights the fundamental chemistry and releasing mechanisms of a range of H_2S donors that have exhibited promising protective effects in models of myocardial ischemia-reperfusion (MI/R) injury and cancer chemotherapy-induced cardiotoxicity, specifically. Thus, in addition to serving as important investigative tools that further advance our knowledge and understanding of H_2S chemical biology, the compounds highlighted in this review have the potential to serve as vital therapeutic agents for the treatment (or prevention) of various cardiomyopathies.

Keywords: hydrogen sulfide; H_2S donors; cardioprotection; MI/R injury; chemotherapy-induced cardiotoxicity; H_2S codrugs

Citation: Hu, Q.; Lukesh, J.C., III H₂S Donors with Cytoprotective Effects in Models of MI/R Injury and Chemotherapy-Induced Cardiotoxicity. *Antioxidants* **2023**, *12*, 650. https://doi.org/10.3390/antiox12030650

Academic Editors: John Toscano and Vinayak Khodade

Received: 26 January 2023
Revised: 21 February 2023
Accepted: 28 February 2023
Published: 5 March 2023

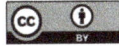

Copyright: © 2023 by the authors. Licensee MDPI, Basel, Switzerland. This article is an open access article distributed under the terms and conditions of the Creative Commons Attribution (CC BY) license (https://creativecommons.org/licenses/by/4.0/).

1. Introduction

Hydrogen sulfide (H_2S) is a malodorous, toxic, and flammable gas that was once disregarded as a mere environmental and industrial pollutant [1–3]. Landmark studies near the turn of the 20th century [4–6], however, revealed that H_2S is also a biologically active gas that is expressed in mammalian systems, primarily via the enzymatic metabolism of cysteine and homocysteine [7]. From these reports, a paradigm shift ensued, and today H_2S is regarded as the third gasotransmitter, alongside nitric oxide (NO) and carbon monoxide (CO) [8–11].

H_2S is soluble in water (~80 mM at 37 °C [12]) and exhibits weak acidity that gives rise to an equilibrium between its diprotic (H_2S) and hydrosulfide (HS^-) forms in an aqueous environment. With a pK_{a1} of 6.98 [12], its HS^- form dominates at physiological pH and begets its high reactivity and strong nucleophilic character under biologically relevant conditions.

In its diprotic form, its lipophilicity, low molecular weight, and gaseous nature enable H_2S to easily traverse the lipid bilayer, allowing it to act on intracellular targets that mediate numerous physiological and pathophysiological processes within the human body [13–16]. Its proven ability to reduce oxidative stress and inflammation [17–19], induce vasodilation [6], and promote angiogenesis [20] underscores the positive influence of H_2S on the cardiovascular system, specifically. Not surprisingly, small molecule donors that improve the exogenous delivery and bioavailability of H_2S are currently being investigated with great enthusiasm as potential cardioprotective agents [21].

This review will summarize the structure, reactivity, and mode of delivery for H$_2$S donors that have displayed promising cardioprotective effects in myocardial ischemia-reperfusion (MI/R) injury and cancer chemotherapeutic-induced cardiotoxicity models, in particular. Thus, the compounds reported on herein not only represent important investigative tools for probing the chemical biology of hydrogen sulfide but may also serve to unlock its vast therapeutic potential for the treatment of cardiovascular-related diseases.

2. H$_2$S Biosynthesis and Metabolism

In mammals, both enzymatic and nonenzymatic pathways are involved in H$_2$S biosynthesis, with the former being the principal route towards its formation. The use of enzymes provides strict spatiotemporal control over the production of H$_2$S, resulting in concentration variances in specific tissues and cellular compartments, and in response to certain physiological and pathophysiological events. The three enzymes primarily responsible for H$_2$S biosynthesis are cystathionine β-synthase (CBS) [22], cystathionine γ-lyase (CSE) [23], and 3-mercaptopyruvate sulfurtransferase (3-MST) [24].

CBS and CSE are ubiquitous enzymes of the transsulfuration pathway that facilitate the conversion of homocysteine to cysteine via the intermediate cystathionine (Figure 1) [25,26]. Both are pyridoxal 5′-phosphate (PLP)-dependent enzymes that are primarily located in the cytosol and generate H$_2$S via the direct desulfhydration of cysteine and homocysteine. In addition to being primarily responsible for H$_2$S biosynthesis in the brain and central nervous system, CBS is amply expressed in the ileum, kidneys, liver, and uterus [5,27,28]. CSE, on the other hand, exhibits low expression levels in the central nervous system but is the principal H$_2$S-producing enzyme of the cardiovascular system [29].

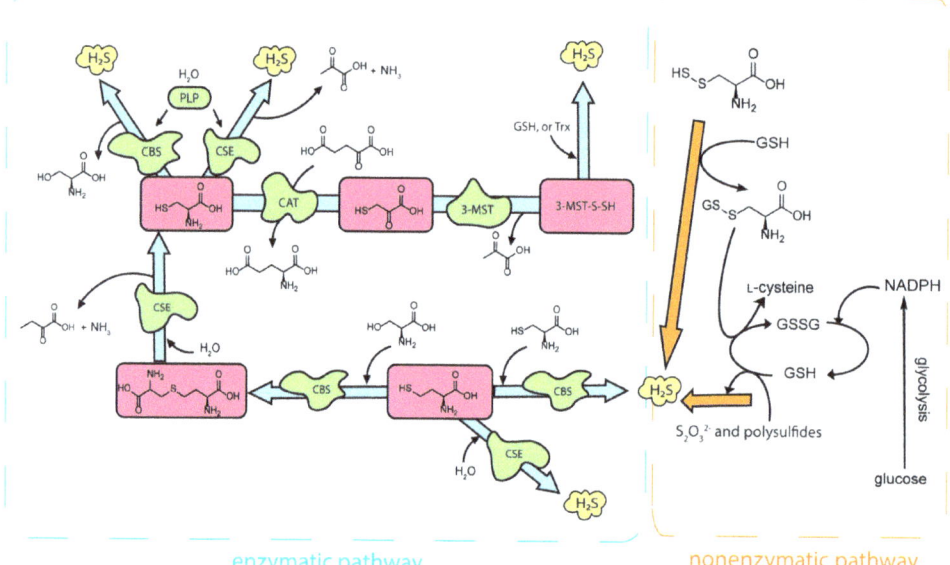

Figure 1. Enzymatic and nonenzymatic production of H$_2$S in mammalian systems. PLP: pyridoxal 5′-phosphate; CBS: cystathionine β-synthase; CSE: cystathionine γ-lyase; CAT: cysteine aminotransferase; 3-MST: 3-mercaptopyruvate sulfurtransferase; NADPH: nicotinamide adenine dinucleotide phosphate.

Unlike CBS and CSE, 3-MST is a PLP-independent enzyme that is chiefly expressed in mitochondria and produces H$_2$S from the indirect desulfhydration of cysteine [30]. As depicted in Figure 1, in this pathway, cysteine must first be transformed into 3-mercaptopyruvate

(3MP) via the enzyme cysteine aminotransferase (CAT). Then, using 3MP as a substrate, 3-MST transfers a sulfur atom onto itself forming a hydropersulfide (3-MST-SSH). In the presence of reductants, 3MST-SSH is reduced, releasing H_2S in the process.

In addition to the enzymatic routes outlined above, nonenzymatic pathways also contribute to the endogenous production of H_2S in mammals. In general, sulfane sulfur and other reactive sulfur species (RSS), including hydropersulfides (RSSH), polysulfides (RSS_nR), and thiosulfate ($S_2O_3^{2-}$), serve as effective H_2S precursors in the presence of glutathione and other reductants (Figure 1) [31–33]. To this end, processes that increase the production of nicotinamide adenine dinucleotide phosphate (NADPH), which facilitates the recycling of oxidized glutathione back to its reduced form, have been shown to enhance this nonenzymatic pathway and promote H_2S biosynthesis [8].

While less is known about the metabolism and removal of H_2S from mammalian systems, the primary pathways are believed to involve mitochondrial oxidation [34,35], cytosolic methylation [36], hemoglobin and metalloprotein binding [37], expiration via the lungs [38], and its storage in proteins as bound sulfane sulfur [39]. The majority of H_2S is ultimately excreted via the kidneys in the form of sulfate (SO_4^{2-}) [40]. This oxidation of H_2S occurs in mitochondria and is facilitated by the enzymes sulfide quinone reductase (SQR) and rhodanese. This metabolic process also accentuates the biological activity of H_2S and its ability to stimulate oxidative phosphorylation and ATP production through its donation of electrons to the mitochondrial electron transport chain through SQR and mitochondrial complex II [41,42].

3. H_2S Bioactivity and Its Attenuation of Myocardial Ischemia-Reperfusion Injury

In addition to serving as a mitochondrial protectant and stimulator of mitochondrial bioenergetics, endogenous H_2S has been shown to play a key role in several other physiological and pathophysiological processes [14–16,43–47]. The cardiovascular system, in particular, appears to be positively influenced by H_2S given its involvement in vasodilation and blood pressure regulation [6,48]; its antioxidative [19], anti-inflammatory [17,49], and cytoprotective properties [50,51]; and its ability to promote angiogenesis [20]. Additionally, recent evidence suggests that the co-release of H_2S (via the transsulfuration pathway) and adenosine (via the methionine cycle) may protect the myocardium from injury [52,53]. For these reasons it is theorized that the exogenous delivery of H_2S may hold therapeutic value for the prevention and treatment of various cardiovascular-related diseases [54,55], including myocardial ischemia-reperfusion (MI/R) injury [56–62] (Figure 2).

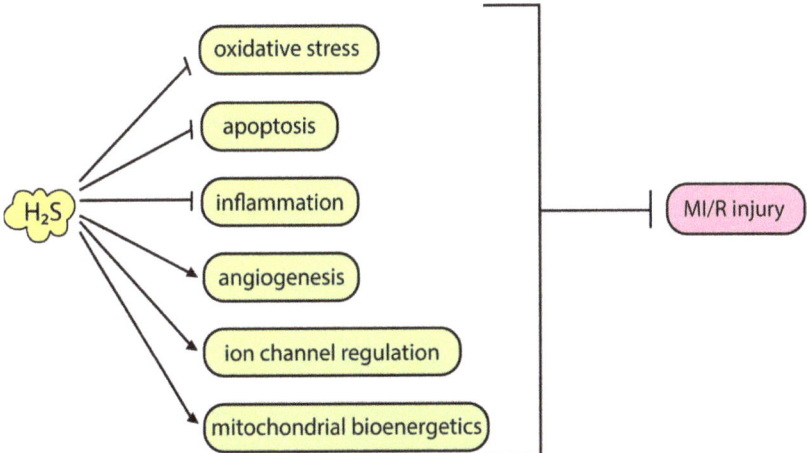

Figure 2. Molecular mechanisms that underscore the cardioprotective effects of H_2S, including its ability to combat MI/R injury.

Myocardial ischemia occurs when blood flow to the heart is restricted due to the buildup of plaque in a coronary artery. If left unchecked, this may lead to myocardial infarction, or heart attack, which is the leading cause of death worldwide [63,64]. To repair myocardial structural damage and prevent ischemic progression, reperfusion therapy is typically employed. This rapid return of blood to ischemic tissue, however, often leads to (MI/R) injury caused by inflammation and oxidative damage [65,66]. Increased levels of reactive oxygen species (ROS), coupled with an overwhelmed antioxidant defense, play a major role in reperfusion injury and can exacerbate cardiac damage that occurs during ischemia [67].

Intracellular calcium overload, a hallmark of reperfusion injury, stimulates the translocation of CSE from the cytosol to mitochondria, which elevates the production of H_2S within that subcellular space [68]. This innate response of the human body is produced in an effort to preserve mitochondrial function and protect the myocardium from oxidative damage, highlighting the potential for therapeutic intervention with H_2S delivery. Indeed, recent studies have highlighted the protective effects of exogenous hydrogen sulfide during MI/R. One of the earliest examples in vitro was a study conducted by Johansen and co-workers [69]. Using an isolated perfused heart assay with rats, preconditioning with 1 µM NaHS (an H_2S equivalent in buffer) 10 min prior to coronary occlusion and up until 10 min post reperfusion, they observed a 20% reduction in infarct size. Pretreatment with Glibenclamide (K_{ATP} blocker) nullified the effect of exogenous H_2S, which supports its involvement in K_{ATP} channel opening as a primary mechanism of alleviation. Later studies have shown that H_2S promotes the persulfidation (protein-SSH) of Cys43 of the K_{ATP} protein, resulting in channel opening, an influx of K^+, and vascular smooth muscle relaxation.

Additionally, sulfide salts have been used to demonstrate the protective effects of H_2S against MI/R injury in vivo. In an early study by Sivarajah et al. [70], mice were exposed to 25 min of regional myocardial ischemia and 2 h of subsequent reperfusion. When NaHS (3 mg/kg) was delivered 15 min prior to ischemia, a 26% reduction in infarct size was reported in comparison to the vehicle control. Subsequently, Elrod and co-workers investigated the impact of exogenous H_2S being delivered at the time of reperfusion rather than prior to the ischemic event [71]. In their study, mice were subjected to 30 min of left coronary artery ischemia followed by a 24 h period of reperfusion in the presence of Na_2S (50 µg/kg). Remarkably, they observed a 72% reduction in infarct size under these conditions.

While sulfide salts, such as NaHS and Na_2S, serve as convenient H_2S precursors, their addition to buffered solutions results in a rapid surge in H_2S concentration, followed by a swift decline due to the instability and transient nature of hydrogen sulfide [72]. Moreover, these characteristics poorly mimic the slow and steady enzymatic production of H_2S, which often leads to adverse side effects when sulfide salts are employed. For these reasons, small molecule donors designed to release H_2S in a controlled fashion, and under biologically relevant conditions, have been sought to harness the medicinal properties of H_2S [73–77].

In the ensuing section, we will highlight examples of small molecule donors that better mimic the natural biosynthesis of H_2S and exhibit promising cardioprotective effects, especially against myocardial ischemia-reperfusion injury.

4. H_2S Donors That Protect against Myocardial Ischemia-Reperfusion Injury

Hydrogen sulfide donors with success at protecting against MI/R injury are highlighted in Table 1 and arranged by their mechanism for H_2S release. In this section, the H_2S releasing mechanism of each donor will be detailed, and their resulting therapeutic effects in various MI/R injury models will be summarized.

Table 1. Synthetic H$_2$S donors with documented protective effects against MI/R injury.

H$_2$S Donor	Release Mechanism	Preclinical Studies
GYY4137	Hydrolysis-Triggered	In vivo rat and diabetic mice models of MI/R injury
DTTs	Hydrolysis-Triggered	Rat isolated perfused heart model of MI/R injury
JK Donors	pH-Triggered	H9c2 cardiomyocyte model of H/R injury and in vivo murine model of MI/R injury
N-Mercaptos	Thiol-Triggered	In vivo murine model of MI/R injury
Acyl Perthiols	Thiol-Triggered	In vivo murine model of MI/R injury
Allyl Thioesters	Thiol-Triggered	In vivo murine model of MI/R injury
Perthiocarbamates	Thiol-Triggered	Mouse isolated perfused heart model of MI/R injury
Aryl Isothiocyanates	Thiol-Triggered	Rat isolated perfused heart model and in vivo murine model of MI/R Injury
Arylthioamides	Thiol-Triggered	In vivo rabbit model of MI/R injury
Hydroxymethyl Persulfide Prodrugs	Enzyme-Triggered	in vivo murine model of MI/R injury
HSDs	ROS-Triggered	H9c2 cardiomyocyte model of H/R injury and in vivo murine model of MI/R injury

4.1. Hydrolysis-Triggered Donors

Morpholin-4-ium 4-methoxyphenyl (morpholino) phosphinodithioate (GYY4137) is the first and most-researched H$_2$S donor ever developed [78,79]. It was accessed by treating Lawesson's reagent with morpholine to impart high water solubility (~30 mg/mL at pH 7.4), which facilitates its use in biological studies. The proposed H$_2$S releasing mechanism for

GYY4137 is depicted in Figure 3. From detailed mechanistic work carried out by Alexander and co-workers [80], a two-step hydrolysis was put forth, which ultimately yields an arylphosphonate and 2 equiv of H_2S. The second hydrolysis step, however, was deemed to be too slow to be responsible for any of its observed biological activity, suggesting that GYY4137 primarily undergoes a single hydrolytic P–S bond cleavage event in water to release 1 equiv of H_2S.

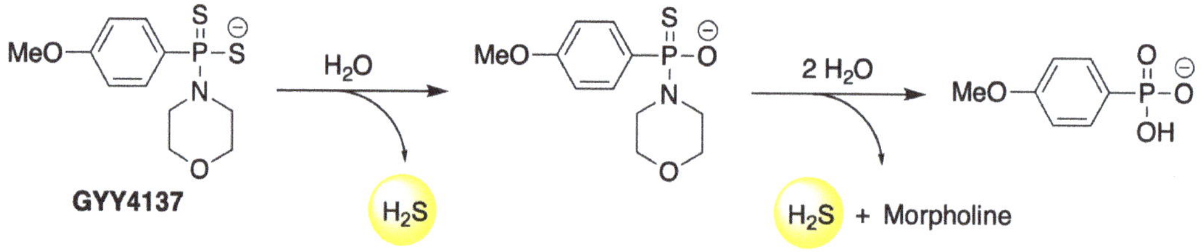

Figure 3. Hydrolysis-triggered H_2S release from GYY4137.

In stark contrast to sulfide salts, GYY4137 is recognized for its ability to provide the slow and continuous release of H_2S for up to a week after its introduction to water. In its first reported study, GYY4137 was shown to relax rat aortic rings due to its activation of vascular smooth muscle K_{ATP} channels [78]. Moreover, unlike sulfide salts whose effects were brief, GYY4137 was found to be a far more potent vasorelaxant, presumably due to its sustained release of H_2S and extended interaction with aortic rings. Perhaps not surprisingly, GYY4137 has also exhibited protective effects against MI/R injury [81–83]. Beyond its activation of vascular smooth muscle K_{ATP} channels [78,84], additional mechanisms have been invoked which include the ability of GYY4137 to attenuate oxidative stress and apoptosis through increased Bcl-2 expression and its activation of the Nrf2 signaling pathway [81,82].

Aside from GYY4137, 1,2-dithiole-3-thiones (DTTs) represent another important H_2S donating scaffold that operates via chemical hydrolysis (Figure 4) [85]. Although detailed mechanistic studies have yet to be carried out, conventional wisdom suggests that, in water, DTTs are converted into their corresponding 1,2-dithiole-3-one structure with the concurrent liberation of H_2S.

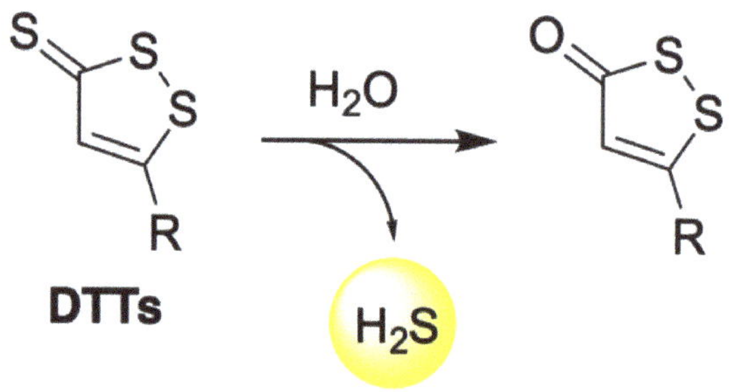

Figure 4. Hydrolysis-triggered H_2S release from DTTs.

ADT and ADT-OH are the most common among this donor class, and their biological properties have been assessed in numerous disease models [86–91]. Perhaps most notably, several interesting H_2S donor hybrids have been obtained by coupling ADT-OH through its phenol onto other therapeutically useful drugs [92], yielding compounds such as MADTOH and ACS14 (Figure 5).

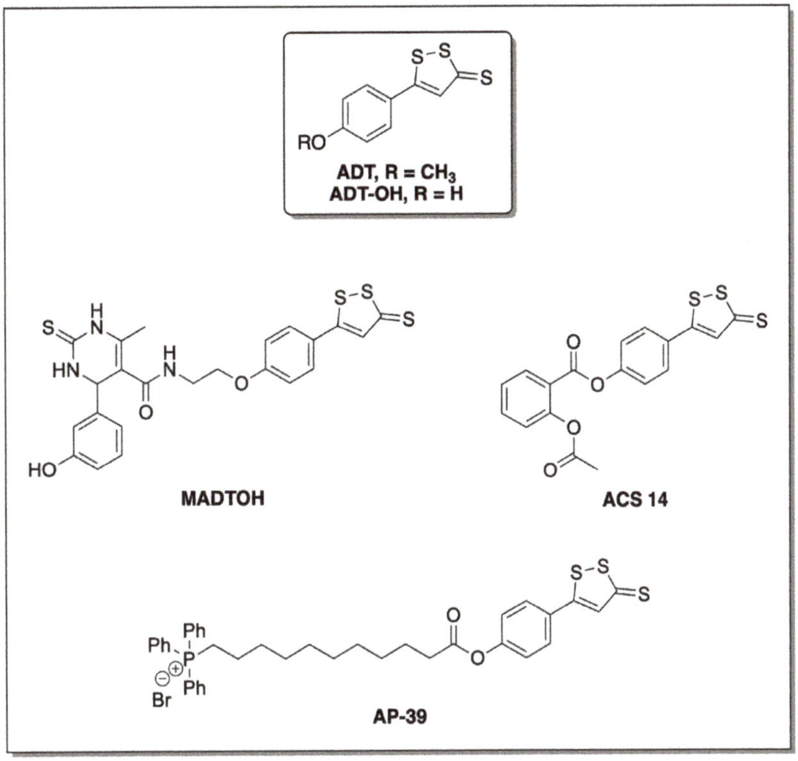

Figure 5. Chemical structures of DTTs and donor hybrids with protective effects against MI/R injury.

Impressive drug synergism was observed with MADTOH, a monastrol-H$_2$S-releasing hybrid, as increased inhibitory effects against L-type calcium channels were observed with this compound in comparison to both monastrol and ADT-OH alone [93]. L-type calcium channel blockers hold promise as an effective therapy for several cardiovascular disorders, including myocardial ischemia [94]. Thus, hybrid molecules, such as MADTOH, may be especially advantageous in treating MI/R injury and warrant further studies.

Along those lines, ACS14 is an H$_2$S-releasing, nonsteroidal anti-inflammatory hybrid that combines aspirin and donor ADT-OH. Originally reported on in 2009 [95], ACS14 was first developed in an effort to reduce the gastric toxicity of aspirin by combatting redox imbalance through its release of H$_2$S and subsequent increase in heme oxygenase-1 expression. Since this initial report, the cardioprotective effects of ACS14 have also been highlighted in later studies, including its ability to reduce MI/R injury in buthionine sulfoximine-treated rats [96,97].

Similarly, AP39 is an ADT-OH conjugate with impressive therapeutic effects in cardiovascular disease models (Figure 5) [98,99]. By combining ADT-OH with a triphenylphosphonium moiety through an ester linkage, AP39 effectively targets mitochondria, which significantly improves its potency. This was first established in a study aimed at assessing its effects on mitochondrial bioenergetics, which noted that only nanomolar concentrations of AP39 were required to observe stimulatory effects whereas micromolar doses of other H$_2$S donors are typically required to evoke similar results. The selective delivery of H$_2$S to mitochondria may also heighten its cardioprotective qualities. Indeed, later studies have showcased the ability of AP39 to protect myocardium from ischemia-reperfusion injury by significantly attenuating mitochondrial ROS production and through its stabilization of mitochondrial membrane potentials [100–102].

4.2. pH-Triggered Donors

JK donors are a class of pH-triggered, H_2S-releasing compounds developed by Xian and co-workers [103]. By appending different amino acids, a series of phosphorothioate-based donors were accessed that undergo an intramolecular cyclization reaction that liberates H_2S with high efficiency in weakly acidic (pH 5–6) environments (Figure 6). This pathway, however, appears to be inoperable under neutral to slightly basic conditions (pH 7–8), which provides greater spatiotemporal control over their delivery of hydrogen sulfide. These observations are likely to stem from the fact that under weakly acidic conditions, the phosphorothiol moiety is protonated and functions as a good leaving group, while the carboxylate component still resides in its deprotonated, nucleophilic form.

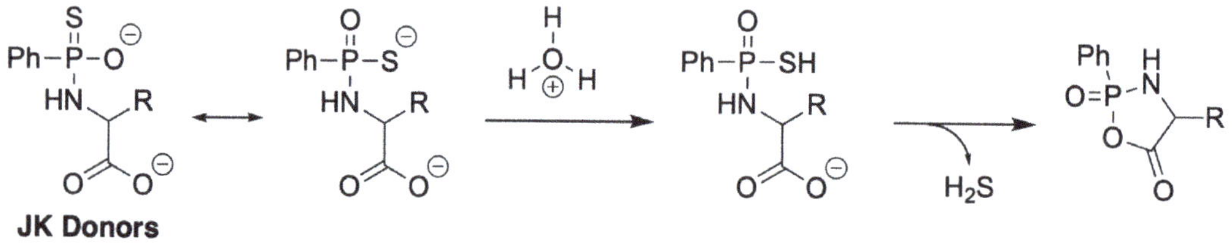

Figure 6. pH-triggered H_2S release from JK donors.

Since numerous pathological conditions are known to lead to a reduction in pH (inflammation, cancer, and cardiovascular disorders), JK donors have the potential to selectively deliver H_2S under conditions in which a therapeutic benefit is likely to arise. In their original study, the authors successfully demonstrated that both JK-1 and JK-2 (Figure 7) could provide significant cardioprotection in both cellular and in vivo murine models of MI/R injury [103].

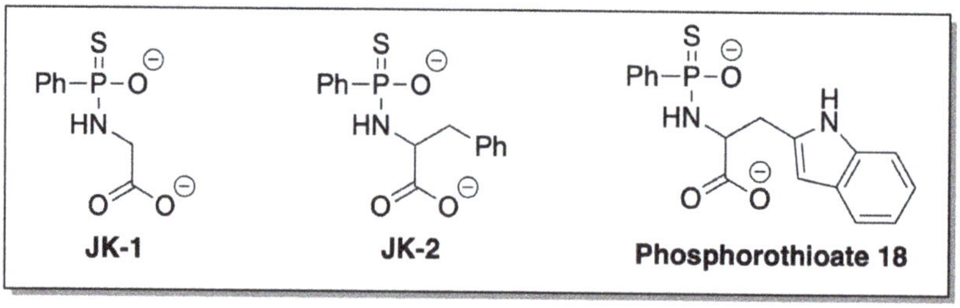

Figure 7. JK donors with established cardioprotective effects in MI/R injury models.

It is worth noting that additional donors of this type have been prepared by further modifying the amino acid substituent. Phosphorothioate 18 (Figure 7), for example, was recently accessed and found to protect H9c2 cardiomyocytes from hypoxia-reoxygenation (H/R) injury [104]. In addition, JK-1 was shown to exhibit low toxicity and good pharmacokinetic properties, accentuating the fact that further structure–activity relationship (SAR) studies and additional therapeutic and preclinical profiling within this series is likely to be advantageous.

4.3. Thiol-Triggered Donors

H_2S donors selectively responsive to biologically abundant thiols, such as cysteine and glutathione, have also exhibited promising cardioprotective effects. Figure 8 outlines specific compounds within this series that have displayed promising protective effects in MI/R injury models.

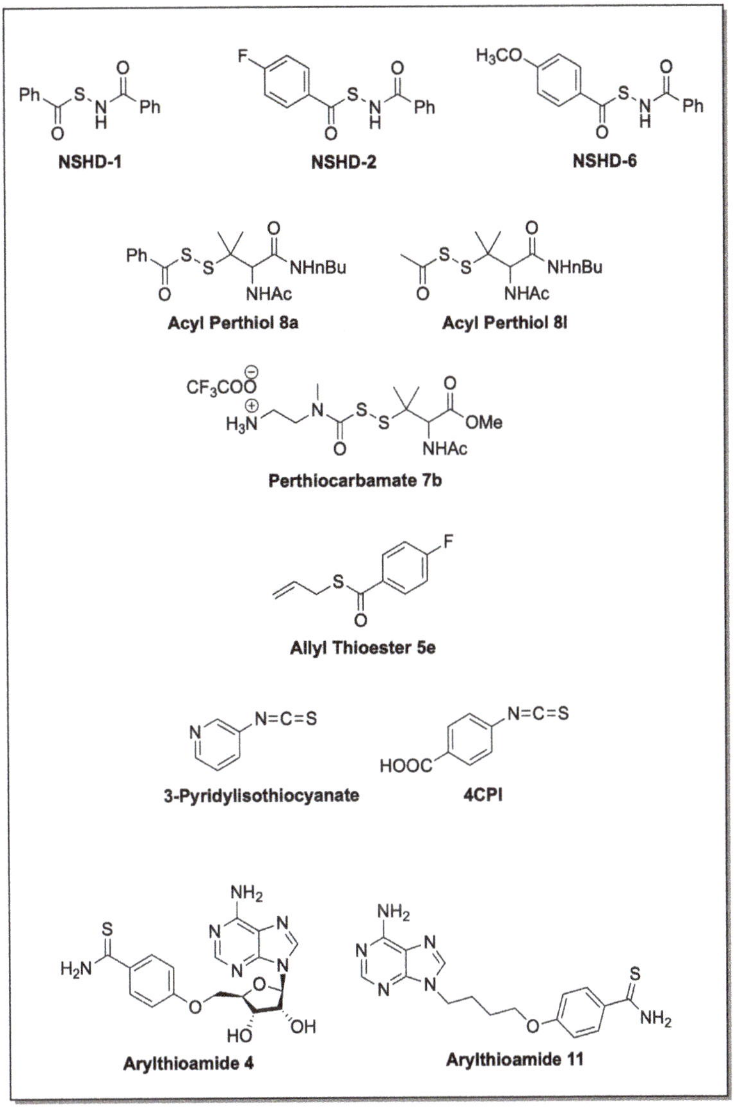

Figure 8. Thiol-triggered donors with established cardioprotective effects in H/R and MI/R injury models.

Among the first to be examined were a series of N-mercapto-based donors (NSHDs) developed by Zhao et al. (Figure 8) [105]. These compounds were shown to be stable in buffer and require the presence of cysteine to effectively deliver H_2S in aqueous media. Specifically, within this donor class, NSHD-1, NSHD-2, and NSHD-6 demonstrated cytoprotective effects against H_2O_2-induced damage in H9c2 cardiomyocytes. Furthermore, NSHD-1 and NSHD-2 also exhibited potent cardioprotective effects in a murine model of MI/R injury.

Additionally, acyl perthiols, allyl thioesters, and perthiocarbamates are responsive to cellular thiols and have established cardioprotective effects in H9c2 cardiomyocytes and other MI/R injury models as a result of their H_2S release. In the case of acyl perthiols, compounds 8a and 8l demonstrated notable reductions in infarct size relative to vehicle-treated mice in a murine MI/R injury model [58]. Moreover, a significant reduction in circulating cardiac troponin I was observed in both 8a- and 8l-treated mice, which supports the involvement of an H$_2$S-related mechanism in their cardioprotection. Within the allyl thioester series, 5e was shown to be the most potent donor in cardiomyocyte (H9c2) models of oxidative damage [106]. It also displayed protective qualities in an in vivo mouse model, reducing infarct size and cardiomyocyte apoptosis. Similarly, perthiocarbamate 7b showcased impressive cardioprotective effects in a Langendorff model of MI/R [107].

Although very electrophilic, isothiocyanates are another class of thiol-activated donors with promising cardioprotective characteristics. In Langendorff-perfused rat hearts, 4CPI was shown to improve post-ischemic recovery through its attenuation of oxidative stress and activation of mitoK$_{ATP}$ channels [108]. Through an extensive SAR study, 3-pyridyl-isothiocynante was identified as another potent donor within this series, exhibiting maximum myocardial protection in an in vivo rat model for acute myocardial infarction at a dose of just 20 µg/kg and from its activation of mitoK$_{ATP}$ channels [109].

Arylthioamides are the final donor class that we will touch upon within this section. What makes arylthioamides distinct from the donors mentioned above is that their release of H$_2$S is extremely slow and inefficient, even with the addition of nucleophilic thiols [110]. Moreover, the release of H$_2$S from this scaffold proceeds through an unidentified mechanistic pathway. Nevertheless, two hybrid adenine-containing donors, arylthioamide 4 and 11, appear to show synergistic cardioprotective effects by activating the PKG/PLN pathway in ischemic myocardium [111].

Pathways for thiol-triggered release of H$_2$S have been explored with these donors. Plausible mechanisms put forth by the authors, based on detailed mechanistic studies, the identification of reaction intermediates, and established organic reactivity, are presented below.

As depicted in Figure 9, NSHDs initially undergo a nucleophilic acyl substitution with cysteine to form a thioester and an N-mercapto (N-SH) species. Although this first step is reversible, the ensuing thioester undergoes a rapid S-to-N-acyl transfer that essentially renders this step irreversible. In the presence of excess cysteine, the N-mercapto species is transformed into a primary amide, forming cysteine persulfide in the process. Cysteine persulfide then reacts further with cysteine to generate cystine and free H$_2$S. From a detailed SAR analysis, it was discovered that both electronic and steric effects at R$_1$ (but not R$_2$) influence the rate of H$_2$S release [105]. In general, NSHDs with smaller electron-withdrawing substituents at this position exhibited faster kinetics.

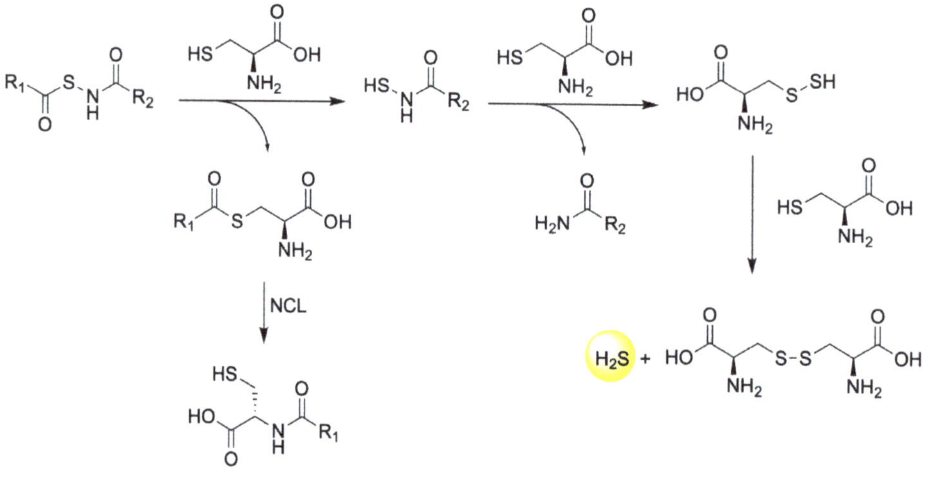

Figure 9. Thiol-triggered H$_2$S release from NSHDs.

H$_2$S can be released from acyl perthiols through an initial thioester exchange reaction that liberates a persulfide [58] (Figure 10). The ensuing hydropersulfide can then undergo an additional thiol exchange reaction to form a disulfide while generating H$_2$S.

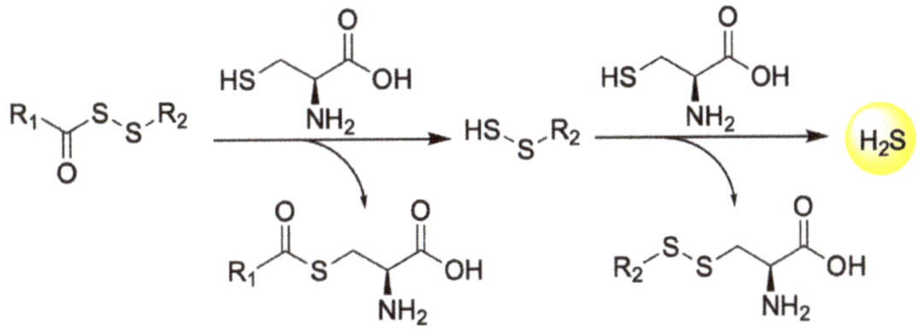

Figure 10. Thiol-triggered H$_2$S release from acyl perthiols.

Similarly, allyl thioesters liberate H$_2$S by undergoing an initial thioester exchange reaction to generate an allylic thiol, which then oxidizes to form a diallyl disulfide (Figure 11). Diallyl disulfides are known H$_2$S donors that are likely to operate through a hydropersulfide intermediate [112–118].

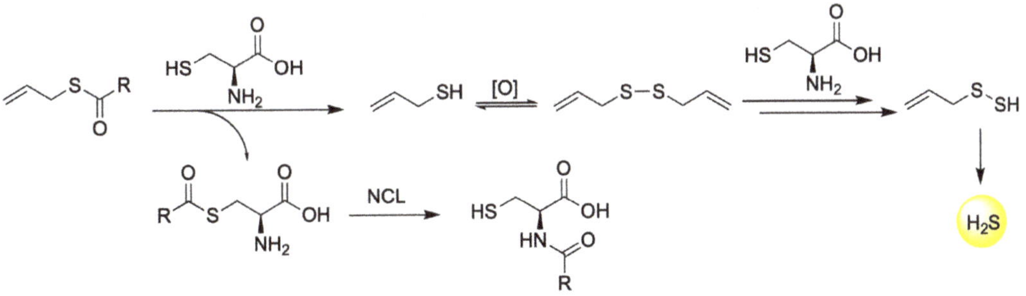

Figure 11. Thiol-triggered H$_2$S release from allyl thioesters.

Within this series of donors, perthiocarbamates are unique in their ability to generate H$_2$S from two distinct pathways: hydropersulfide formation and carbonyl sulfide (COS) liberation [107]. As outlined in Figure 12, the COS delivery pathway is initiated by a thiol–disulfide exchange reaction that yields an unstable carbamic thioacid that quickly decomposes and gives rise to COS. In the presence of the ubiquitous enzyme carbonic anhydrase (CA), COS is quickly transformed into H$_2$S [119]. Alternatively, perthiocarbamates can liberate H$_2$S from a hydropersulfide intermediate that is generated from an intramolecular cyclization reaction that bypasses the need for a specific stimulus to trigger the event.

The mechanism of H$_2$S liberation from isothiocyanates has been carefully investigated by Lin and co-workers [120]. As delineated in Figure 13, they propose that the reaction commences with the nucleophilic attack by cysteine to form a dithiocarbamate. This intermediate then undergoes an intramolecular cyclization that forms a 5-membered ring and assists in the elimination of H$_2$S.

4.4. Enzyme-Triggered Donors

Hydrogen sulfide donors that are selectively responsive to specific enzymes have also been developed. Those that have displayed promising protective effects in MI/R injury models are featured below.

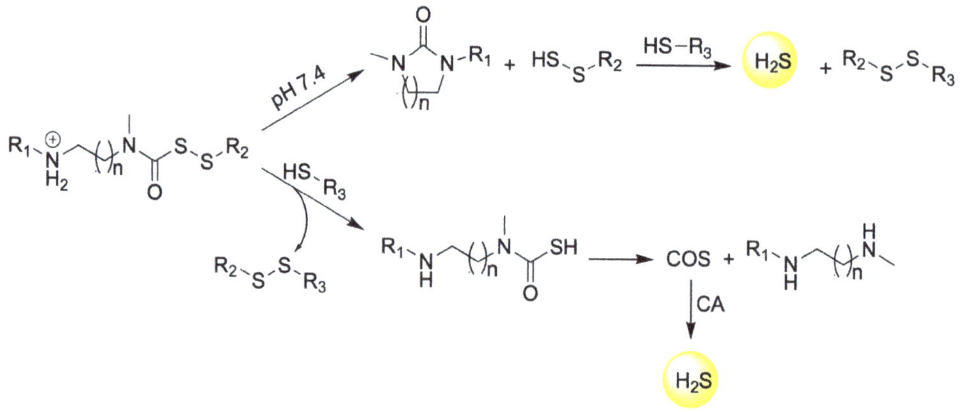

Figure 12. Thiol-triggered H$_2$S release from perthiocarbamates.

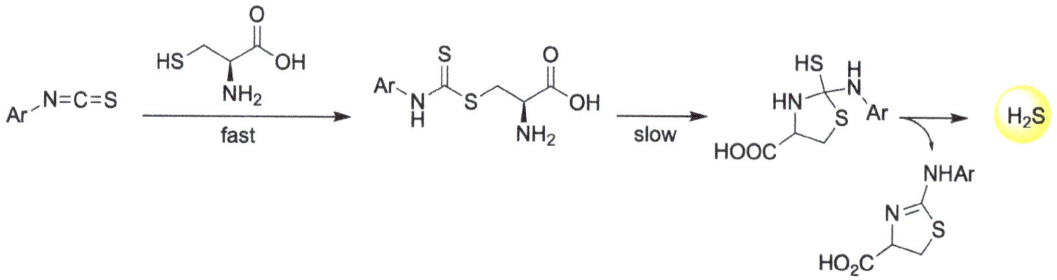

Figure 13. Thiol-triggered H$_2$S release from isothiocyanates.

Esterase enzymes are omnipresent in human cells and, as their name implies, catalyze the hydrolysis of esters [121]. Not surprisingly, H$_2$S liberation from a donor that is initiated by esterase-catalyzed hydrolysis is a common approach [122–127]. In general, the molecular framework is designed in such a way that upon ester hydrolysis, the resultant alcohol undergoes a self-immolative step that results in the eventual release of H$_2$S. Donor P2 (Figure 14) illustrates this approach, as an unstable hydroxymethyl persulfide is unveiled after esterase-catalyzed hydrolysis [128]. This intermediate quickly decomposes to generate acetaldehyde and a hydropersulfide, which serves as an effective H$_2$S precursor under biological conditions. Donor P2 was used in a murine model of MI/R injury and displayed promising protective effects with a bell-shaped therapeutic profile.

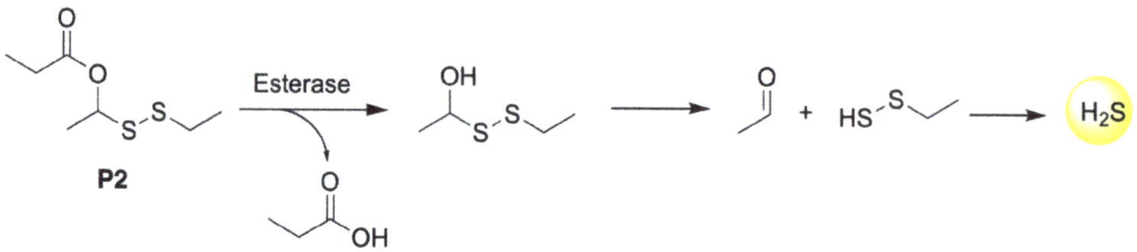

Figure 14. Esterase-triggered H$_2$S release from P2, a donor with cardioprotective effects in MI/R injury models.

Donors selectively responsive to the enzyme β-galactosidase have also displayed favorable cardioprotective effects. The NO-H$_2$S donor hybrid depicted in Figure 15 is an example of such a design [129]. In the presence of β-galactosidase, the glycosidic bonds in the molecule are cleaved, producing an unstable intermediate that further unravels to liberate H_2S (via COS hydrolysis) and nitric oxide (NO). To underline its cardioprotective effects, this hybrid prodrug was used in a rat model of heart failure. In general, it was shown that administration of the NO-H_2S donor hybrid noticeably improved cardiac function post myocardial infarction, and especially in comparison to NO or H_2S treatment alone, highlighting the effectiveness of a hybrid approach.

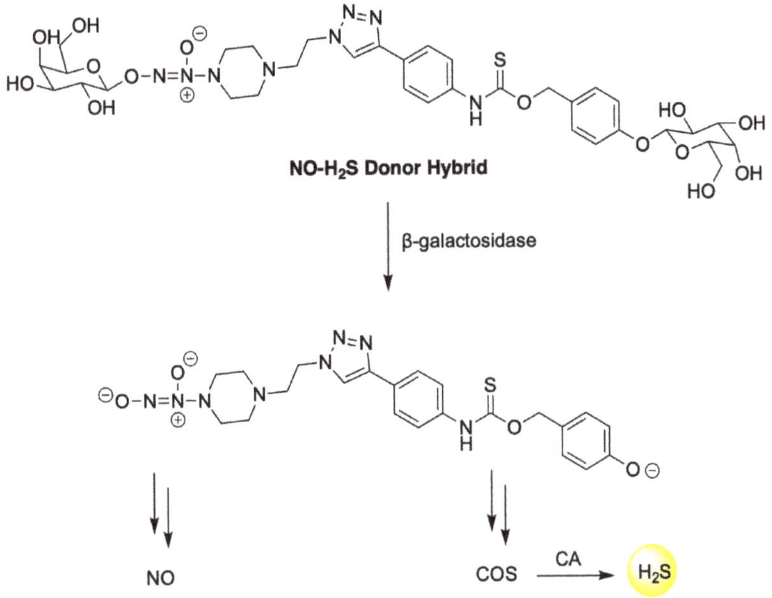

Figure 15. β-galactosidase-triggered H_2S release from an NO-H_2S donor hybrid, a compound with cardioprotective effects in MI/R injury models.

4.5. ROS-Triggered Donors

H_2S donors selectively responsive to elevated levels of ROS have been shown to be especially advantageous at combatting oxidative stress-related diseases [130–134], including MI/R injury. Within the structural framework of these donors, an O- or S-alkyl thiocarbamate is often linked to an aryl boronate ester, which serves as an ROS-responsive trigger [135–137]. In the presence of ROS (especially hydrogen peroxide or peroxynitrite), the aryl boronate ester is quickly oxidized to an unstable phenol that undergoes a 1,6-elimination to provide H_2S through carbonic anhydrase catalyzed COS hydrolysis (Figure 16).

An advantage of donors that proceed through the COS/H_2S pathway is their concurrent release of an aryl amine (or aryl alcohol) which affords an easy opportunity to access self-reporting donors that can track their H_2S delivery via fluorescence spectroscopy and other imaging techniques [134,138–140]. HSD-B and HSD-R (Figure 17) serve as examples of this, due to there being a latent fluorescent reporter embedded within their O-alkyl thiocarbamate framework. Moreover, these compounds were rationally designed to target mitochondria, thanks to their lipophilicity and cationic charge, which are likely to contribute to their pronounced cardioprotective effects that have been observed in H/R injury models [139,140]. HSD-B, for example, was shown to provide protection in a H9c2 cellular model of H/R injury, while HSD-R exhibited anti-apoptotic (inhibition of pro-apoptotic genes, including Bid, Apaf-1, and P53), anti-inflammatory, and pro-angiogenic effects in a rat MI/R injury model.

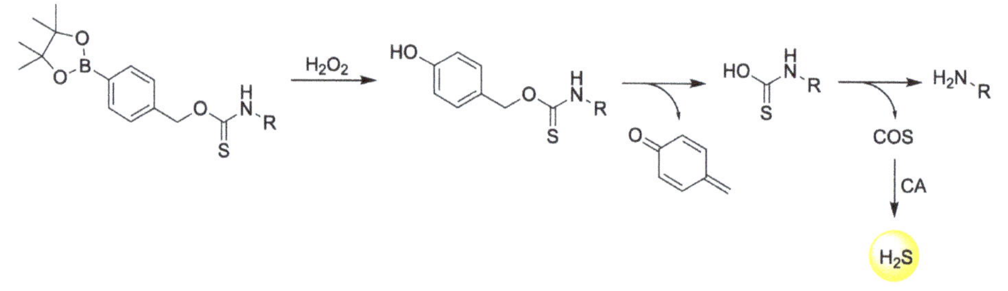

Figure 16. General mechanism for H₂S release from ROS-triggered, O-alkyl thiocarbamate-based donors.

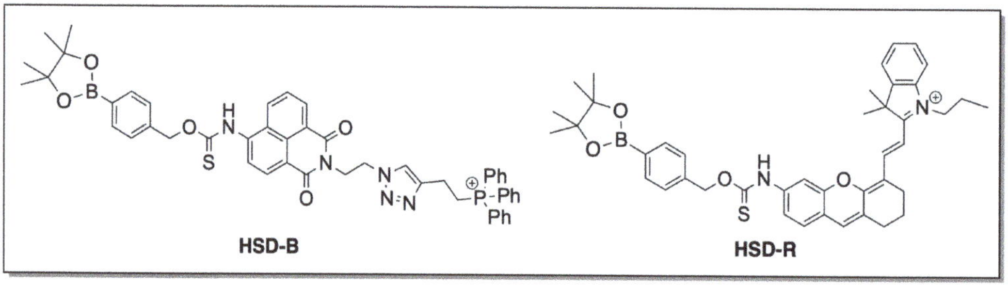

Figure 17. ROS-triggered donors with cardioprotective effects in H/R and MI/R injury models.

5. Chemotherapy-Induced Cardiotoxicity

Chemotherapy-induced cardiotoxicity is a serious complication that affects the long-term survival of cancer patients and often manifests itself several years to several decades after the completion of treatment [141,142]. By convention, chemotherapy-induced cardiotoxicity is sorted into two distinct categories: type I, which is more severe, dose-dependent, and triggered by anthracycline-based drugs [143–145], and type II, which is less severe, believed to be reversible upon the cessation of treatment, and associated with cisplatin, alkylating agents, antimetabolites, and other non-anthracycline-based chemotherapeutics [146].

Anthracyclines, such as doxorubicin (DOX) and daunorubicin, are among the most effective anticancer agents in clinical use [147]. Their planar anthraquinone tetracyclic structure allows them to insert between DNA base pairs and interfere with the enzyme topoisomerase II, which, in turn, prevents the DNA unwinding and replication that ultimately induces apoptosis in proliferating cancer cells [148]. However, the same chemical features that give rise to DNA intercalation also predispose anthracyclines to redox cycling that generates superfluous levels of ROS within a cellular environment and, specifically, in mitochondria [149,150]. With increased mitochondrial density and a relatively deficient antioxidant defense system in place, cardiomyocytes are especially susceptible to oxidative injury [151,152]. Therefore, while other mechanisms may be in play, the uncontrolled production of ROS is believed to be primarily responsible for the dose-dependent, irreversible heart damage that is observed with anthracycline-based chemotherapeutics [153–155].

Given the significance of anthracyclines in the fight against cancer, it comes as no surprise that new therapeutic strategies are being extensively explored in an effort to diminish their cardiotoxic side effects. To this end, it has been suggested that the co-administration of H₂S—with its impressive antioxidative, anti-inflammatory, and anti-apoptotic effects—may offer an effective solution [156]. This hypothesis was first explored by Su and co-workers in 2009, using a DOX-treated rat model [157]. Employing NaHS as an H₂S donor, the attenuation of DOX-induced mitochondrial injury was in fact observed, along with significant improvements in overall cardiac function. Subsequent investigations have corroborated these initial findings, and the beneficial effects of H₂S are now well-established for combatting chemotherapy-induced cardiotoxicity of both type 1 and type 2 through various mechanisms (Figure 18) [158–162].

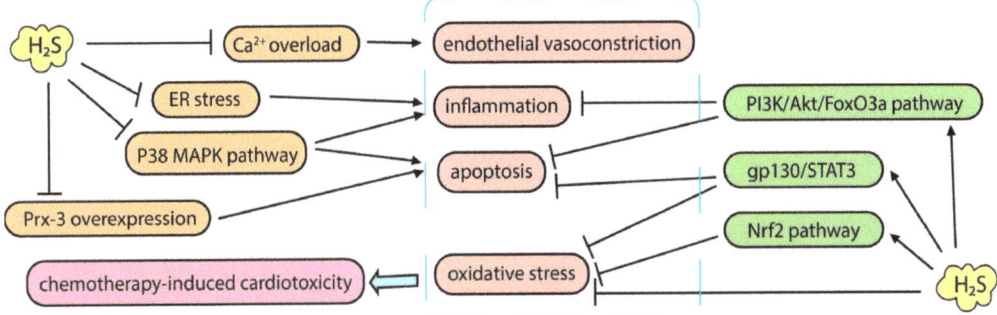

Figure 18. Protective mechanisms of H₂S against chemotherapy-induced cardiotoxicity.

While the co-administration of H₂S appears to be a promising approach for reducing the cardiotoxic profile of drug molecules, efforts to improve absorption and target delivery have led to the emergence of a new codrug design in which a known H₂S-donating moiety is directly linked to a chemotherapeutic agent of interest. This strategy is akin to the ABT-OH donor hybrids discussed earlier (Section 4.1) and has proven to be especially beneficial for mitigating DOX-induced cardiotoxicity, in particular. Therefore, given their obvious translational potential and clever chemical design, these hybrid DOX molecules are detailed below.

6. H₂S Conjugated Codrugs That Combat Anthracycline-Induced Cardiotoxicity

Chegaev and co-workers were the first to synthesize and assess a series of H₂S-releasing, DOX hybrid codrugs (termed H₂S-DOXOs) [163]. To accomplish this, they appended known H₂S-donating motifs via an ester bond at C-14 of DOX. As seen in Figure 19, the affixed H₂S-donating moieties included DTT derivative (H₂S-DOXOs 10–13), allyl sulfide (H₂S-DOXO 14), allyl disulfide (H₂S-DOXO 15), and an aryl thioamide (H₂S-DOXO 16).

After verifying H₂S liberation from H₂S-DOXOs in cell culture media, an LDH assay was used to assess their cytotoxic effects in H9c2 cardiomyocytes in culture. Compared to DOX, H₂S-DOXOs 10–14 were found to be significantly less cytotoxic, and the addition of the H₂S scavenger hydroxocobalamin confirmed that their release of hydrogen sulfide was responsible for their reduced cardiotoxicity.

Perhaps most notably, however, H₂S-DOXOs 10 and 11 simultaneously displayed impressive anticancer activity in human osteosarcoma cells (U-20S), even compared to the parent drug. Follow-up studies with H₂S-DOXO 10 indicated that the increased potency is likely to stem from their disruption of drug efflux by Pgp [164], which increases their cellular concentration. Thus, the appendage of an H₂S donor to DOX appears to impart several distinct advantages, including improved functional activity against multidrug-resistant cancers in addition to a reduced cardiotoxic profile.

Since this initial study, H₂S-DOXO 10 (or Sdox) has undergone additional preclinical studies (Table 2) [165–167]. In a DOX-resistant prostate cancer mouse model, treatment with Sdox led to significantly reduced tumor volumes and improved safety. Conversely, DOX-treated mice exhibited reduced body weight and cardiotoxicity, which was assessed by measuring troponin plasma levels and left-ventricular-wall thickness.

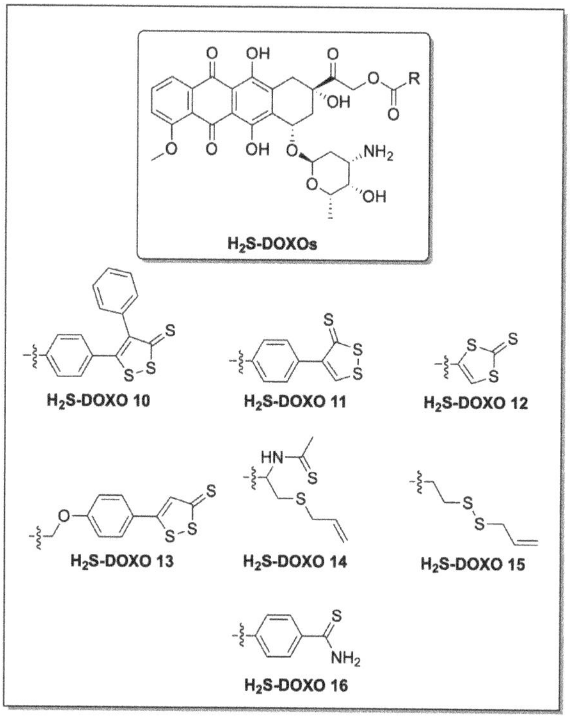

Figure 19. H$_2$S-donating, doxorubicin hybrid codrugs with protective effects against anthracycline-induced cardiotoxicity.

Table 2. H$_2$S-releasing hybrid codrugs with protective effects against anthracycline-induced cardiotoxicity.

H2S Hybrid	Release Mechanism	Preclinical Studies
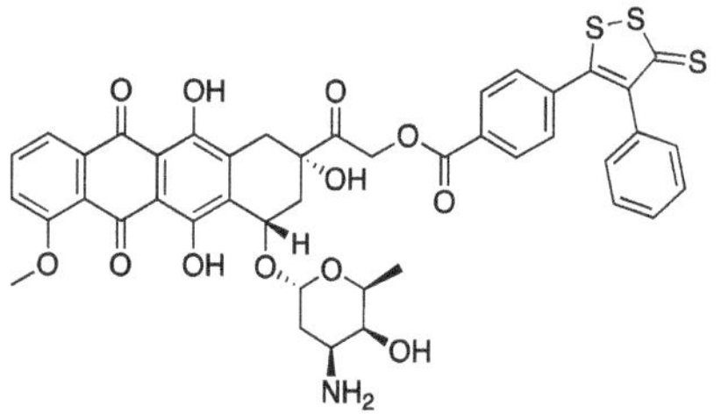 H$_2$S-DOXO 10	Hydrolysis-Triggered	H9c2 cardiomyocytes, U-2OS osteosarcoma cells, DU-145 prostate cancer cells, and in vivo DOX-resistant mouse models
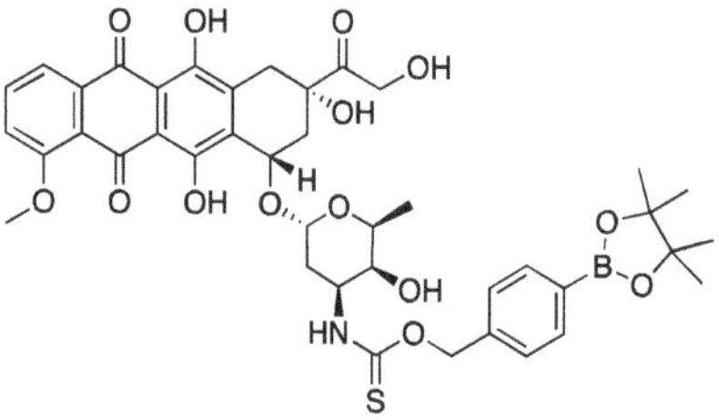 c1	ROS-Triggered	H9c2 cardiomyocytes and 4T1 breast cancer cells

In a similar fashion, Hu et al. recently reported on an H$_2$S-releasing, DOX hybrid codrug (c1, Figure 20) [168]. However, unlike H$_2$S-DOXOs, c1 is a prodrug that only liberates active DOX and H$_2$S under conditions of oxidative stress.

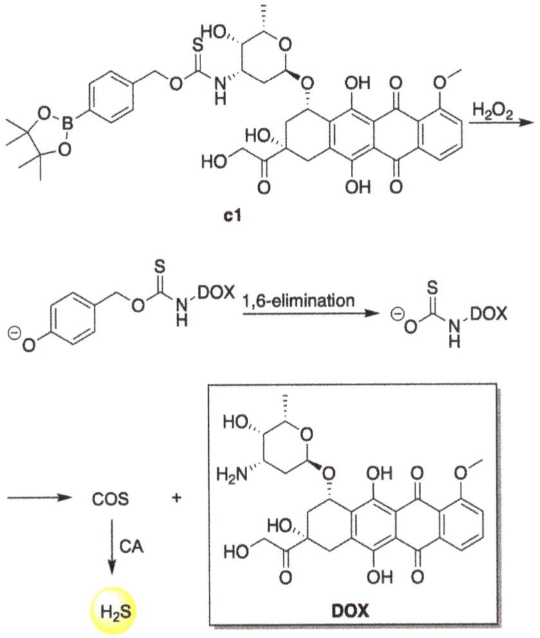

Figure 20. ROS-triggered H$_2$S release from c1, an ROS-responsive DOX hybrid prodrug with reduced cardiotoxicity in rat cardiomyocytes in culture.

Elevated levels of ROS are found in most cancers for a variety of reasons [169]. Consequently, ROS-inducible anticancer prodrugs have emerged as a promising design strategy for improving the therapeutic index of anticancer chemotherapeutic agents [170–173]. Thus, the design of c1 represents a novel strategy that imparts both tumor-selective activation and H$_2$S delivery in combination to further reduce the cardiotoxic side effects of DOX.

As highlighted in Figure 20, c1 utilizes an aryl boronate ester as an H$_2$O$_2$-selective trigger. Upon its oxidation by peroxide, the ensuing phenol undergoes a 1,6-elimination that releases both H$_2$S (by way of COS hydrolysis) and DOX. The authors confirmed this mechanism through LCMS studies and verified the selective release of both DOX and H$_2$S in response to H$_2$O$_2$.

The toxicity of c1 was assessed in rat cardiomyocytes in culture (Table 2). Using this model, c1 exhibited reduced cardiotoxicity compared to that of DOX. By enlisting an H$_2$O$_2$-activated DOX prodrug as a control, which provided CO$_2$ release rather than COS, it was concluded that the protective effects of c1 are likely to stem from its co-release of H$_2$S. Cells treated with c1 also evinced significantly higher Nrf2 activation and heme oxygenase-1 expression compared to controls, providing a likely mechanism of cellular protection [174–177].

Notably, c1 also appeared to maintain the antitumor effects of DOX in a 4T1 mouse breast-cancer cell line. Therefore, while further preclinical profiling—especially in vivo—is required, the selective tumor activation and H$_2$S liberation provided by c1 offer further promising options for overcoming DOX-derived cardiotoxicity in the clinic.

7. Conclusions

Once regarded as merely a toxic and foul-smelling gas, H_2S has more recently been recognized as a key signaling molecule and important endogenous mediator of numerous physiological and pathophysiological processes within mammalian systems. Its positive influence on the cardiovascular system, in particular, is rooted in its involvement in vasodilation (activation of K_{ATP} channels and the PI3K/Akt signaling pathway) [178–181], as well as its anti-inflammatory (inhibition of the p38 MAPK/NF-κB pathway) [182,183], antioxidative (activation of the Nrf2 signaling pathway) [59,168,184], and anti-apoptotic (suppression of pro-apoptotic genes Bid, Apaf-1, and p53) [140] properties, which have been extensively reviewed elsewhere in the literature [54,55,116,185].

Exogenous supplementation with H_2S has been shown to vastly improve outcomes in various in vitro and in vivo cardiovascular disease models. In this review, its effectiveness at combating MI/R injury and chemotherapy-induced cardiotoxicity was explored, along with the fundamental chemistry and H_2S releasing mechanism of the donor molecules that were utilized in these studies. The continued development and refinement of H_2S-releasing compounds is critical to unlocking the translational therapeutic potential of hydrogen sulfide, by augmenting its delivery and bioavailability while better mimicking its natural and prolonged enzymatic production. Thus, the compounds reported on herein not only represent important investigative tools for probing the chemical biology of hydrogen sulfide but may also one day serve as important therapeutic agents for the treatment of MI/R injury and anthracycline-induced cardiotoxicity.

Author Contributions: Conceptualization, Q.H. and J.C.L.III; writing—original draft preparation, Q.H.; writing—review and editing, J.C.L.III; supervision, J.C.L.III. All authors have read and agreed to the published version of the manuscript.

Funding: This research was funded by the National Science Foundation, grant number 2143826.

Conflicts of Interest: The authors declare no conflict of interest.

References

1. Beauchamp, R.O.; Bus, J.S.; Popp, J.A.; Boreiko, C.J.; Andjelkovich, D.A.; Leber, P. A Critical Review of the Literature on Hydrogen Sulfide Toxicity. *CRC Crit. Rev. Toxicol.* **1984**, *13*, 25–97. [CrossRef]
2. Tomlin, S. Smelly Cats. *Nature* **1998**, *396*, 628. [CrossRef]
3. Fiedler, N.; Kipen, H.; Ohman-Strickland, P.; Zhang, J.; Weisel, C.; Laumbach, R.; Kelly-McNeil, K.; Olejeme, K.; Lioy, P. Sensory and Cognitive Effects of Acute Exposure to Hydrogen Sulfide. *Environ. Health Perspect.* **2008**, *116*, 78–85. [CrossRef] [PubMed]
4. Abe, K.; Kimura, H. The Possible Role of Hydrogen Sulfide as an Endogenous Neuromodulator. *J. Neurosci.* **1996**, *16*, 1066–1071. [CrossRef] [PubMed]
5. Kimura, H. Hydrogen Sulfide as a Neuromodulator. *Mol. Neurobiol.* **2002**, *26*, 013–020. [CrossRef] [PubMed]
6. Bhatia, M. Hydrogen Sulfide as a Vasodilator. *IUBMB Life Int. Union Biochem. Mol. Biol. Life* **2005**, *57*, 603–606. [CrossRef] [PubMed]
7. Kabil, O.; Banerjee, R. Redox Biochemistry of Hydrogen Sulfide. *J. Biol. Chem.* **2010**, *285*, 21903–21907. [CrossRef]
8. Wang, R. Two's Company, Three's a Crowd: Can H_2S Be the Third Endogenous Gaseous Transmitter? *FASEB J.* **2002**, *16*, 1792–1798. [CrossRef]
9. Wang, R. The Gasotransmitter Role of Hydrogen Sulfide. *Antioxid. Redox Signal.* **2003**, *5*, 493–501. [CrossRef]
10. Wang, R. Shared Signaling Pathways among Gasotransmitters. *Proc. Natl. Acad. Sci. USA* **2012**, *109*, 8801–8802. [CrossRef]
11. Papapetropoulos, A.; Foresti, R.; Ferdinandy, P. Pharmacology of the 'Gasotransmitters' NO, CO and H_2S: Translational Opportunities. *Br. J. Pharmacol.* **2015**, *172*, 1395–1396. [CrossRef]
12. Hughes, M.N.; Centelles, M.N.; Moore, K.P. Making and Working with Hydrogen Sulfide. *Free Radic. Biol. Med.* **2009**, *47*, 1346–1353. [CrossRef]
13. Fukuto, J.M.; Carrington, S.J.; Tantillo, D.J.; Harrison, J.G.; Ignarro, L.J.; Freeman, B.A.; Chen, A.; Wink, D.A. Small Molecule Signaling Agents: The Integrated Chemistry and Biochemistry of Nitrogen Oxides, Oxides of Carbon, Dioxygen, Hydrogen Sulfide, and Their Derived Species. *Chem. Res. Toxicol.* **2012**, *25*, 769–793. [CrossRef]
14. Cao, X.; Ding, L.; Xie, Z.; Yang, Y.; Whiteman, M.; Moore, P.K.; Bian, J.-S. A Review of Hydrogen Sulfide Synthesis, Metabolism, and Measurement: Is Modulation of Hydrogen Sulfide a Novel Therapeutic for Cancer? *Antioxid. Redox Signal.* **2019**, *31*, 1–38. [CrossRef] [PubMed]
15. Kimura, H. Hydrogen Sulfide: Its Production, Release and Functions. *Amino Acids* **2011**, *41*, 113–121. [CrossRef] [PubMed]

16. Filipovic, M.R.; Zivanovic, J.; Alvarez, B.; Banerjee, R. Chemical Biology of H$_2$S Signaling through Persulfidation. *Chem. Rev.* **2018**, *118*, 1253–1337. [CrossRef]
17. Li, M.; Mao, J.; Zhu, Y. New Therapeutic Approaches Using Hydrogen Sulfide Donors in Inflammation and Immune Response. *Antioxid. Redox Signal.* **2021**, *35*, 341–356. [CrossRef]
18. Whiteman, M.; Winyard, P.G. Hydrogen Sulfide and Inflammation: The Good, the Bad, the Ugly and the Promising. *Expert Rev. Clin. Pharmacol.* **2011**, *4*, 13–32. [CrossRef] [PubMed]
19. Zhang, H.-X.; Liu, S.-J.; Tang, X.-L.; Duan, G.-L.; Ni, X.; Zhu, X.-Y.; Liu, Y.-J.; Wang, C.-N. H$_2$S Attenuates LPS-Induced Acute Lung Injury by Reducing Oxidative/Nitrative Stress and Inflammation. *Cell. Physiol. Biochem.* **2016**, *40*, 1603–1612. [CrossRef]
20. Papapetropoulos, A.; Pyriochou, A.; Altaany, Z.; Yang, G.; Marazioti, A.; Zhou, Z.; Jeschke, M.G.; Branski, L.K.; Herndon, D.N.; Wang, R.; et al. Hydrogen Sulfide Is an Endogenous Stimulator of Angiogenesis. *Proc. Natl. Acad. Sci. USA* **2009**, *106*, 21972–21977. [CrossRef] [PubMed]
21. Corvino, A.; Frecentese, F.; Magli, E.; Perissutti, E.; Santagada, V.; Scognamiglio, A.; Caliendo, G.; Fiorino, F.; Severino, B. Trends in H$_2$S-Donors Chemistry and Their Effects in Cardiovascular Diseases. *Antioxidants* **2021**, *10*, 429. [CrossRef] [PubMed]
22. Miles, E.W.; Kraus, J.P. Cystathionine β-Synthase: Structure, Function, Regulation, and Location of Homocystinuria-Causing Mutations. *J. Biol. Chem.* **2004**, *279*, 29871–29874. [CrossRef] [PubMed]
23. Pan, L.L.; Liu, X.H.; Gong, Q.H.; Yang, H.B.; Zhu, Y.Z. Role of Cystathionine γ -Lyase/Hydrogen Sulfide Pathway in Cardiovascular Disease: A Novel Therapeutic Strategy? *Antioxid. Redox Signal.* **2012**, *17*, 106–118. [CrossRef]
24. Shibuya, N.; Tanaka, M.; Yoshida, M.; Ogasawara, Y.; Togawa, T.; Ishii, K.; Kimura, H. 3-Mercaptopyruvate Sulfurtransferase Produces Hydrogen Sulfide and Bound Sulfane Sulfur in the Brain. *Antioxid. Redox Signal.* **2009**, *11*, 703–714. [CrossRef]
25. Sbodio, J.I.; Snyder, S.H.; Paul, B.D. Regulators of the Transsulfuration Pathway: Modulating the Transsulfuration Pathway in Disease. *Br. J. Pharmacol.* **2019**, *176*, 583–593. [CrossRef] [PubMed]
26. Kabil, O.; Vitvitsky, V.; Xie, P.; Banerjee, R. The Quantitative Significance of the Transsulfuration Enzymes for H$_2$S Production in Murine Tissues. *Antioxid. Redox Signal.* **2011**, *15*, 363–372. [CrossRef] [PubMed]
27. Kaneko, Y.; Kimura, Y.; Kimura, H.; Niki, I. L-Cysteine Inhibits Insulin Release from the Pancreatic β-Cell. *Diabetes* **2006**, *55*, 1391–1397. [CrossRef] [PubMed]
28. Patel, P.; Vatish, M.; Heptinstall, J.; Wang, R.; Carson, R.J. The Endogenous Production of Hydrogen Sulphide in Intrauterine Tissues. *Reprod. Biol. Endocrinol.* **2009**, *7*, 10. [CrossRef] [PubMed]
29. Hosoki, R.; Matsuki, N.; Kimura, H. The Possible Role of Hydrogen Sulfide as an Endogenous Smooth Muscle Relaxant in Synergy with Nitric Oxide. *Biochem. Biophys. Res. Commun.* **1997**, *237*, 527–531. [CrossRef] [PubMed]
30. Nagahara, N.; Ito, T.; Kitamura, H.; Nishino, T. Tissue and Subcellular Distribution of Mercaptopyruvate Sulfurtransferase in the Rat: Confocal Laser Fluorescence and Immunoelectron Microscopic Studies Combined with Biochemical Analysis. *Histochem. Cell Biol.* **1998**, *110*, 243–250. [CrossRef]
31. Olson, K.R.; DeLeon, E.R.; Gao, Y.; Hurley, K.; Sadauskas, V.; Batz, C.; Stoy, G.F. Thiosulfate: A Readily Accessible Source of Hydrogen Sulfide in Oxygen Sensing. *Am. J. Physiol.-Regul. Integr. Comp. Physiol.* **2013**, *305*, R592–R603. [CrossRef]
32. Kolluru, G.K.; Shen, X.; Bir, S.C.; Kevil, C.G. Hydrogen Sulfide Chemical Biology: Pathophysiological Roles and Detection. *Nitric Oxide* **2013**, *35*, 5–20. [CrossRef]
33. Zuhra, K.; Augsburger, F.; Majtan, T.; Szabo, C. Cystathionine-β-Synthase: Molecular Regulation and Pharmacological Inhibition. *Biomolecules* **2020**, *10*, 697. [CrossRef] [PubMed]
34. Jackson, M.R.; Melideo, S.L.; Jorns, M.S. Human Sulfide:Quinone Oxidoreductase Catalyzes the First Step in Hydrogen Sulfide Metabolism and Produces a Sulfane Sulfur Metabolite. *Biochemistry* **2012**, *51*, 6804–6815. [CrossRef] [PubMed]
35. Jackson, M.R.; Melideo, S.L.; Jorns, M.S. Role of Human Sulfide. In *Methods in Enzymology*; Elsevier: Amsterdam, The Netherlands, 2015; Volume 554, pp. 255–270, ISBN 978-0-12-801512-4.
36. Weisiger, R.A.; Pinkus, L.M.; Jakoby, W.B. Thiol S-Methyltransferase: Suggested Role in Detoxication of Intestinal Hydrogen Sulfide. *Biochem. Pharmacol.* **1980**, *29*, 2885–2887. [CrossRef]
37. Cerda-Colón, J.F.; Silfa, E.; López-Garriga, J. Unusual Rocking Freedom of the Heme in the Hydrogen Sulfide-Binding Hemoglobin from *Lucina pectinata*. *J. Am. Chem. Soc.* **1998**, *120*, 9312–9317. [CrossRef]
38. Insko, M.A.; Deckwerth, T.L.; Hill, P.; Toombs, C.F.; Szabo, C. Detection of Exhaled Hydrogen Sulphide Gas in Rats Exposed to Intravenous Sodium Sulphide. *Br. J. Pharmacol.* **2009**, *157*, 944–951. [CrossRef] [PubMed]
39. Ishigami, M.; Hiraki, K.; Umemura, K.; Ogasawara, Y.; Ishii, K.; Kimura, H. A Source of Hydrogen Sulfide and a Mechanism of Its Release in the Brain. *Antioxid. Redox Signal.* **2009**, *11*, 205–214. [CrossRef]
40. Bartholomew, T.C.; Powell, G.M.; Dodgson, K.S.; Curtis, C.G. Oxidation of Sodium Sulphide by Rat Liver, Lungs and Kidney. *Biochem. Pharmacol.* **1980**, *29*, 2431–2437. [CrossRef]
41. Módis, K.; Ju, Y.; Ahmad, A.; Untereiner, A.A.; Altaany, Z.; Wu, L.; Szabo, C.; Wang, R. S-Sulfhydration of ATP Synthase by Hydrogen Sulfide Stimulates Mitochondrial Bioenergetics. *Pharmacol. Res.* **2016**, *113*, 116–124. [CrossRef]
42. Szabo, C. Hydrogen Sulfide, an Endogenous Stimulator of Mitochondrial Function in Cancer Cells. *Cells* **2021**, *10*, 220. [CrossRef]
43. Kimura, H. Hydrogen Sulfide (H$_2$S) and Polysulfide (H$_2$S$_n$) Signaling: The First 25 Years. *Biomolecules* **2021**, *11*, 896. [CrossRef] [PubMed]

44. Filipovic, M.R. Persulfidation (S-Sulfhydration) and H$_2$S. In *Chemistry, Biochemistry and Pharmacology of Hydrogen Sulfide*; Moore, P.K., Whiteman, M., Eds.; Handbook of Experimental Pharmacology; Springer International Publishing: Cham, Switzerland, 2015; Volume 230, pp. 29–59, ISBN 978-3-319-18143-1.
45. Kabil, O.; Motl, N.; Banerjee, R. H$_2$S and Its Role in Redox Signaling. *Biochim. Biophys. Acta BBA Proteins Proteomics* **2014**, *1844*, 1355–1366. [CrossRef] [PubMed]
46. di Masi, A.; Ascenzi, P. H$_2$S: A "Double Face" Molecule in Health and Disease. *BioFactors* **2013**, *39*, 186–196. [CrossRef]
47. Paul, B.D.; Snyder, S.H. H$_2$S: A Novel Gasotransmitter That Signals by Sulfhydration. *Trends Biochem. Sci.* **2015**, *40*, 687–700. [CrossRef] [PubMed]
48. Benavides, G.A.; Squadrito, G.L.; Mills, R.W.; Patel, H.D.; Isbell, T.S.; Patel, R.P.; Darley-Usmar, V.M.; Doeller, J.E.; Kraus, D.W. Hydrogen Sulfide Mediates the Vasoactivity of Garlic. *Proc. Natl. Acad. Sci. USA* **2007**, *104*, 17977–17982. [CrossRef]
49. Benedetti, F.; Curreli, S.; Krishnan, S.; Davinelli, S.; Cocchi, F.; Scapagnini, G.; Gallo, R.C.; Zella, D. Anti-Inflammatory Effects of H$_2$S during Acute Bacterial Infection: A Review. *J. Transl. Med.* **2017**, *15*, 100. [CrossRef]
50. Gemici, B.; Elsheikh, W.; Feitosa, K.B.; Costa, S.K.P.; Muscara, M.N.; Wallace, J.L. H$_2$S-Releasing Drugs: Anti-Inflammatory, Cytoprotective and Chemopreventative Potential. *Nitric Oxide* **2015**, *46*, 25–31. [CrossRef]
51. Gemici, B.; Wallace, J.L. Anti-Inflammatory and Cytoprotective Properties of Hydrogen Sulfide. In *Methods in Enzymology*; Elsevier: Amsterdam, The Netherlands, 2015; Volume 555, pp. 169–193, ISBN 978-0-12-801511-7.
52. Paganelli, F.; Mottola, G.; Fromonot, J.; Marlinge, M.; Deharo, P.; Guieu, R.; Ruf, J. Hyperhomocysteinemia and Cardiovascular Disease: Is the Adenosinergic System the Missing Link? *Int. J. Mol. Sci.* **2021**, *22*, 1690. [CrossRef]
53. Fromonot, J.; Deharo, P.; Bruzzese, L.; Cuisset, T.; Quilici, J.; Bonatti, S.; Fenouillet, E.; Mottola, G.; Ruf, J.; Guieu, R. Adenosine Plasma Level Correlates with Homocysteine and Uric Acid Concentrations in Patients with Coronary Artery Disease. *Can. J. Physiol. Pharmacol.* **2016**, *94*, 272–277. [CrossRef]
54. Szabó, G.; Veres, G.; Radovits, T.; Gerő, D.; Módis, K.; Miesel-Gröschel, C.; Horkay, F.; Karck, M.; Szabó, C. Cardioprotective Effects of Hydrogen Sulfide. *Nitric Oxide* **2011**, *25*, 201–210. [CrossRef]
55. Shen, Y.; Shen, Z.; Luo, S.; Guo, W.; Zhu, Y.Z. The Cardioprotective Effects of Hydrogen Sulfide in Heart Diseases: From Molecular Mechanisms to Therapeutic Potential. *Oxid. Med. Cell. Longev.* **2015**, *2015*, 1–13. [CrossRef]
56. Chen, Y.; Zhang, F.; Yin, J.; Wu, S.; Zhou, X. Protective Mechanisms of Hydrogen Sulfide in Myocardial Ischemia. *J. Cell. Physiol.* **2020**, *235*, 9059–9070. [CrossRef]
57. Wen, Y.-D.; Wang, H.; Zhu, Y.-Z. The Drug Developments of Hydrogen Sulfide on Cardiovascular Disease. *Oxid. Med. Cell. Longev.* **2018**, *2018*, 1–21. [CrossRef] [PubMed]
58. Zhao, Y.; Bhushan, S.; Yang, C.; Otsuka, H.; Stein, J.D.; Pacheco, A.; Peng, B.; Devarie-Baez, N.O.; Aguilar, H.C.; Lefer, D.J.; et al. Controllable Hydrogen Sulfide Donors and Their Activity against Myocardial Ischemia-Reperfusion Injury. *ACS Chem. Biol.* **2013**, *8*, 1283–1290. [CrossRef] [PubMed]
59. Calvert, J.W.; Jha, S.; Gundewar, S.; Elrod, J.W.; Ramachandran, A.; Pattillo, C.B.; Kevil, C.G.; Lefer, D.J. Hydrogen Sulfide Mediates Cardioprotection Through Nrf2 Signaling. *Circ. Res.* **2009**, *105*, 365–374. [CrossRef] [PubMed]
60. Sodha, N.R.; Clements, R.T.; Feng, J.; Liu, Y.; Bianchi, C.; Horvath, E.M.; Szabo, C.; Sellke, F.W. The Effects of Therapeutic Sulfide on Myocardial Apoptosis in Response to Ischemia–Reperfusion Injury. *Eur. J. Cardiothorac. Surg.* **2008**, *33*, 906–913. [CrossRef] [PubMed]
61. Osipov, R.M.; Robich, M.P.; Feng, J.; Liu, Y.; Clements, R.T.; Glazer, H.P.; Sodha, N.R.; Szabo, C.; Bianchi, C.; Sellke, F.W. Effect of Hydrogen Sulfide in a Porcine Model of Myocardial Ischemia-Reperfusion: Comparison of Different Administration Regimens and Characterization of the Cellular Mechanisms of Protection. *J. Cardiovasc. Pharmacol.* **2009**, *54*, 287–297. [CrossRef]
62. Ji, Y.; Pang, Q.; Xu, G.; Wang, L.; Wang, J.; Zeng, Y. Exogenous Hydrogen Sulfide Postconditioning Protects Isolated Rat Hearts against Ischemia-Reperfusion Injury. *Eur. J. Pharmacol.* **2008**, *587*, 1–7. [CrossRef]
63. Ahmed, N. Myocardial Ischemia. In *Pathophysiology of Ischemia Reperfusion Injury and Use of Fingolimod in Cardioprotection*; Elsevier: Amsterdam, The Netherlands, 2019; pp. 41–56, ISBN 978-0-12-818023-5.
64. Crossman, D.C. The Pathophysiology of Myocardial Ischaemia. *Heart* **2004**, *90*, 576–580. [CrossRef]
65. Heusch, G. Myocardial Ischaemia–Reperfusion Injury and Cardioprotection in Perspective. *Nat. Rev. Cardiol.* **2020**, *17*, 773–789. [CrossRef] [PubMed]
66. Parlakpinar, H.; Orum, M.; Sagir, M. Pathophysiology of Myocardial Ischemia Reperfusion Injury: A Review. *Med. Sci. Int. Med. J.* **2013**, *2*, 935. [CrossRef]
67. Pei, H.; Yang, Y.; Zhao, H.; Li, X.; Yang, D.; Li, D.; Yang, Y. The Role of Mitochondrial Functional Proteins in ROS Production in Ischemic Heart Diseases. *Oxid. Med. Cell. Longev.* **2016**, *2016*, 1–8. [CrossRef]
68. Andreadou, I.; Schulz, R.; Papapetropoulos, A.; Turan, B.; Ytrehus, K.; Ferdinandy, P.; Daiber, A.; Di Lisa, F. The Role of Mitochondrial Reactive Oxygen Species, NO and H$_2$S in Ischemia/Reperfusion Injury and Cardioprotection. *J. Cell. Mol. Med.* **2020**, *24*, 6510–6522. [CrossRef] [PubMed]
69. Johansen, D.; Ytrehus, K.; Baxter, G.F. Exogenous Hydrogen Sulfide (H$_2$S) Protects against Regional Myocardial Ischemia–Reperfusion Injury: Evidence for a Role of KATP Channels. *Basic Res. Cardiol.* **2006**, *101*, 53–60. [CrossRef]
70. Sivarajah, A.; McDonald, M.C.; Thiemermann, C. The production of hydrogen sulfide limits myocardial ischemia and reperfusion injury and contributes to the cardioprotective effects of preconditioning with endotoxin, but not ischemia in the rat. *Shock* **2006**, *26*, 154–161. [CrossRef]

71. Elrod, J.W.; Calvert, J.W.; Morrison, J.; Doeller, J.E.; Kraus, D.W.; Tao, L.; Jiao, X.; Scalia, R.; Kiss, L.; Szabo, C.; et al. Hydrogen Sulfide Attenuates Myocardial Ischemia-Reperfusion Injury by Preservation of Mitochondrial Function. *Proc. Natl. Acad. Sci. USA* **2007**, *104*, 15560–15565. [CrossRef]
72. Moore, P.K.; Whiteman, M. (Eds.) Chemistry, Biochemistry and Pharmacology of Hydrogen Sulfide. In *Handbook of Experimental Pharmacology*, 1st ed.; Springer International Publishing: Cham, Switzerland, 2015; ISBN 978-3-319-18144-8.
73. Bora, P.; Chauhan, P.; Pardeshi, K.A.; Chakrapani, H. Small Molecule Generators of Biologically Reactive Sulfur Species. *RSC Adv.* **2018**, *8*, 27359–27374. [CrossRef]
74. Hartle, M.D.; Pluth, M.D. A Practical Guide to Working with H_2S at the Interface of Chemistry and Biology. *Chem. Soc. Rev.* **2016**, *45*, 6108–6117. [CrossRef]
75. Levinn, C.M.; Cerda, M.M.; Pluth, M.D. Activatable Small-Molecule Hydrogen Sulfide Donors. *Antioxid. Redox Signal.* **2020**, *32*, 96–109. [CrossRef]
76. Powell, C.R.; Dillon, K.M.; Matson, J.B. A Review of Hydrogen Sulfide (H_2S) Donors: Chemistry and Potential Therapeutic Applications. *Biochem. Pharmacol.* **2018**, *149*, 110–123. [CrossRef] [PubMed]
77. Xu, S.; Hamsath, A.; Neill, D.L.; Wang, Y.; Yang, C.; Xian, M. Strategies for the Design of Donors and Precursors of Reactive Sulfur Species. *Chem.-Eur. J.* **2019**, *25*, 4005–4016. [CrossRef]
78. Li, L.; Whiteman, M.; Guan, Y.Y.; Neo, K.L.; Cheng, Y.; Lee, S.W.; Zhao, Y.; Baskar, R.; Tan, C.-H.; Moore, P.K. Characterization of a Novel, Water-Soluble Hydrogen Sulfide–Releasing Molecule (GYY4137): New Insights Into the Biology of Hydrogen Sulfide. *Circulation* **2008**, *117*, 2351–2360. [CrossRef] [PubMed]
79. Rose, P.; Dymock, B.W.; Moore, P.K. GYY4137, a Novel Water-Soluble, H_2S-Releasing Molecule. In *Methods in Enzymology*; Elsevier: Amsterdam, The Netherlands, 2015; Volume 554, pp. 143–167, ISBN 978-0-12-801512-4.
80. Alexander, B.E.; Coles, S.J.; Fox, B.C.; Khan, T.F.; Maliszewski, J.; Perry, A.; Pitak, M.B.; Whiteman, M.; Wood, M.E. Investigating the Generation of Hydrogen Sulfide from the Phosphonamidodithioate Slow-Release Donor GYY4137. *MedChemComm* **2015**, *6*, 1649–1655. [CrossRef]
81. GYY4137 Protects against Myocardial Ischemia and Reperfusion Injury by Attenuating Oxidative Stress and Apoptosis in Rats. *J. Biomed. Res.* **2015**, *29*, 203–213. [CrossRef]
82. Qiu, Y.; Wu, Y.; Meng, M.; Luo, M.; Zhao, H.; Sun, H.; Gao, S. GYY4137 Protects against Myocardial Ischemia/Reperfusion Injury via Activation of the PHLPP-1/Akt/Nrf2 Signaling Pathway in Diabetic Mice. *J. Surg. Res.* **2018**, *225*, 29–39. [CrossRef]
83. Karwi, Q.G.; Whiteman, M.; Wood, M.E.; Torregrossa, R.; Baxter, G.F. Pharmacological Postconditioning against Myocardial Infarction with a Slow-Releasing Hydrogen Sulfide Donor, GYY4137. *Pharmacol. Res.* **2016**, *111*, 442–451. [CrossRef]
84. Robinson, H.; Wray, S. A New Slow Releasing, H_2S Generating Compound, GYY4137 Relaxes Spontaneous and Oxytocin-Stimulated Contractions of Human and Rat Pregnant Myometrium. *PLoS ONE* **2012**, *7*, e46278. [CrossRef]
85. Landis, P.S. The Chemistry of 1,2-Dithiole-3-Thiones. *Chem. Rev.* **1965**, *65*, 237–245. [CrossRef]
86. Hamada, T.; Nakane, T.; Kimura, T.; Arisawa, K.; Yoneda, K.; Yamamoto, T.; Osaki, T. Treatment of Xerostomia with the Bile Secretion-Stimulating Drug Anethole Trithione: A Clinical Trial. *Am. J. Med. Sci.* **1999**, *318*, 146–151. [CrossRef]
87. Perrino, E.; Cappelletti, G.; Tazzari, V.; Giavini, E.; Soldato, P.D.; Sparatore, A. New Sulfurated Derivatives of Valproic Acid with Enhanced Histone Deacetylase Inhibitory Activity. *Bioorg. Med. Chem. Lett.* **2008**, *18*, 1893–1897. [CrossRef]
88. Tazzari, V.; Cappelletti, G.; Casagrande, M.; Perrino, E.; Renzi, L.; Del Soldato, P.; Sparatore, A. New Aryldithiolethione Derivatives as Potent Histone Deacetylase Inhibitors. *Bioorg. Med. Chem.* **2010**, *18*, 4187–4194. [CrossRef] [PubMed]
89. Sen, C.K.; Traber, K.E.; Packer, L. Inhibition of NF-KB Activation in Human T-Cell Lines by Anetholdithiolthione. *Biochem. Biophys. Res. Commun.* **1996**, *218*, 148–153. [CrossRef] [PubMed]
90. Zanatta, S.D.; Jarrott, B.; Williams, S.J. Synthesis and Preliminary Pharmacological Evaluation of Aryl Dithiolethiones with Cyclooxygenase-2-Selective Inhibitory Activity and Hydrogen Sulfide-Releasing Properties. *Aust. J. Chem.* **2010**, *63*, 946. [CrossRef]
91. Qandil, A. Prodrugs of Nonsteroidal Anti-Inflammatory Drugs (NSAIDs), More Than Meets the Eye: A Critical Review. *Int. J. Mol. Sci.* **2012**, *13*, 17244–17274. [CrossRef]
92. Caliendo, G.; Cirino, G.; Santagada, V.; Wallace, J.L. Synthesis and Biological Effects of Hydrogen Sulfide (H_2S): Development of H_2S-Releasing Drugs as Pharmaceuticals. *J. Med. Chem.* **2010**, *53*, 6275–6286. [CrossRef]
93. Braga, T.C.; de Jesus, I.C.G.; Soares, K.V.; Guatimosim, S.; da Silva Neto, L.; da-Silva, C.J.; Modolo, L.V.; Menezes Filho, J.E.R.; Rhana, P.; Cruz, J.S.; et al. A Novel H_2S Releasing-Monastrol Hybrid (MADTOH) Inhibits L-Type Calcium Channels. *New J. Chem.* **2021**, *45*, 671–678. [CrossRef]
94. Majid, P.A.; De Jong, J. Acute Hemodynamic Effects of Nifedipine in Patients with Ischemic Heart Disease. *Circulation* **1982**, *65*, 1114–1118. [CrossRef]
95. Sparatore, A.; Perrino, E.; Tazzari, V.; Giustarini, D.; Rossi, R.; Rossoni, G.; Erdman, K.; Schröder, H.; Soldato, P.D. Pharmacological Profile of a Novel H_2S-Releasing Aspirin. *Free Radic. Biol. Med.* **2009**, *46*, 586–592. [CrossRef]
96. Huang, Q.; Sparatore, A.; Del Soldato, P.; Wu, L.; Desai, K. Hydrogen Sulfide Releasing Aspirin, ACS14, Attenuates High Glucose-Induced Increased Methylglyoxal and Oxidative Stress in Cultured Vascular Smooth Muscle Cells. *PLoS ONE* **2014**, *9*, e97315. [CrossRef]

97. Rossoni, G.; Manfredi, B.; Tazzari, V.; Sparatore, A.; Trivulzio, S.; Del Soldato, P.; Berti, F. Activity of a New Hydrogen Sulfide-Releasing Aspirin (ACS14) on Pathological Cardiovascular Alterations Induced by Glutathione Depletion in Rats. *Eur. J. Pharmacol.* **2010**, *648*, 139–145. [CrossRef] [PubMed]
98. Gerő, D.; Torregrossa, R.; Perry, A.; Waters, A.; Le-Trionnaire, S.; Whatmore, J.L.; Wood, M.; Whiteman, M. The Novel Mitochondria-Targeted Hydrogen Sulfide (H_2S) Donors AP123 and AP39 Protect against Hyperglycemic Injury in Microvascular Endothelial Cells in Vitro. *Pharmacol. Res.* **2016**, *113*, 186–198. [CrossRef] [PubMed]
99. Szczesny, B.; Módis, K.; Yanagi, K.; Coletta, C.; Le Trionnaire, S.; Perry, A.; Wood, M.E.; Whiteman, M.; Szabo, C. AP39, a Novel Mitochondria-Targeted Hydrogen Sulfide Donor, Stimulates Cellular Bioenergetics, Exerts Cytoprotective Effects and Protects against the Loss of Mitochondrial DNA Integrity in Oxidatively Stressed Endothelial Cells in Vitro. *Nitric Oxide* **2014**, *41*, 120–130. [CrossRef] [PubMed]
100. Ikeda, K.; Marutani, E.; Hirai, S.; Wood, M.E.; Whiteman, M.; Ichinose, F. Mitochondria-Targeted Hydrogen Sulfide Donor AP39 Improves Neurological Outcomes after Cardiac Arrest in Mice. *Nitric Oxide* **2015**, *49*, 90–96. [CrossRef]
101. Ahmad, A.; Olah, G.; Szczesny, B.; Wood, M.E.; Whiteman, M.; Szabo, C. AP39, a Mitochondrially Targeted Hydrogen Sulfide Donor, Exerts Protective Effects in Renal Epithelial Cells Subjected to Oxidative Stress in Vitro and in Acute Renal Injury in Vivo. *Shock* **2016**, *45*, 88–97. [CrossRef]
102. Karwi, Q.G.; Bornbaum, J.; Boengler, K.; Torregrossa, R.; Whiteman, M.; Wood, M.E.; Schulz, R.; Baxter, G.F. AP39, a Mitochondria-Targeting Hydrogen Sulfide (H_2S) Donor, Protects against Myocardial Reperfusion Injury Independently of Salvage Kinase Signalling: Cardioprotection with AP39. *Br. J. Pharmacol.* **2017**, *174*, 287–301. [CrossRef]
103. Kang, J.; Li, Z.; Organ, C.L.; Park, C.-M.; Yang, C.; Pacheco, A.; Wang, D.; Lefer, D.J.; Xian, M. PH-Controlled Hydrogen Sulfide Release for Myocardial Ischemia-Reperfusion Injury. *J. Am. Chem. Soc.* **2016**, *138*, 6336–6339. [CrossRef]
104. Zhang, J.; Zhang, Q.; Wang, Y.; Li, J.; Bai, Z.; Zhao, Q.; He, D.; Wang, Z.; Zhang, J.; Chen, Y. Toxicity, Bioactivity, Release of H_2S in Vivo and Pharmaco-Kinetics of H_2S-Donors with Thiophosphamide Structure. *Eur. J. Med. Chem.* **2019**, *176*, 456–475. [CrossRef]
105. Zhao, Y.; Yang, C.; Organ, C.; Li, Z.; Bhushan, S.; Otsuka, H.; Pacheco, A.; Kang, J.; Aguilar, H.C.; Lefer, D.J.; et al. Design, Synthesis, and Cardioprotective Effects of *N*-Mercapto-Based Hydrogen Sulfide Donors. *J. Med. Chem.* **2015**, *58*, 7501–7511. [CrossRef]
106. Yao, H.; Luo, S.; Liu, J.; Xie, S.; Liu, Y.; Xu, J.; Zhu, Z.; Xu, S. Controllable Thioester-Based Hydrogen Sulfide Slow-Releasing Donors as Cardioprotective Agents. *Chem. Commun.* **2019**, *55*, 6193–6196. [CrossRef]
107. Khodade, V.S.; Pharoah, B.M.; Paolocci, N.; Toscano, J.P. Alkylamine-Substituted Perthiocarbamates: Dual Precursors to Hydropersulfide and Carbonyl Sulfide with Cardioprotective Actions. *J. Am. Chem. Soc.* **2020**, *142*, 4309–4316. [CrossRef] [PubMed]
108. Testai, L.; Marino, A.; Piano, I.; Brancaleone, V.; Tomita, K.; Di Cesare Mannelli, L.; Martelli, A.; Citi, V.; Breschi, M.C.; Levi, R.; et al. The Novel H_2S-Donor 4-Carboxyphenyl Isothiocyanate Promotes Cardioprotective Effects against Ischemia/Reperfusion Injury through Activation of MitoK ATP Channels and Reduction of Oxidative Stress. *Pharmacol. Res.* **2016**, *113*, 290–299. [CrossRef]
109. Citi, V.; Corvino, A.; Fiorino, F.; Frecentese, F.; Magli, E.; Perissutti, E.; Santagada, V.; Brogi, S.; Flori, L.; Gorica, E.; et al. Structure-Activity Relationships Study of Isothiocyanates for H_2S Releasing Properties: 3-Pyridyl-Isothiocyanate as a New Promising Cardioprotective Agent. *J. Adv. Res.* **2021**, *27*, 41–53. [CrossRef] [PubMed]
110. Hu, Q.; Suarez, S.I.; Hankins, R.A.; Lukesh, J.C. Intramolecular Thiol- and Selenol-Assisted Delivery of Hydrogen Sulfide. *Angew. Chem. Int. Ed.* **2022**, *61*, e202210754. [CrossRef] [PubMed]
111. Lougiakis, N.; Papapetropoulos, A.; Gikas, E.; Toumpas, S.; Efentakis, P.; Wedmann, R.; Zoga, A.; Zhou, Z.; Iliodromitis, E.K.; Skaltsounis, A.-L.; et al. Synthesis and Pharmacological Evaluation of Novel Adenine–Hydrogen Sulfide Slow Release Hybrids Designed as Multitarget Cardioprotective Agents. *J. Med. Chem.* **2016**, *59*, 1776–1790. [CrossRef]
112. Ried, K.; Frank, O.R.; Stocks, N.P. Aged Garlic Extract Reduces Blood Pressure in Hypertensives: A Dose–Response Trial. *Eur. J. Clin. Nutr.* **2013**, *67*, 64–70. [CrossRef]
113. Jacob, C.; Anwar, A.; Burkholz, T. Perspective on Recent Developments on Sulfur-Containing Agents and Hydrogen Sulfide Signaling. *Planta Med.* **2008**, *74*, 1580–1592. [CrossRef]
114. Kashfi, K.; Olson, K.R. Biology and Therapeutic Potential of Hydrogen Sulfide and Hydrogen Sulfide-Releasing Chimeras. *Biochem. Pharmacol.* **2013**, *85*, 689–703. [CrossRef]
115. Li, L.; Hsu, A.; Moore, P.K. Actions and Interactions of Nitric Oxide, Carbon Monoxide and Hydrogen Sulphide in the Cardiovascular System and in Inflammation—A Tale of Three Gases! *Pharmacol. Ther.* **2009**, *123*, 386–400. [CrossRef]
116. Nicholson, C.K.; Calvert, J.W. Hydrogen Sulfide and Ischemia–Reperfusion Injury. *Pharmacol. Res.* **2010**, *62*, 289–297. [CrossRef]
117. Olson, K.R. The Therapeutic Potential of Hydrogen Sulfide: Separating Hype from Hope. *Am. J. Physiol.-Regul. Integr. Comp. Physiol.* **2011**, *301*, R297–R312. [CrossRef] [PubMed]
118. Predmore, B.L.; Lefer, D.J.; Gojon, G. Hydrogen Sulfide in Biochemistry and Medicine. *Antioxid. Redox Signal.* **2012**, *17*, 119–140. [CrossRef] [PubMed]
119. Levinn, C.M.; Cerda, M.M.; Pluth, M.D. Development and Application of Carbonyl Sulfide-Based Donors for H_2S Delivery. *Acc. Chem. Res.* **2019**, *52*, 2723–2731. [CrossRef]
120. Lin, Y.; Yang, X.; Lu, Y.; Liang, D.; Huang, D. Isothiocyanates as H_2S Donors Triggered by Cysteine: Reaction Mechanism and Structure and Activity Relationship. *Org. Lett.* **2019**, *21*, 5977–5980. [CrossRef] [PubMed]
121. Wang, D.; Zou, L.; Jin, Q.; Hou, J.; Ge, G.; Yang, L. Human Carboxylesterases: A Comprehensive Review. *Acta Pharm. Sin. B* **2018**, *8*, 699–712. [CrossRef]

122. Chauhan, P.; Bora, P.; Ravikumar, G.; Jos, S.; Chakrapani, H. Esterase Activated Carbonyl Sulfide/Hydrogen Sulfide (H_2S) Donors. *Org. Lett.* **2017**, *19*, 62–65. [CrossRef]
123. Fosnacht, K.G.; Cerda, M.M.; Mullen, E.J.; Pigg, H.C.; Pluth, M.D. Esterase-Activated Perthiocarbonate Persulfide Donors Provide Insights into Persulfide Persistence and Stability. *ACS Chem. Biol.* **2022**, *17*, 331–339. [CrossRef]
124. Shyaka, C.; Xian, M.; Park, C.-M. Esterase-Sensitive Trithiane-Based Hydrogen Sulfide Donors. *Org. Biomol. Chem.* **2019**, *17*, 9999–10003. [CrossRef]
125. Steiger, A.K.; Marcatti, M.; Szabo, C.; Szczesny, B.; Pluth, M.D. Inhibition of Mitochondrial Bioenergetics by Esterase-Triggered COS/H_2S Donors. *ACS Chem. Biol.* **2017**, *12*, 2117–2123. [CrossRef]
126. Yuan, Z.; Zheng, Y.; Yu, B.; Wang, S.; Yang, X.; Wang, B. Esterase-Sensitive Glutathione Persulfide Donor. *Org. Lett.* **2018**, *20*, 6364–6367. [CrossRef]
127. Zheng, Y.; Yu, B.; Ji, K.; Pan, Z.; Chittavong, V.; Wang, B. Esterase-Sensitive Prodrugs with Tunable Release Rates and Direct Generation of Hydrogen Sulfide. *Angew. Chem. Int. Ed.* **2016**, *55*, 4514–4518. [CrossRef]
128. Zheng, Y.; Yu, B.; Li, Z.; Yuan, Z.; Organ, C.L.; Trivedi, R.K.; Wang, S.; Lefer, D.J.; Wang, B. An Esterase-Sensitive Prodrug Approach for Controllable Delivery of Persulfide Species. *Angew. Chem.* **2017**, *129*, 11911–11915. [CrossRef]
129. Liu, Q.; Ji, G.; Chu, Y.; Hao, T.; Qian, M.; Zhao, Q. Enzyme-Responsive Hybrid Prodrug of Nitric Oxide and Hydrogen Sulfide for Heart Failure Therapy. *Chem. Commun.* **2022**, *58*, 7396–7399. [CrossRef] [PubMed]
130. Zhao, Y.; Pluth, M.D. Hydrogen Sulfide Donors Activated by Reactive Oxygen Species. *Angew. Chem.* **2016**, *128*, 14858–14862. [CrossRef]
131. Powell, C.R.; Dillon, K.M.; Wang, Y.; Carrazzone, R.J.; Matson, J.B. A Persulfide Donor Responsive to Reactive Oxygen Species: Insights into Reactivity and Therapeutic Potential. *Angew. Chem. Int. Ed.* **2018**, *57*, 6324–6328. [CrossRef] [PubMed]
132. Bora, P.; Chauhan, P.; Manna, S.; Chakrapani, H. A Vinyl-Boronate Ester-Based Persulfide Donor Controllable by Hydrogen Peroxide, a Reactive Oxygen Species (ROS). *Org. Lett.* **2018**, *20*, 7916–7920. [CrossRef]
133. Hankins, R.A.; Suarez, S.I.; Kalk, M.A.; Green, N.M.; Harty, M.N.; Lukesh, J.C. An Innovative Hydrogen Peroxide-Sensing Scaffold and Insight Towards Its Potential as an ROS-Activated Persulfide Donor. *Angew. Chem. Int. Ed.* **2020**, *59*, 22238–22245. [CrossRef]
134. Zhu, C.; Suarez, S.I.; Lukesh, J.C. Illuminating and Alleviating Cellular Oxidative Stress with an ROS-Activated, H_2S-Donating Theranostic. *Tetrahedron Lett.* **2021**, *69*, 152944. [CrossRef]
135. Lippert, A.R.; Van de Bittner, G.C.; Chang, C.J. Boronate Oxidation as a Bioorthogonal Reaction Approach for Studying the Chemistry of Hydrogen Peroxide in Living Systems. *Acc. Chem. Res.* **2011**, *44*, 793–804. [CrossRef]
136. Bezner, B.J.; Ryan, L.S.; Lippert, A.R. Reaction-Based Luminescent Probes for Reactive Sulfur, Oxygen, and Nitrogen Species: Analytical Techniques and Recent Progress. *Anal. Chem.* **2020**, *92*, 309–326. [CrossRef]
137. Ye, H.; Zhou, Y.; Liu, X.; Chen, Y.; Duan, S.; Zhu, R.; Liu, Y.; Yin, L. Recent Advances on Reactive Oxygen Species-Responsive Delivery and Diagnosis System. *Biomacromolecules* **2019**, *20*, 2441–2463. [CrossRef] [PubMed]
138. Hu, Y.; Li, X.; Fang, Y.; Shi, W.; Li, X.; Chen, W.; Xian, M.; Ma, H. Reactive Oxygen Species-Triggered off-on Fluorescence Donor for Imaging Hydrogen Sulfide Delivery in Living Cells. *Chem. Sci.* **2019**, *10*, 7690–7694. [CrossRef]
139. Zhang, N.; Hu, P.; Wang, Y.; Tang, Q.; Zheng, Q.; Wang, Z.; He, Y. A Reactive Oxygen Species (ROS) Activated Hydrogen Sulfide (H_2S) Donor with Self-Reporting Fluorescence. *ACS Sens.* **2020**, *5*, 319–326. [CrossRef] [PubMed]
140. Yao, M.; Lu, Y.; Shi, L.; Huang, Y.; Zhang, Q.; Tan, J.; Hu, P.; Zhang, J.; Luo, G.; Zhang, N. A ROS-Responsive, Self-Immolative and Self-Reporting Hydrogen Sulfide Donor with Multiple Biological Activities for the Treatment of Myocardial Infarction. *Bioact. Mater.* **2022**, *9*, 168–182. [CrossRef] [PubMed]
141. Buzdar, A.U.; Marcus, C.; Blumenschein, G.R.; Smith, T.L. Early and Delayed Clinical Cardiotoxicity of Doxorubicin. *Cancer* **1985**, *55*, 2761–2765. [CrossRef]
142. Swain, S.M.; Whaley, F.S.; Ewer, M.S. Congestive Heart Failure in Patients Treated with Doxorubicin: A Retrospective Analysis of Three Trials. *Cancer* **2003**, *97*, 2869–2879. [CrossRef] [PubMed]
143. Ai, D.; Banchs, J.; Owusu-Agyemang, P.; Cata, J.P. Chemotherapy-Induced Cardiovascular Toxicity: Beyond Anthracyclines. *Minerva Anestesiol.* **2014**, *80*, 586–594. [PubMed]
144. Lipshultz, S.E.; Franco, V.I.; Cochran, T.R. Cardiotoxicity in Childhood Cancer Survivors: A Problem with Long-Term Consequences in Need of Early Detection and Prevention: Cardiotoxicity in Childhood Cancer Survivors. *Pediatr. Blood Cancer* **2013**, *60*, 1395–1396. [CrossRef]
145. Zamorano, J.L.; Lancellotti, P.; Rodriguez Muñoz, D.; Aboyans, V.; Asteggiano, R.; Galderisi, M.; Habib, G.; Lenihan, D.J.; Lip, G.Y.H.; Lyon, A.R.; et al. 2016 ESC Position Paper on Cancer Treatments and Cardiovascular Toxicity Developed under the Auspices of the ESC Committee for Practice Guidelines: The Task Force for Cancer Treatments and Cardiovascular Toxicity of the European Society of Cardiology (ESC). *Eur. Heart J.* **2016**, *37*, 2768–2801. [CrossRef]
146. O'Hare, M.; Sharma, A.; Murphy, K.; Mookadam, F.; Lee, H. Cardio-Oncology Part I: Chemotherapy and Cardiovascular Toxicity. *Expert Rev. Cardiovasc. Ther.* **2015**, *13*, 511–518. [CrossRef]
147. Minotti, G.; Menna, P.; Salvatorelli, E.; Cairo, G.; Gianni, L. Anthracyclines: Molecular Advances and Pharmacologic Developments in Antitumor Activity and Cardiotoxicity. *Pharmacol. Rev.* **2004**, *56*, 185–229. [CrossRef] [PubMed]
148. Gewirtz, D. A Critical Evaluation of the Mechanisms of Action Proposed for the Antitumor Effects of the Anthracycline Antibiotics Adriamycin and Daunorubicin. *Biochem. Pharmacol.* **1999**, *57*, 727–741. [CrossRef] [PubMed]

149. Doroshow, J.H.; Davies, K.J. Redox Cycling of Anthracyclines by Cardiac Mitochondria. II. Formation of Superoxide Anion, Hydrogen Peroxide, and Hydroxyl Radical. *J. Biol. Chem.* **1986**, *261*, 3068–3074. [CrossRef] [PubMed]
150. Wallace, K.B.; Sardão, V.A.; Oliveira, P.J. Mitochondrial Determinants of Doxorubicin-Induced Cardiomyopathy. *Circ. Res.* **2020**, *126*, 926–941. [CrossRef]
151. Granados-Principal, S.; Quiles, J.L.; Ramirez-Tortosa, C.L.; Sanchez-Rovira, P.; Ramirez-Tortosa, M.C. New Advances in Molecular Mechanisms and the Prevention of Adriamycin Toxicity by Antioxidant Nutrients. *Food Chem. Toxicol.* **2010**, *48*, 1425–1438. [CrossRef]
152. Doroshow, J.H.; Locker, G.Y.; Myers, C.E. Enzymatic Defenses of the Mouse Heart Against Reactive Oxygen Metabolites. *J. Clin. Investig.* **1980**, *65*, 128–135. [CrossRef]
153. Octavia, Y.; Tocchetti, C.G.; Gabrielson, K.L.; Janssens, S.; Crijns, H.J.; Moens, A.L. Doxorubicin-Induced Cardiomyopathy: From Molecular Mechanisms to Therapeutic Strategies. *J. Mol. Cell. Cardiol.* **2012**, *52*, 1213–1225. [CrossRef]
154. Upadhayay, S.; Sharma, N.; Mantha, A.K.; Dhiman, M. Anti-Cancer Drug Doxorubicin Induced Cardiotoxicity: Understanding The Mechanisms Involved In Ros Generation Resulting In Mitochondrial Dysfunction. *Rasayan J. Chem.* **2020**, *13*, 1042–1053. [CrossRef]
155. Rawat, P.S.; Jaiswal, A.; Khurana, A.; Bhatti, J.S.; Navik, U. Doxorubicin-Induced Cardiotoxicity: An Update on the Molecular Mechanism and Novel Therapeutic Strategies for Effective Management. *Biomed. Pharmacother.* **2021**, *139*, 111708. [CrossRef]
156. Du, S.; Huang, Y.; Jin, H.; Wang, T. Protective Mechanism of Hydrogen Sulfide against Chemotherapy-Induced Cardiotoxicity. *Front. Pharmacol.* **2018**, *9*, 32. [CrossRef]
157. Su, Y.-W.; Liang, C.; Jin, H.-F.; Tang, X.-Y.; Han, W.; Chai, L.-J.; Zhang, C.-Y.; Geng, B.; Tang, C.-S.; Du, J.-B. Hydrogen Sulfide Regulates Cardiac Function and Structure in Adriamycin-Induced Cardiomyopathy. *Circ. J.* **2009**, *73*, 741–749. [CrossRef]
158. Guo, R.; Lin, J.; Xu, W.; Shen, N.; Mo, L.; Zhang, C.; Feng, J. Hydrogen Sulfide Attenuates Doxorubicin-Induced Cardiotoxicity by Inhibition of the P38 MAPK Pathway in H9c2 Cells. *Int. J. Mol. Med.* **2013**, *31*, 644–650. [CrossRef] [PubMed]
159. Wang, X.-Y.; Yang, C.-T.; Zheng, D.-D.; Mo, L.-Q.; Lan, A.-P.; Yang, Z.-L.; Hu, F.; Chen, P.-X.; Liao, X.-X.; Feng, J.-Q. Hydrogen Sulfide Protects H9c2 Cells against Doxorubicin-Induced Cardiotoxicity through Inhibition of Endoplasmic Reticulum Stress. *Mol. Cell. Biochem.* **2012**, *363*, 419–426. [CrossRef]
160. Liu, M.-H.; Lin, X.-L.; Zhang, Y.; He, J.; Tan, T.-P.; Wu, S.-J.; Liu, J.; Tian, W.; Chen, L.; Yu, S.; et al. Hydrogen Sulfide Attenuates Doxorubicin-Induced Cardiotoxicity by Inhibiting Reactive Oxygen Species-Activated Extracellular Signal-Regulated Kinase 1/2 in H9c2 Cardiac Myocytes. *Mol. Med. Rep.* **2015**, *12*, 6841–6848. [CrossRef]
161. Waz, S.; Heeba, G.H.; Hassanin, S.O.; Abdel-latif, R.G. Nephroprotective Effect of Exogenous Hydrogen Sulfide Donor against Cyclophosphamide-Induced Toxicity Is Mediated by Nrf2/HO-1/NF-KB Signaling Pathway. *Life Sci.* **2021**, *264*, 118630. [CrossRef]
162. Azarbarz, N.; Shafiei Seifabadi, Z.; Moaiedi, M.Z.; Mansouri, E. Assessment of the Effect of Sodium Hydrogen Sulfide (Hydrogen Sulfide Donor) on Cisplatin-Induced Testicular Toxicity in Rats. *Environ. Sci. Pollut. Res.* **2020**, *27*, 8119–8128. [CrossRef]
163. Chegaev, K.; Rolando, B.; Cortese, D.; Gazzano, E.; Buondonno, I.; Lazzarato, L.; Fanelli, M.; Hattinger, C.M.; Serra, M.; Riganti, C.; et al. H_2S-Donating Doxorubicins May Overcome Cardiotoxicity and Multidrug Resistance. *J. Med. Chem.* **2016**, *59*, 4881–4889. [CrossRef]
164. Persidis, A. Cancer Multidrug Resistance. *Nat. Biotechnol.* **1999**, *17*, 94–95. [CrossRef] [PubMed]
165. Bigagli, E.; Luceri, C.; De Angioletti, M.; Chegaev, K.; D'Ambrosio, M.; Riganti, C.; Gazzano, E.; Saponara, S.; Longini, M.; Luceri, F.; et al. New NO- and H_2S-Releasing Doxorubicins as Targeted Therapy against Chemoresistance in Castration-Resistant Prostate Cancer: In Vitro and in Vivo Evaluations. *Invest. New Drugs* **2018**, *36*, 985–998. [CrossRef] [PubMed]
166. Durante, M.; Frosini, M.; Chiaino, E.; Fusi, F.; Gamberucci, A.; Gorelli, B.; Chegaev, K.; Riganti, C.; Saponara, S. Sdox, a H_2S Releasing Anthracycline, with a Safer Profile than Doxorubicin toward Vasculature. *Vascul. Pharmacol.* **2022**, *143*, 106969. [CrossRef]
167. Gazzano, E.; Buondonno, I.; Marengo, A.; Rolando, B.; Chegaev, K.; Kopecka, J.; Saponara, S.; Sorge, M.; Hattinger, C.M.; Gasco, A.; et al. Hyaluronated Liposomes Containing H_2S-Releasing Doxorubicins Are Effective against P-Glycoprotein-Positive/Doxorubicin-Resistant Osteosarcoma Cells and Xenografts. *Cancer Lett.* **2019**, *456*, 29–39. [CrossRef]
168. Hu, Q.; Yammani, R.D.; Brown-Harding, H.; Soto-Pantoja, D.R.; Poole, L.B.; Lukesh, J.C. Mitigation of Doxorubicin-Induced Cardiotoxicity with an H_2O_2-Activated, H_2S-Donating Hybrid Prodrug. *Redox Biol.* **2022**, *53*, 102338. [CrossRef]
169. Liou, G.-Y.; Storz, P. Reactive Oxygen Species in Cancer. *Free Radic. Res.* **2010**, *44*, 479–496. [CrossRef]
170. Wang, L.; Xie, S.; Ma, L.; Chen, Y.; Lu, W. 10-Boronic Acid Substituted Camptothecin as Prodrug of SN-38. *Eur. J. Med. Chem.* **2016**, *116*, 84–89. [CrossRef] [PubMed]
171. Kuang, Y.; Balakrishnan, K.; Gandhi, V.; Peng, X. Hydrogen Peroxide Inducible DNA Cross-Linking Agents: Targeted Anticancer Prodrugs. *J. Am. Chem. Soc.* **2011**, *133*, 19278–19281. [CrossRef] [PubMed]
172. Ai, Y.; Obianom, O.N.; Kuser, M.; Li, Y.; Shu, Y.; Xue, F. Enhanced Tumor Selectivity of 5-Fluorouracil Using a Reactive Oxygen Species-Activated Prodrug Approach. *ACS Med. Chem. Lett.* **2019**, *10*, 127–131. [CrossRef] [PubMed]
173. Skarbek, C.; Serra, S.; Maslah, H.; Rascol, E.; Labruère, R. Arylboronate Prodrugs of Doxorubicin as Promising Chemotherapy for Pancreatic Cancer. *Bioorganic Chem.* **2019**, *91*, 103158. [CrossRef]
174. Mirzaei, S.; Zarrabi, A.; Hashemi, F.; Zabolian, A.; Saleki, H.; Azami, N.; Hamzehlou, S.; Farahani, M.V.; Hushmandi, K.; Ashrafizadeh, M.; et al. Nrf2 Signaling Pathway in Chemoprotection and Doxorubicin Resistance: Potential Application in Drug Discovery. *Antioxidants* **2021**, *10*, 349. [CrossRef]

175. Nordgren, K.K.S.; Wallace, K.B. Disruption of the Keap1/Nrf2-Antioxidant Response System After Chronic Doxorubicin Exposure In Vivo. *Cardiovasc. Toxicol.* **2020**, *20*, 557–570. [CrossRef]
176. Alzahrani, A.M.; Rajendran, P.; Veeraraghavan, V.P.; Hanieh, H. Cardiac Protective Effect of Kirenol against Doxorubicin-Induced Cardiac Hypertrophy in H9c2 Cells through Nrf2 Signaling via PI3K/AKT Pathways. *Int. J. Mol. Sci.* **2021**, *22*, 3269. [CrossRef]
177. Gu, J.; Huang, H.; Liu, C.; Jiang, B.; Li, M.; Liu, L.; Zhang, S. Pinocembrin Inhibited Cardiomyocyte Pyroptosis against Doxorubicin-Induced Cardiac Dysfunction via Regulating Nrf2/Sirt3 Signaling Pathway. *Int. Immunopharmacol.* **2021**, *95*, 107533. [CrossRef]
178. Pan, T.-T.; Feng, Z.-N.; Lee, S.W.; Moore, P.K.; Bian, J.-S. Endogenous Hydrogen Sulfide Contributes to the Cardioprotection by Metabolic Inhibition Preconditioning in the Rat Ventricular Myocytes. *J. Mol. Cell. Cardiol.* **2006**, *40*, 119–130. [CrossRef] [PubMed]
179. Mazza, R.; Pasqua, T.; Cerra, M.C.; Angelone, T.; Gattuso, A. Akt/ENOS Signaling and PLN S-Sulfhydration Are Involved in H_2S-Dependent Cardiac Effects in Frog and Rat. *Am. J. Physiol.-Regul. Integr. Comp. Physiol.* **2013**, *305*, R443–R451. [CrossRef] [PubMed]
180. Hu, Y.; Chen, X.; Pan, T.-T.; Neo, K.L.; Lee, S.W.; Khin, E.S.W.; Moore, P.K.; Bian, J.-S. Cardioprotection Induced by Hydrogen Sulfide Preconditioning Involves Activation of ERK and PI3K/Akt Pathways. *Pflüg. Arch.—Eur. J. Physiol.* **2007**, *455*, 607–616. [CrossRef] [PubMed]
181. Liu, M.-H.; Zhang, Y.; He, J.; Tan, T.-P.; Wu, S.-J.; Guo, D.-M.; He, H.; Peng, J.; Tang, Z.-H.; Jiang, Z.-S. Hydrogen Sulfide Protects H9c2 Cardiac Cells against Doxorubicin-Induced Cytotoxicity through the PI3K/Akt/FoxO3a Pathway. *Int. J. Mol. Med.* **2016**, *37*, 1661–1668. [CrossRef] [PubMed]
182. Guo, R.; Wu, K.; Chen, J.; Mo, L.; Hua, X.; Zheng, D.; Chen, P.; Chen, G.; Xu, W.; Feng, J. Exogenous Hydrogen Sulfide Protects against Doxorubicin-Induced Inflammation and Cytotoxicity by Inhibiting P38MAPK/NFκB Pathway in H9c2 Cardiac Cells. *Cell. Physiol. Biochem.* **2013**, *32*, 1668–1680. [CrossRef]
183. Xu, W.; Chen, J.; Lin, J.; Liu, D.; Mo, L.; Pan, W.; Feng, J.; Wu, W.; Zheng, D. Exogenous H_2S Protects H9c2 Cardiac Cells against High Glucose-Induced Injury and Inflammation by Inhibiting the Activation of the NF-κB and IL-1β Pathways. *Int. J. Mol. Med.* **2015**, *35*, 177–186. [CrossRef]
184. Yarmohammadi, F.; Hayes, A.W.; Karimi, G. The Cardioprotective Effects of Hydrogen Sulfide by Targeting Endoplasmic Reticulum Stress and the Nrf2 Signaling Pathway: A Review. *BioFactors* **2021**, *47*, 701–712. [CrossRef]
185. Wu, D.; Gu, Y.; Zhu, D. Cardioprotective Effects of Hydrogen Sulfide in Attenuating Myocardial Ischemia-reperfusion Injury (Review). *Mol. Med. Rep.* **2021**, *24*, 875. [CrossRef]

Disclaimer/Publisher's Note: The statements, opinions and data contained in all publications are solely those of the individual author(s) and contributor(s) and not of MDPI and/or the editor(s). MDPI and/or the editor(s) disclaim responsibility for any injury to people or property resulting from any ideas, methods, instructions or products referred to in the content.

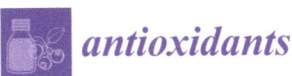

Review

Organelle-Targeted Fluorescent Probes for Sulfane Sulfur Species

Biswajit Roy [†], Meg Shieh [†], Geat Ramush and Ming Xian *

Department of Chemistry, Brown University, Providence, RI 02912, USA
* Correspondence: ming_xian@brown.edu
† These authors contributed equally to this work.

Abstract: Sulfane sulfurs, which include hydropersulfides (RSSH), hydrogen polysulfides (H_2S_n, n > 1), and polysulfides (RS_nR, n > 2), play important roles in cellular redox biology and are closely linked to hydrogen sulfide (H_2S) signaling. While most studies on sulfane sulfur detection have focused on sulfane sulfurs in the whole cell, increasing the recognition of the effects of reactive sulfur species on the functions of various subcellular organelles has emerged. This has driven a need for organelle-targeted detection methods. However, the detection of sulfane sulfurs, particularly of RSSH and H_2S_n, in biological systems is still a challenge due to their low endogenous concentrations and instabilities. In this review, we summarize the development and design of organelle-targeted fluorescent sulfane sulfur probes, examine their organelle-targeting strategies and choices of fluorophores (e.g., ratiometric, near-infrared, etc.), and discuss their mechanisms and ability to detect endogenous and exogenous sulfane sulfur species. We also present the advantages and limitations of the probes and propose directions for future work on this topic.

Keywords: sulfane sulfur; fluorescent probe; organelle; chemistry

1. Introduction

Biological sulfane sulfurs (S^0), including hydropersulfides (RSSH), polysulfides (RSS_nSR), hydrogen polysulfides (H_2S_n, n ≥ 2), and protein-bound elemental sulfurs (S_8), have become increasingly recognized as important reactive sulfur species (RSS) with distinct functions in redox biology that are closely linked to hydrogen sulfide (H_2S) signaling [1]. Sulfane sulfurs are sulfur atoms with six valence electrons and no charge that are covalently bonded to other sulfur atoms. Significantly, sulfane sulfurs have been discovered to influence various physiological and pathological processes, including activating the transient receptor potential ankyrin 1 (TRPA1) channel, relaxing vascular smooth muscles, mediating neurotransmission, and regulating inflammation [2–5]. Yet, due to their instabilities, sulfane sulfurs such as RSSH and H_2S_n are understudied despite their active involvement in redox signaling. Considering the importance of sulfane sulfurs in biological systems, the development of detection methods for these species is important to better understand their biological mechanisms of action and potential therapeutic applications.

Some of the most popular detection methods for sulfane sulfurs or other biologically important analytes are fluorescence spectroscopy and fluorescence microscopy [6–15]. These methods involve the usage of fluorescent probes, which are important tools in the study of biological systems because they allow researchers to visualize and track specific molecules or processes within cells and tissues. By emitting light when excited by a specific wavelength of light, fluorescent probes allow scientists to detect and even quantify the presence of specific molecules in real time [13–15]. Thus, fluorescent probes can answer fundamental questions regarding the production and mechanisms of action for sulfane sulfurs in biological samples, making these probes essential for medical diagnosis, treatment, and basic biomedical research.

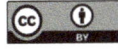

Most reported fluorescent probes and studies for sulfane sulfur detection examine cellular sulfane sulfur levels rather than those in subcellular microenvironments. Yet, organelles are specialized subunits within cells that perform specific functions that are essential for the overall health and survival of the cell. In events of stress or malfunction, disease can result. For example, the mitochondria are involved in many critical processes, including the regulation of cell signaling and differentiation, cell death pathways, and the cell cycle [16]. Mitochondrial oxidative damage has been found to contribute to a wide range of human disorders, including ischemia-reperfusion injury and aging-associated dysfunction [17]. While studies have found that H_2S offers cardioprotective effects by preserving mitochondrial function, sulfane sulfurs are less well-studied. It has been reported, however, that the majority of bound sulfane sulfurs in cells are in the mitochondria, suggesting the importance of this organelle in maintaining cardiovascular homeostasis [18]. It is also known that the mitochondrial enzyme sulfide quinone oxidoreductase (SQOR) rapidly converts H_2S into sulfane sulfurs (persulfides and polysulfides) which are then stored in the mitochondria until they are released in response to physiological signals [19]. Considering that this organelle has been found to play key roles in diseases and sulfane sulfurs have been found as actual signaling species in a range of biological activities previously attributed to H_2S, an accurate, sensitive, and real-time method for detecting sulfane sulfurs in the mitochondria is essential to understand their mechanisms.

Other subcellular organelles also have specific functions that contribute to the operation of a cell and can result in disease in the event of dysfunction. For example, lysosomes are single-layered membrane organelles that are responsible for cellular waste digestion and contain acidic environments and hydrolases. RSS plays a role in the regulation of lysosomal activity and membrane permeability, thus affecting many biological processes [20]. The rough endoplasmic reticulum (ER) is responsible for protein synthesis, while the smooth ER is primarily involved in calcium signaling, lipid synthesis, and carbohydrate metabolism. ER stress and protein misfolding have been associated with diseases, including myocardial ischemia-reperfusion (MI/R) injury, cardiomyopathy, heart failure, hypertension, and diabetes [21–24]. The Golgi apparatus processes, packages, and transports proteins and lipids. The lysosomes, ER, and Golgi apparatus have connected functions as part of a secretory pathway with the cell membrane; therefore, the subcellular targeting of sulfane sulfurs in these organelles using fluorescent probes is critical for better understanding the physiological and pathological impacts of sulfane sulfurs on various diseases. This greater knowledge may even have potential implications for clinical diagnosis and improved therapeutics.

Due to the rising interest in organelles, sulfane sulfurs, and the role of sulfane sulfurs in maintaining intracellular redox homeostasis, developments in organelle-targeted fluorescent probes for sulfane sulfurs have been made in recent years. In this article, we reviewed the popular strategies for organelle-targeted probe design and discussed the reported organelle-targeted fluorescent probes for sulfane sulfurs along with their properties and potential limitations. A summary of these molecules is shown in Figure 1.

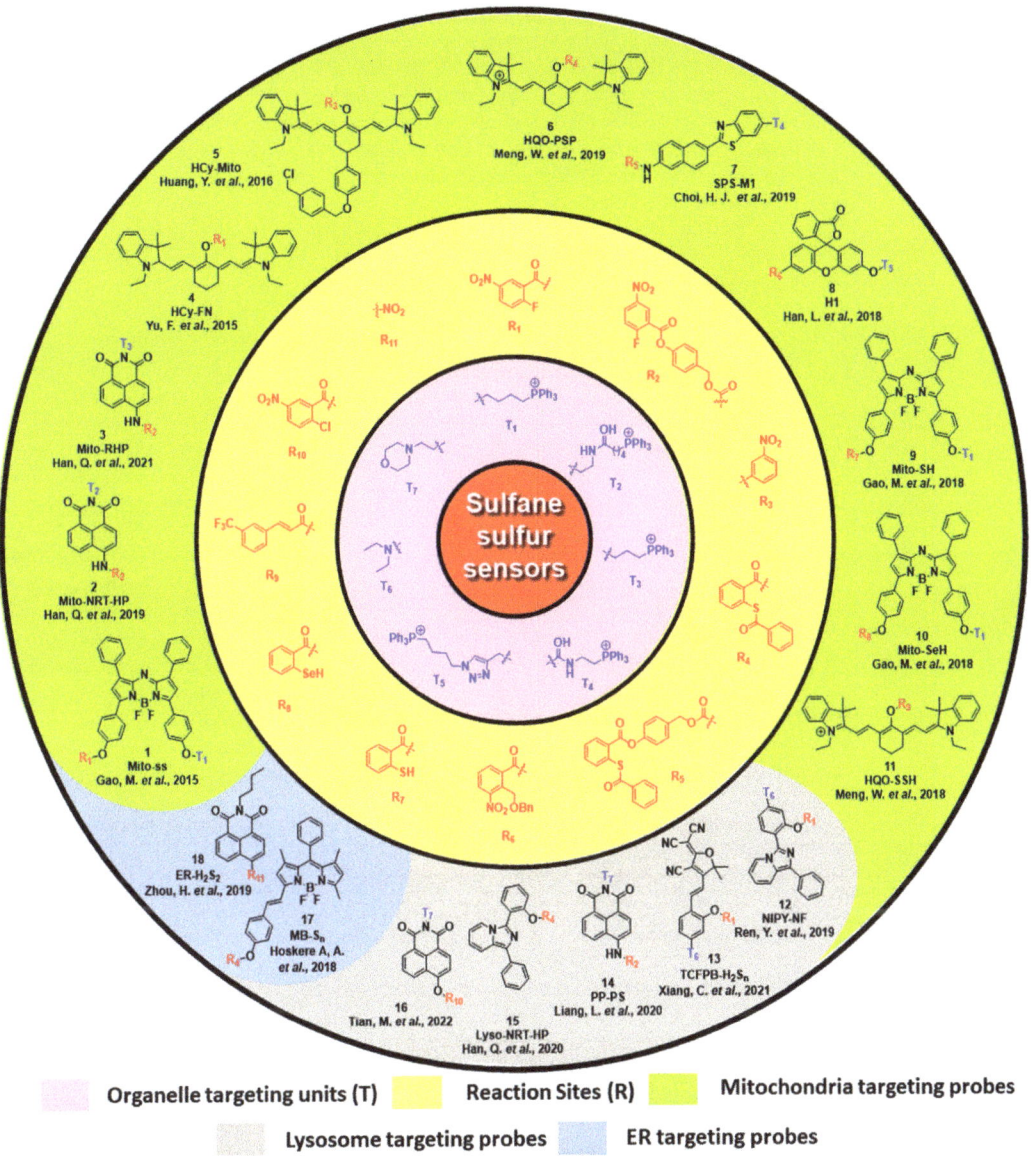

Figure 1. A summary of reported organelle-targeted fluorescent probes for sulfane sulfurs.

2. Mitochondria-Targeting Probes

Mitochondria are the major source of reactive oxygen species (ROS). During mitochondrial respiration, nearly 0.1–4% of oxygen is reduced to the superoxide ion ($O_2^{\bullet-}$) due to electron leakage from the respiratory chain. This species is then transformed into other ROSs via enzymatic or non-enzymatic pathways [25]. Meanwhile, endogenously produced H_2S is oxidized in the presence of mitochondrial ROS to form sulfane sulfurs, which can also be formed directly via enzymes such as 3MST. Thus, to better understand redox homeostasis, monitoring sulfane sulfurs via fluorescence imaging is useful. Mitochondria possess a unique double-layered membrane structure with a negative membrane potential (as high as −180 mV) [26]. Hence, in most cases, mitochondria-targeted probes possess at least one lipophilic cation [27]. Non-cationic probes can be functionalized by attaching triphenyl phosphonium [20] or pyridinium [28–30] as the anchor. However, functionalized cationic dyes are also known to target other organelles [31–35]. Based on colocalization experiments with commercially available mitochondria-targeting dyes, some non-cationic dyes have been reported to selectively target the mitochondria due to their unique structures [36]. Here, we summarize the reported cationic and non-cationic mitochondria-targeted probes for sulfane sulfur detection.

In 2015, Chen and coworkers developed a reaction-based near-infrared (NIR) fluorescent probe (Mito-ss) for the detection of mitochondrial hydrogen polysulfides (H_2S_n, n > 1) [37]. Mito-ss consists of (i) a NIR dye based on the azo-BODIPY chromophore, (ii) a lipophilic triphenyl phosphonium group, and (iii) an H_2S_n-reactive nitrofluorobenzoate moiety (Scheme 1a). They chose a NIR fluorophore because NIR lights possess certain advantages, including deep tissue penetration, low cytotoxicity, and minimum background noise. Nitrofluorobenzoate is a commonly used functional group for the design of H_2S_n sensors [38]. Nitrofluorobenzoate bears two electrophilic sites. H_2S_n first reacts with it via nucleophilic aromatic substitution (S_NAr) to replace the F atom and form a persulfide (-SSH) intermediate, which then undergoes a spontaneous intramolecular cyclization with the ester group to uncage the fluorophore. Due to its electron with-drawing nature, nitrofluorobenzoate quenches the fluorescence of the azo-BODIPY chromophore via a donor-excited photoinduced electron transfer (d-PET) process. As such, Mito-ss is a reaction-based 'turn-on' sensor for H_2S_n. Mito-ss reacts rapidly (~30 s) with H_2S_n and exhibits a 24-fold fluorescence increase at an emission of 730 nm. The probe was examined with various ROS, reactive nitrogen species (RNS), and other RSS and demonstrated no fluorescence turn-on. Biothiols such as glutathione (GSH), cysteine (Cys), N-acetyl-L-cysteine, etc., could react with Mito-ss. However, as the reaction stopped at the S_NAr step, no fluorescence was observed. The limit of detection (LOD) for Mito-ss was calculated to be 25 nM. The probe was used for the real-time detection of exogenous and endogenous H_2S_n using six different cell lines. Mito-ss was also found to be suitable for the in vivo detection of exogenously injected H_2S_n in BALB/c mice.

Using the same nitrofluorobenzoate reaction site, Han et al. developed a ratiometric fluorescent probe, Mito-NRT-HP, for the detection of mitochondrial H_2S_n in 2019 [39]. The structure of Mito-NRT-HP is similar to Mito-ss, though with a two-photon responsive naphthalimide fluorophore instead of a single-photon responsive fluorophore. The naphthalimide fluorophore has the advantage of easily tunable photophysical properties by blocking and/or unblocking the internal charge transfer (ICT) process. It is highly photostable, resistant to pH interference, and possesses a large two-photon absorption cross-section. Importantly, 1,8-naphthalimide can be easily functionalized by simple synthetic tailoring [40]. The main advantages of two-photon excitation over single-photon excitation include deep tissue penetration, lesser damage, poor scattering, etc. In the case of two-photon excitation, a femto second pulsed laser is used, and the molecule can be excited only at the focal point of the laser. Three-dimensional imaging can be obtained [41]. Upon titrating with different concentrations of Na_2S_2, it was found that Mito-NRT-HP gave ratiometric responses with a changing fluorescence color from blue to green. When the solution of Mito-NRT-HP was treated with H_2S_n, the initial emission maximum at 478 nm decreased gradually, with a concomitant peak increase at 546 nm. The detection limit was 10 nM which suggests that Mito-NRT-HP could have the relevant sensitivity needed for the quantitative detection of H_2S_n under physiological conditions. The two-photon absorption cross-section values (δ) of Mito-NRT-HP and its fluorophore Mito-NRT (Scheme 1b) were recorded in a buffer using a pulsed laser, and fluorescein was used as the reference molecule. Their δ values were measured over a range of wavelengths starting from 750 nm to 825 nm. The highest δ was 290 GM [1 GM (Goeppert-Mayer) = 10^{-50} cm^4 s $photon^{-1}$] for Mito-NRT-HP and ~190 GM for Mito-NRT at 810 nm. Mito-NRT-HP was found to exhibit good cell permeability and weak cytotoxicity, which was suitable for the ratiometric imaging of endogenous H_2S_2 in cells. Mito-NRT-HP was colocalized with MitoTracker Red (MTR) and LysoTracker Red (LTR), and the colocalization coefficients were found to be 0.94 and 0.42, respectively, indicating that Mito-NRT-HP was specifically localized in the mitochondria. Using two-photon microscopy, images of the tissue slices from mice with lipopolysaccharide (LPS)-induced acute organ injury were taken and compared with the control tissues. The enhanced fluorescence in the former case was observed. In 2021, Han et al. reported a similar probe for the detection of mitochondrial H_2S_n during H_2O_2-induced redox imbalance [42]. The structure of this probe (Mito-RHP) only differed from Mito-NRT-HP in the linker between naphthalimide and the triphenylphosphonium unit. Upon the addition of Na_2S_2 to the solution of Mito-RHP, the initial emission spectra of Mito-RHP at 485 nm gradually decreased, and a continuous increase in the new peak to 550 nm was observed, along with a change in fluorescence color from blue to yellowish green. In this case, the Stokes shift was 109 nm, which was higher than that of Mito-NRT-HP. The detection limit was calculated to be 20 nM. Other properties, such as photostability, solubility, permeability, and cytotoxicity, were similar. However, the mitochondria-targeting ability of the new probe (overlap coefficient = 0.836) was not as good as that of Mito-NRT-HP (overlap coefficient = 0.94). The in vivo imaging of exogenous H_2S_n (using Na_2S_2) was performed in zebrafish using Mito-RHP.

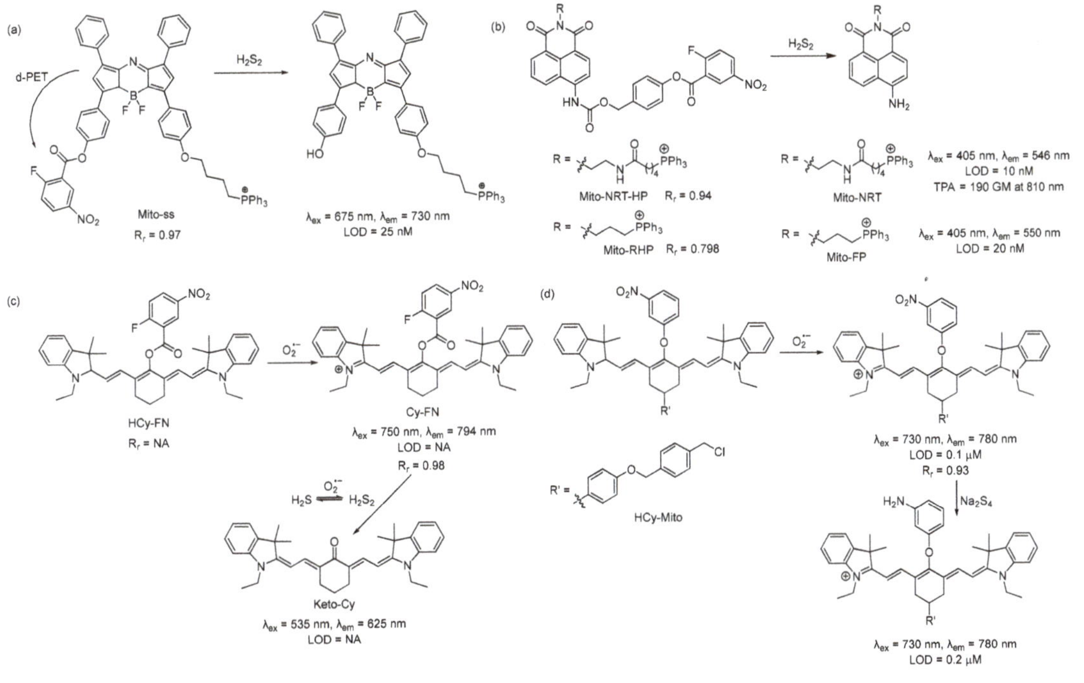

Scheme 1. Structures and reactions of probes (**a**) Mito-ss, (**b**) Mito-NRT-HP, (**c**) HCy-FN, and (**d**) HCy-Mito.

An interesting single-component multi analyte responsive NIR fluorescent probe was reported by Chen and coworkers in 2015 for the detection of the superoxide ion ($O_2^{\bullet-}$) and H_2S_n to understand redox homeostasis in the mitochondria [43]. Both $O_2^{\bullet-}$ and H_2S_n are short-lived reactive species, and their concentrations change quickly. To solve this problem, they developed a cyanine-based NIR probe, HCy-FN. This probe consists of two different reaction sites: one for the abstraction of hydrogen to detect $O_2^{\bullet-}$ and the other for the detection of H_2S_n using nitrofluorobenzoate (Scheme 1c). Both sensing steps were monitored by two different channels. Upon reacting with $O_2^{\bullet-}$, HCy-FN was oxidized to Cy-FN, and this transformation was monitored by an increase in the emission intensity from channel 1 at 794 nm (λ_{ex} = 750 nm). Next, the nitrofluorobenzoate part of Cy-FN reacted with H_2S_n to result in a decrease in the emission intensity of channel 1 followed by an increase in the emission intensity in channel 2 at 625 nm (λ_{ex} = 535 nm) due to the formation of Keto-Cy. They examined different ROS with HCy-FN and found that only $O_2^{\bullet-}$ was able to oxidize the probe. Similarly, the reactivity of other RSS towards Cy-FN was also evaluated, and no changes in emission spectra were noted. HCy-FN was used for the detection of exogenous and endogenous H_2S_n with the macrophage cell line RAW264.7 to monitor both sensing steps by dual channel emission. It was found that the Pearson correlation coefficient (R_r) of Cy-FN and mitochondria-localizing Rhodamine 123 was 0.98, confirming that Cy-FN was localized in the mitochondria. Moreover, HCy-FN could detect endogenously produced $O_2^{\bullet-}/H_2S_n$ in BALB/c mice. This work represents an interesting way to detect $O_2^{\bullet-}/H_2S_n$ in the biological system. However, the claim that the probe is capable of monitoring mitochondrial $O_2^{\bullet-}/H_2S_n$ may not be accurate. The authors only provided the R_r value for the intermediate compound Cy-FN and not for the actual probe. The structure of HCy-FN suggests that it may not be a suitable candidate to target the mitochondria because of the lack of a lipophilic cationic moiety.

In 2016, Chen and coworkers developed a probe (HCy-Mito) for the selective detection of superoxide anion ($O_2^{\bullet-}$) and H_2S_n in the mitochondria [44]. The reaction sites for $O_2^{\bullet-}$ and H_2S_n were the reduced cyanine dye (similar to HCy-FN) and m-nitrophenyl ether (Scheme 1d). In the presence of $O_2^{\bullet-}$, Hcy-Mito was oxidized to form a cyanine derivative, and the reduced nature of H_2S_n converted the nitro group to -NH_2, which terminated the d-PET process and resulted in an increase in emission intensity to 780 nm. The detection limits for $O_2^{\bullet-}$ and H_2S_n by HCy-Mito were found to be 0.1 μM and 0.2 μM, respectively. In vitro experiments with RAW264.7 cells by HCy-Mito suggest that it could image exogenous and endogenous $O_2^{\bullet-}/H_2S_n$ and localize specifically in the mitochondria (R_r = 0.93). This probe was further utilized for the in vivo detection of $O_2^{\bullet-}$ (generated from phorbol myristate acetate (PMA) and H_2S_n (via injected Na_2S_4) in BALB/c mice.

In 2019, Meng et al., used a different reaction site based on the 2-(acylthio)benzoate for the design of a mitochondria-targeted probe for H_2S_n [45]. This template utilized both the nucleophilic and electrophilic nature of H_2S_n for its recognition (Scheme 2a) [46]. Briefly, the thioester exchange between the H_2S_n and 2-(acylthio)benzoate produced a thiophenol derivative, which, in turn, reacted with H_2S_n to form an -SSH intermediate. This intermediate underwent an intramolecular cyclization to release the fluorophore. This template was attached to a red-emitting fluorophore to develop the probe, HQO-PSP. HQO-PSP itself was non-fluorescent but, upon sensing H_2S_n, exhibited a fluorescence turn-on (86-fold) at an emission of 633 nm due to the formation of the keto derivative HQO. The probe was found to be relatively fast (7 min) and highly selective to H_2S_n, with a detection limit of 95.2 nM. In vitro studies with A549 cells revealed that HQO-PSP could specifically localize within the mitochondria (R_r = 0.98) and selectively image exogenously added H_2S_n in the live cells.

In the same year, Choi et al. reported that the ratiometric probe SPS-M1 for mitochondrial H_2S_n detection was based on a two-photon excitable naphthalene fluorophore [47]. The reaction site was the same as that of HQO-PSP except for an additional self-immolating carbamate linker (Scheme 2b). The probe exhibited a blue fluorescence (λ_{em} = 429 nm) but produced the deprotected yellow fluorescent dye M1 (λ_{em} = 506 nm) upon sensing H_2S_n. Interestingly, the two-photon absorption (TPA) cross-section (δ) of SPS-M1 and M1 was found to be 11 and 108 GM, respectively, at 750 nm. The large TPA cross-section resulted from the strong ICT process in M1. SPS-M1 was found to be suitable for the quantification of H_2S_n in live cells, and the in vitro detection limit was 1 μM. The two-photon microscopic imaging with SPS-M1 for endogenous H_2S_n using the wild-type and Parkinson's disease (PD) model neurons and brain tissues of mice revealed that H_2S_n concentrations were higher in the PD model.

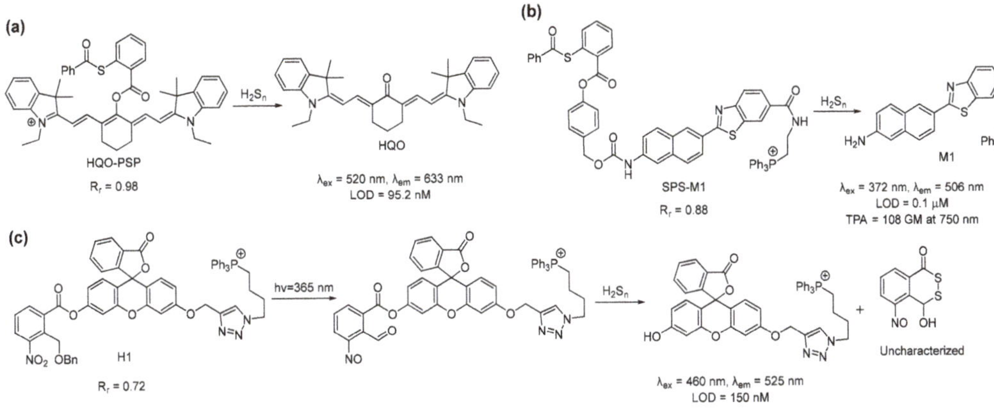

Scheme 2. Structures and reactions of probes (**a**) HQO-PSP, (**b**) SPS-M1, and (**c**) H1.

Another interesting approach for the spatiotemporal detection of mitochondrial H_2S_n was reported by Han et al. in 2018 [48]. Probe H1 consisted of a fluorescein dye attached to a triphenylphosphonium group and a nitrobenzyl photoactivable protecting group (Scheme 2c). Upon irradiation with UV light (365 nm), the nitrobenzyl part produced an aldehyde derivative, which served as the H_2S_n recognition site. H_2S_n attacks the aldehyde group to form a persulfide intermediate, which then should undergo cyclization to liberate the fluorophore and generate a side product (4-hydroxybenzo[d][1,2]dithiin-1(4H)-one). H1 showed a turn-on of fluorescence at 525 nm only when it was irradiated with UV light along with H_2S_2 in the solutions. The detection limit was calculated to be 150 nM. The targeting ability of H1 was confirmed by counterstaining with MitoTracker Green (MTG) (R_r = 0.72). Although this photo-triggered probe was interesting, the authors did not provide experimental support for the proposed detection mechanism. This aldehyde-based intermediate may also possess some problems as 2-formyl carboxylate is a well-known H_2S recognition site [49,50], and the aldehyde group has a high reactivity towards free cysteine [51–53].

In addition to specific probes for H_2S_n, general probes for sulfane sulfurs in the mitochondria have also been reported. Chen and coworkers reported the sulfane sulfur-responsive probe Mito-SH based on the azo-BODIPY fluorophore with a sulfane sulfur reaction site-thiosalicylate (Scheme 3a) in 2018 [54]. The sensing mechanism was based on the nucleophilicity of the thiol group toward the electrophilic sulfane sulfurs [55,56]. Upon reacting with sulfane sulfurs, the probe formed an -SSH intermediate, which immediately underwent an intermolecular cyclization to release the fluorophore. Mito-SH was found to be highly selective, highly responsive (100 s), and free from pH interference (range pH 4–7.8). It exhibited a 10-fold enhancement in the emission intensity upon sensing sulfane sulfurs in the NIR region (723 nm). The detection limit was 73 nM. Mito-SH exhibited mitochondria-specific localization as verified by a colocalization experiment with MTG (R_r = 0.91). In vitro imaging of exogenous (with Na_2S_4 as the source) and endogenous (generated from CSE) sulfane sulfurs were performed with this probe using SH-SY5Y cells. This was then further utilized for imaging sulfane sulfur changes caused by acute ischemia in mice. The same group reported a different approach in 2018, utilizing the reactivity of the selenol (-SeH) group towards sulfane sulfurs [57]. The probe Mito-SeH is the same as Mito-SH except for the replacement of -SH by -SeH. Due to the difference in the pK_a value of SeH (pK_a 5.9) vs. SH (pK_a 6.5), the former was found to be more reactive towards sulfane sulfurs. Mito-SeH ratiometrically reacted with sulfane sulfurs and exhibited fluorescence when turned on at 720 nm with a detection limit of 3.1 nM. In vitro experimentation using smooth muscle cells (SMCs) revealed that this probe could sense both exogenous (using Na_2S_4, thiophosphates, or 3H-1, 2-dithiole-3-thione as the source of sulfane sulfurs) and endogenous sulfane sulfurs (using LPS to induce cystathionine γ-lyase (CSE) production). Mito-SeH was utilized for the in vivo detection of sulfane sulfurs in the acute ischemia of mice, and it was concluded that sulfane sulfurs exhibited cytoprotective effects against hypoxia. While this selenol-based probe showed interesting activities, its stability could be a problem as -SeH groups are known to be highly sensitive to oxidation under air.

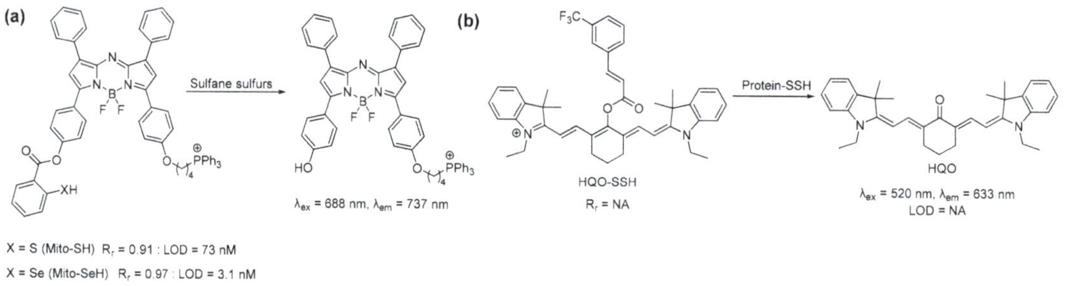

Scheme 3. Structures and reactions of probes (a) Mito-SH/Mito-SeH and (b) HQO-SSH.

In 2018, Meng et al. reported an 'off-on' fluorescent probe HQO-SSH for the detection of protein persulfidation. This probe appeared to also target mitochondria (presumably due to the cationic nature of the cyanine dye) [58]. The authors claimed that this probe was selected by screening a library of compounds to identify a suitable functional group to specifically react with persulfides. However, it is unclear what compounds were screened. It was suggested that persulfides could remove the acryloyl group and release the cyanine dye while other species, such as H_2S, biothiols, ROS, etc., could not. Persulfidated papain and glyceraldehyde-3-phosphate dehydrogenase (GAPDH) were used as models to validate the probe. Upon sensing persulfides, it exhibited a turn-on of fluorescence at ~635 nm. The probe was used for the imaging of mitochondrial protein persulfide changes in A549 and BEAS-2B lung cells (persulfidation induced by propargylglycine and Na_2S), as well as in sulfur mustard-induced lung injury tissues. However, those studies did not rule out the possibility of the probe turn-on by non-protein persulfides, such as small molecule persulfides or other sulfane sulfur species.

3. Lysosome-Targeted Probes

Lysosomes are membrane-bound organelles with acidic pH values which could reach as low as 4.5–4.7 [59]. A popular method to target these vesicles involves exploiting their low pH by incorporating a moiety (normally lipophilic amines) that can become easily protonated on a fluorescent sensor upon entering the lysosome. [60] The resulting compound is membrane impermeable and can then accumulate in the acidic lysosomal matrix. However, it must be noted that not all lysosome-targeted fluorescent probes contain a pH-sensing moiety [61–63].

One of the first lysosome-targeted fluorescent probes for sulfane sulfur detection was reported by Ren et al. in 2019 [64]. They utilized diethylamine to direct the probe to the lysosomes. The previously reported imidazo [1,5-α] pyridine derivative NIPY-OH fluorophore was chosen for its large Stokes shift (215 nm) due to its excited-state intramolecular proton transfer (ESIPT) process [65]. This property decreases the issues of self-quenching and autofluorescence, which can impact probe performance. The popular 2-fluoro-5-nitrobenzoic ester moiety was selected as the analyte recognition site. The combination of these three groups resulted in the probe NIPY-NF (Scheme 4). Due to photoinduced electron transfer (PET), the probe itself was non-fluorescent. UV-vis and fluorescence analyses determined that NIPY-NF, after responding to H_2S_2, had an excitation wavelength of 340 nm, an emission of 520 nm, a detection limit of 84 nM, and a quick response time (<6 min). It was also observed that NIPY-NF was applied to A549 cells with low cytotoxicity. Bioimaging studies in this cell line determined that the probe could exogenously detect H_2S_n in the cells after treatment with Na_2S_2 as well as after LPS stimulation to increase endogenous levels of H_2S_n. The probe's ability to localize in the lysosomes was confirmed through a colocalization study with the probe and LysoTracker Green.

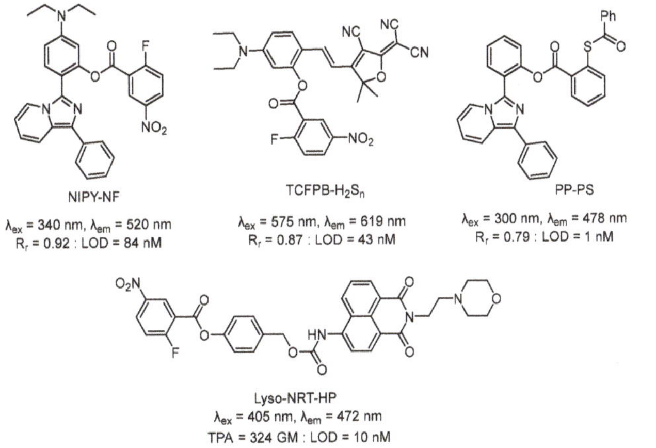

NIPY-NF
λ_{ex} = 340 nm, λ_{em} = 520 nm
R_r = 0.92 : LOD = 84 nM

TCFPB-H_2S_n
λ_{ex} = 575 nm, λ_{em} = 619 nm
R_r = 0.87 : LOD = 43 nM

PP-PS
λ_{ex} = 300 nm, λ_{em} = 478 nm
R_r = 0.79 : LOD = 1 nM

Lyso-NRT-HP
λ_{ex} = 405 nm, λ_{em} = 472 nm
TPA = 324 GM : LOD = 10 nM

Scheme 4. Structures of lysosome-targeted probes.

The same lysosome targeting and H_2S_n detection strategies were employed by Xiang et al. in 2021 to develop a ratiometric fluorescent probe, TCFPB-H_2S_n, with aggregation-induced emission (AIE) characteristics for in vitro and in vivo applications [66]. The benefits of sensors with AIE include the ability to overcome aggregation-induced quenching (ACQ) issues (i.e., decreased fluorescence, autofluorescence in vivo, etc.) that are common to ratiometric probes. This probe employed a tricyanofuranyl imino-salicylaldehyde (TCFIS) as the fluorophore with the incorporation of the 2-fluoro-5-nitrobenzoate to allow for an ICT. Weak ICT effects were expected due to the ester group's weaker electron-donating ability compared to that of the phenol. While the probe itself was expected to be somewhat fluorescent due to π-conjugation in the chain despite the addition of the 2-fluoro-5-nitrobenzoate, the presence of H_2S_n was expected to yield strong ICT effects and lead to an enhanced fluorescence based on DFT calculations. The AIE characteristic, mechanism of the probe, and ICT occurrence (ex: 575 nm; em: 619 nm increase after Na_2S_4 addition; em: 751 nm decrease after Na_2S_4 addition) were verified. Further analyses determined the limit of detection (43 nM) along with a fast reaction time (2 min) and the specificity of the probe for H_2S_n. The intensity of the ratio for the fluorescence signal (I_{619}/I_{751}) decreased at lower pHs (3–5) relative to those at pHs 5–10. Considering the weakly acidic environment of the lysosome, this had the potential to affect probe efficacy. The authors also determined TCFPB-H_2S_n's applicability in biological systems. It was found that the probe had low cytotoxicity (5–25 μM) in HeLa cells, and TCFIS could localize in the lysosomes though with some fluorescence in other areas of the cell (R_r ~0.87217). Significantly, the probe was capable of the real-time imaging of H_2S_n in mice models of acute ulcerative colitis.

Though the 2-fluoro-5-nitrobenzoate-based probes demonstrated good selectivity, the high reactivity of the fluorobenzene had the potential to cause the probes to be consumed in the presence of biothiols. In 2020, Liang et al. reported PP-PS (2-(1-phenylimidazo[1,5-α]pyridin-3-yl)phenyl-2-(benzoylthio)benzoate): [67] a turn-on probe using a previously reported fluorophore PP-OH [68] and a known 2-(acylthio)benzoate reaction site for H_2S_n [46]. The fluorophore could likely be protonated due to its increased stability from aromaticity, thus promoting its aggregation in acidic environments such as the lysosome. The quantum yield of PP-PS was found to be 0.0132 (weak fluorescence signal), which increased to 0.12549 (em: 478 nm, ex: 300 nm) upon the addition of Na_2S_2. Fluorescence analyses determined the limit of detection (1 nM) and a 1 min response time. The probe was found to have low cytotoxicity in A549, MCF-7, and U87 cancer cells, and the fluorescence cell imaging of H$_2$S$_n$ was successful in these cell lines. The probe was also applied in xenograft mouse tumor tissues and LPS-induced inflammation in excised mouse tissues. Colocalization studies using LPS-treated A549 cells, PP-PS, and LysoRed confirmed the presence of the dye in the lysosomes (R$_r$ = 0.79192).

In 2020, Han et al. utilized 4-(2-aminoethyl)-morpholine to prepare Lyso-NRT-HP: a lysosomal-targeted ratiometric two-photon fluorescent probe for H$_2$S$_n$ [69]. Their design also included a 1,8-naphthalimide based fluorophore and a 2-fluoro-5-nitrobenzoyl group to serve as the H$_2$S$_n$ receptor. The former is known for its effective ICT fluorescence and photophysical properties, such as photostability and large Stokes shift, and has been successfully used in the design of other ratiometric two-photon H$_2$S$_n$ probes [70]. The latter allows the probe to specifically react with H$_2$S$_n$ to release the fluorophore Lyso-NRT with a fluorescence emission of 548 nm in contrast to the 472 nm emission of Lyso-NRT-HP. Similarly, the absorption band of the probe was 384 nm, while Lyso-NRT's was 432 nm. The two-photon (TP) induced fluorescence property of Lyso-NRT-HP was confirmed by determining the TPA cross sections of the probe itself and its product after it reacted with Na$_2$S$_2$ (δ = 324 GM). Analyses of the probe determined its selectivity towards H$_2$S$_n$ over other biologically relevant RSS, including stability, quick turn-on (5 min), and limit of detection (10 nM). Lyso-NRT-HP was then applied in HeLa cells and demonstrated its ability to image H$_2$S$_n$. A co-localization study was also carried out to determine whether the probe could be lysosome targeting. HeLa cells were treated with either the probe, LysoTracker Red DND-99, or both, and it was determined that Lyso-NRT could be observed in the lysosomes. Imaging studies were also performed on fresh kidney slices. A similar design was used by Tian et al. in 2022 with a 4-hydroxy-1,8-naphthalimide fluorophore, 2-chloro-5-nitrobenzoate group as the H$_2$S$_n$ recognition site, and the same morpholine moiety [71]. This probe was applied in HeLa cells for H$_2$S$_n$ detection.

4. ER-Targeted Probes

The redox state of the ER was dominated by RSS as the main location for protein disulfide bond formation [72]. Hence, targeting the ER for sulfane sulfur is important to understand the sulfane sulfur dynamics of living systems. Normally, the phenyl sulfonamide moiety is used as the ER-targeting unit because it can bind to cyclooxygenase (COX), which is abundant in the ER membrane [60]. To date, only two probes have been reported for containing imaging sulfane sulfurs within the ER [72,73]. However, neither of the probes is linked to any specific ER-targeting units. Based on colocalization experiments, they were found to be selectively localized within the ER. The first probe, MB-S$_n$, was reported in 2018 by Das et al. and was found to detect H$_2$S$_n$ in the ER (Scheme 5a) [73]. This probe consisted of the well-known thiosalicylate recognition site for H$_2$S$_n$ and a BODIPY-based fluorophore. Upon sensing H$_2$S$_n$, MB-S$_n$ exhibited a turn-on at an emission of 584 nm due to the formation of MB-OH with a detection limit of 26 nM. In vitro studies with MB-S$_n$ using RAW264.7 cells confirmed its ability to sense LPS-induced endogenous sulfane sulfurs and exogenous Na$_2$S$_2$. The colocalization study of MB-S$_n$ with ER-Tracker Green confirmed its ability to target the ER (R$_r$ = 0.944).

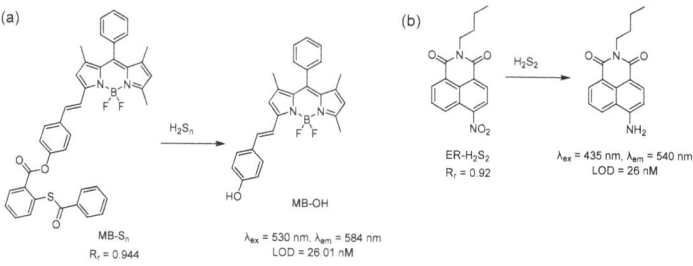

Scheme 5. Structures and reactions of probes (**a**) MB-S$_n$ and (**b**) ER-H$_2$S$_2$.

Zhou et al. utilized the stronger reducing power of H_2S_2 compared to H_2S towards the nitro group and developed a naphthalimide-based probe, ER-H_2S_2, in 2019 (Scheme 5b) [72]. Due to the presence of -NO_2 in the probe, the fluorescence of the probe was masked. ER-H_2S_2 exhibited an enhanced fluorescence at 540 nm with a large Stokes shift of 105 nm in the presence of Na_2S_2. The observed fluorescence could be attributed to the reduction from -NO_2 to -NH_2, which then participated in the ICT process. The detection limit was 26 nM. The selectivity of ER-H_2S_2 was checked against different ROS, RNS, and RSS, including H_2S, and all yielded little to no fluorescence. It should be noted that very similar nitro-containing naphthalimide-based probes have been reported to sense H_2S [74,75]. Thus, these results may appear controversial. It was reported that lipophilic compounds such as alkyl chain-appended naphthalimides tended to accumulate in the lipid-dense ER region. The ER-targeting ability of ER-H_2S_2 was confirmed by a tracking experiment with ER-Tracker Red (R_r = 0.92). This probe was used to detect exogenous H_2S_2 in zebrafish.

5. H_2S_2-Triggered Drug Delivery

Considering the increasingly recognized role of sulfane sulfurs in maintaining cellular redox homeostasis and the recently developed approaches that can specifically sense these analytes in biological systems, it may be possible to utilize elevated sulfane sulfur levels as markers for disease diagnostics and targeted drug delivery. For example, Kim et al. developed a theranostic agent (TA1) in 2021 that could selectively sense H_2S_n while simultaneously releasing an anti-inflammatory drug (Scheme 6) because H_2S_n is an inflammatory site biomarker that can be stored in the mitochondria [76]. TA1 consists of an H_2S_n recognition site (2-(acylthio)benzoate), a two-photon responsive rhodol fluorophore-appended triphenylphosphonium unit (Rhodol-TPP), the anti-inflammatory cyclooxygenase enzyme (COX) inhibitor (indomethacin), and a self-immolating linker. Upon reacting with H_2S_n, TA1 released both the fluorophore and drug. This step was monitored by the increase in TA1's fluorescence intensity at 542 nm, which provided real-time information about the release of indomethacin. In H_2S_n overexpressed models, TA1 suppressed both the COX-2 level in live cells and the prostaglandin E_2 (PGE_2) level in blood serum. Thus, TA1 may be considered an inflammation site-selective theranostic agent for precise diagnosis and anti-inflammatory therapy.

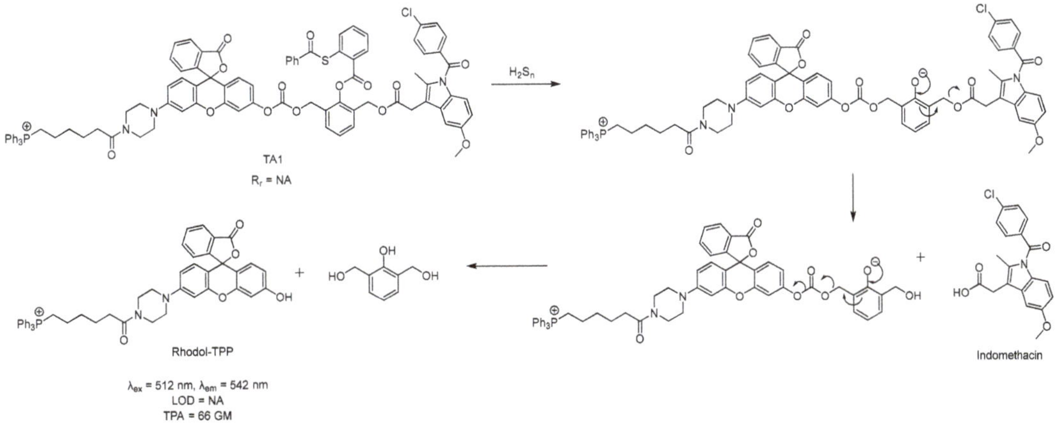

Scheme 6. The structure and mechanism of TA1.

6. Conclusions

The development of fluorescent spectroscopy and fluorescent microscopy technologies over the years has enabled advancement in the understanding of various biochemical processes that occur in biological systems. For example, cellular sulfane sulfurs have received increasing recognition as an important class of RSS that play key roles in multiple physiological and pathological processes [2–5]. Yet, despite the generally acknowledged functional importance of subcellular organelles to the health of the overall cell, organelle-targeted fluorescent probes for sulfane sulfur detection are underexplored. Major challenges include the inherent instabilities of RSSH and H_2S_n, the difficulties of specifically targeting individual organelles, and the sensitivities required to detect sulfane sulfurs at the subcellular level with the expectation that various organelles have different levels of endogenous sulfane sulfurs. In this review, we summarized the sulfane sulfur sensing mechanisms of reported organelle-targeted sensors, their targeting abilities as demonstrated through colocalization studies (based on the calculated Pearson correlation coefficient), sensitivities (by the limit of detection), applicability towards sensing endogenous and exogenous sulfane sulfurs under physiological conditions, and their advantages/disadvantages for the chosen fluorophores. While most of the reported (yet admittedly limited) organelle-targeted sulfane sulfur sensors were designed to target the mitochondria, only a few were synthesized to target the lysosomes and ER. Most of the reported sensors were rationally designed, but some sensors lacked organelle-targeting anchors. As such, the accumulation of these sensors and fluorophores in their desired organelles may possibly be attributed to their unique structural characteristics rather than their targeting ability. Increased development of more diverse and selective organelle-targeting groups that can couple to fluorescent sensors would greatly enhance knowledge in the field. Additionally, to the best of our knowledge, organelle-targeted sulfane sulfur probes for other organelles (i.e., Golgi apparatus, nucleus, etc.) have yet to be developed and provide a potential direction for future work.

Other concerns with some of the probes mentioned in this review involve their sulfane sulfur reaction sites because they have been used for the detection of other analytes, such as H_2S. This raises issues regarding the specificity of the sensors for sulfane sulfurs. The sensing mechanisms of some probes were also not reported. As such, areas of exploration for future work include the discovery of novel and more specific reactions for sulfane sulfur. Through the development and improvement of chemical tools to detect sulfane sulfurs in subcellular organelles, we expect to gain an increased understanding of the role sulfane sulfurs play in the biological system. This may, in turn, lead to the advancement of highly valuable sulfane sulfur-based theranostics. In summary, we expect to see more interesting works from this field in the near future.

Funding: This work was supported by NSF (CHE2100870) and NIH (R01HL151398, R01GM125968). The content is solely the responsibility of the authors and does not necessarily represent the official views of NSF and NIH.

Conflicts of Interest: The authors declare no conflict of interest.

References

1. Kimura, H. Physiological Roles of Hydrogen Sulfide and Polysulfides. *Handb. Exp. Pharmacol.* **2015**, *230*, 61–81. [PubMed]
2. Miyamoto, R.; Koike, S.; Takano, Y.; Shibuya, N.; Kimura, Y.; Hanaoka, K.; Urano, Y.; Ogasawara, Y.; Kimura, H. Polysulfides (H_2S_n) produced from the interaction of hydrogen sulfide (H_2S) and nitric oxide (NO) activate TRPA1 channels. *Sci. Rep.* **2017**, *7*, 45995. [CrossRef] [PubMed]
3. Giovinazzo, D.; Bursac, B.; Sbodio, J.I.; Nalluru, S.; Vignane, T.; Snowman, A.M.; Albacarys, L.M.; Sedlak, T.W.; Torregrossa, R.; Whiteman, M.; et al. Hydrogen sulfide is neuroprotective in Alzheimer's disease by sulfhydrating $GSK_3\beta$ and inhibiting Tau hyperphosphorylation. *Proc. Natl. Acad. Sci. USA* **2021**, *118*, e2017225118. [CrossRef] [PubMed]
4. Paul, B.D.; Snyder, S.H. H_2S signalling through protein sulfhydration and beyond. *Nat. Rev. Mol. Cell Biol.* **2012**, *13*, 499–507. [CrossRef]
5. Ida, T.; Sawa, T.; Ihara, H.; Tsuchiya, Y.; Watanabe, Y.; Kumagai, Y.; Suematsu, M.; Motohashi, H.; Fujii, S.; Matsunaga, T.; et al. Reactive cysteine persulfides and S-polythiolation regulate oxidative stress and redox signaling. *Proc. Natl. Acad. Sci. USA* **2014**, *111*, 7606–7611. [CrossRef]
6. Shieh, M.; Xu, S.; Lederberg, O.L.; Xian, M. Detection of sulfane sulfur species in biological systems. *Redox Biol.* **2022**, *57*, 102502. [CrossRef]
7. Echizen, H.; Sasaki, E.; Hanaoka, K. Recent Advances in Detection, Isolation, and Imaging Techniques for Sulfane Sulfur-Containing Biomolecules. *Biomolecules* **2021**, *11*, 1553. [CrossRef]
8. Takano, Y.; Echizen, H.; Hanaoka, K. Fluorescent Probes and Selective Inhibitors for Biological Studies of Hydrogen Sulfide- and Polysulfide-Mediated Signaling. *Antioxid. Redox Signal.* **2017**, *27*, 669–683. [CrossRef]

9. Zhu, H.; Fan, J.; Du, J.; Peng, X. Fluorescent Probes for Sensing and Imaging within Specific Cellular Organelles. *Acc. Chem. Res.* **2016**, *49*, 2115–2126. [CrossRef]
10. Abeywickrama, C.S. Large Stokes shift benzothiazolium cyanine dyes with improved intramolecular charge transfer (ICT) for cell imaging applications. *Chem. Commun.* **2022**, *58*, 9855–9869. [CrossRef]
11. Han, X.; Wang, Y.; Huang, Y.; Wang, X.; Choo, J.; Chen, L. Fluorescent probes for biomolecule detection under environmental stress. *J. Hazard. Mater.* **2022**, *431*, 128527. [CrossRef] [PubMed]
12. Antina, E.; Bumagina, N.; Marfin, Y.; Guseva, G.; Nikitina, L.; Sbytov, D.; Telegin, F. BODIPY Conjugates as Functional Compounds for Medical Diagnostics and Treatment. *Molecules* **2022**, *27*, 1396. [CrossRef] [PubMed]
13. Rogers, M.L.; Boutelle, M.G. Real-Time Clinical Monitoring of Biomolecules. *Annu. Rev. Anal. Chem.* **2013**, *6*, 427–453. [CrossRef]
14. Shrivastava, S.; Sohn, I.-Y.; Son, Y.-M.; Lee, W.-I.; Lee, N.-E. Real-time label-free quantitative fluorescence microscopy-based detection of ATP using a tunable fluorescent nano-aptasensor platform. *Nanoscale* **2015**, *7*, 19663–19672. [CrossRef]
15. Nie, S.; Chiu, D.T.; Zare, R.N. Real-Time Detection of Single Molecules in Solution by Confocal Fluorescence Microscopy. *Anal. Chem.* **1995**, *67*, 2849–2857. [CrossRef]
16. Osellame, L.D.; Blacker, T.S.; Duchen, M.R. Cellular and molecular mechanisms of mitochondrial function. *Best Pract. Res. Clin. Endocrinol. Metab.* **2012**, *26*, 711–723. [CrossRef] [PubMed]
17. Smith, R.A.; Porteous, C.M.; Coulter, C.V.; Murphy, M.P. Selective targeting of an antioxidant to mitochondria. *Eur. J. Biochem.* **1999**, *263*, 709–716. [CrossRef]
18. Shibuya, N.; Tanaka, M.; Yoshida, M.; Ogasawara, Y.; Togawa, T.; Ishii, K.; Kimura, H. 3-Mercaptopyruvate sulfurtransferase produces hydrogen sulfide and bound sulfane sulfur in the brain. *Antioxid. Redox Signal.* **2009**, *11*, 703–714. [CrossRef]
19. Jackson, M.R.; Melideo, S.L.; Jorns, M.S. Human Sulfide:Quinone Oxidoreductase Catalyzes the First Step in Hydrogen Sulfide Metabolism and Produces a Sulfane Sulfur Metabolite. *Biochemistry* **2012**, *51*, 6804–6815. [CrossRef] [PubMed]
20. Gao, P.; Pan, W.; Li, N.; Tang, B. Fluorescent probes for organelle-targeted bioactive species imaging. *Chem. Sci.* **2019**, *10*, 6035–6071. [CrossRef] [PubMed]
21. Zhong, H.; Yu, H.; Chen, J.; Sun, J.; Guo, L.; Huang, P.; Zhong, Y. Hydrogen Sulfide and Endoplasmic Reticulum Stress: A Potential Therapeutic Target for Central Nervous System Degeneration Diseases. *Front. Pharmacol.* **2020**, *11*, 702. [CrossRef] [PubMed]
22. Li, C.; Hu, M.; Wang, Y.; Lu, H.; Deng, J.; Yan, X. Hydrogen sulfide preconditioning protects against myocardial ischemia/reperfusion injury in rats through inhibition of endo/sarcoplasmic reticulum stress. *Int. J. Clin. Exp. Pathol.* **2015**, *8*, 7740–7751. [PubMed]
23. Wang, H.; Shi, X.; Qiu, M.; Lv, S.; Liu, H. Hydrogen Sulfide Plays an Important Protective Role through Influencing Endoplasmic Reticulum Stress in Diseases. *Int. J. Biol. Sci.* **2020**, *16*, 264–271. [CrossRef]
24. Chen, L.; Ma, K.; Fan, H.; Wang, X.; Cao, T. Exogenous hydrogen sulfide protects against hepatic ischemia/reperfusion injury by inhibiting endoplasmic reticulum stress and cell apoptosis. *Exp. Ther. Med.* **2021**, *22*, 799. [CrossRef] [PubMed]
25. Halliwell, B.; Gutteridge, J.M.C. *Free Radicals in Biology and Medicine*, 3rd ed.; Oxford University Press Inc.: New York, NY, USA, 1999.
26. Kühlbrandt, W. Structure and Function of Mitochondrial Membrane Protein Complexes. *BMC Biol.* **2015**, *13*, 89. [CrossRef]
27. Lin, J.; Yang, K.; New, E.J. Strategies for Organelle Targeting of Fluorescent Probes. *Org. Biomol. Chem.* **2021**, *19*, 9339–9357. [CrossRef]
28. Gong, S.; Zheng, Z.; Guan, X.; Feng, S.; Feng, G. Near-Infrared Mitochondria-Targetable Fluorescent Probe for High-Contrast Bioimaging of H_2S. *Anal. Chem.* **2021**, *93*, 5700–5708. [CrossRef]
29. Xu, J.; Wang, C.; Ma, Q.; Zhang, H.; Tian, M.; Sun, J.; Wang, B.; Chen, Y. Novel Mitochondria-Targeting and Naphthalimide-Based Fluorescent Probe for Detecting HClO in Living Cells. *ACS Omega* **2021**, *6*, 14399–14409. [CrossRef]
30. Xu, G.; Wu, H.; Liu, X.; Feng, R.; Liu, Z. A Simple Pyrene-Pyridinium-Based Fluorescent Probe for Colorimetric and Ratiometric Sensing of Sulfite. *Dyes Pigm.* **2015**, *120*, 322–327. [CrossRef]
31. Zhang, H.; Liu, J.; Wang, L.; Sun, M.; Yan, X.; Wang, J.; Guo, J.-P.; Guo, W. Amino-Si-Rhodamines: A New Class of Two-Photon Fluorescent Dyes with Intrinsic Targeting Ability for Lysosomes. *Biomaterials* **2018**, *158*, 10–22. [CrossRef]
32. Ma, W.; Xu, B.; Sun, R.; Xu, Y.-J.; Ge, J.-F. The Application of Amide Units in the Construction of Neutral Functional Dyes for Mitochondrial Staining. *J. Mater. Chem. B* **2021**, *9*, 2524–2531. [CrossRef] [PubMed]
33. Ding, S.; Yang, M.; Lv, J.; Li, H.; Wei, G.; Gao, J.; Yuan, Z. Novel Lysosome-Targeting Fluorescence Off-On Photosensitizer for Near-Infrared Hypoxia Imaging and Photodynamic Therapy In Vitro and In Vivo. *Molecules* **2022**, *27*, 3457. [CrossRef] [PubMed]
34. Yadav, A.; Rao, C.; Nandi, C.K. Fluorescent Probes for Super-Resolution Microscopy of Lysosomes. *ACS Omega* **2020**, *5*, 26967–26977. [CrossRef] [PubMed]
35. He, H.; Ye, Z.; Zheng, Y.; Xu, X.; Guo, C.; Xiao, Y.; Yang, W.; Qian, X.; Yang, Y. Super-Resolution Imaging of Lysosomes with a Nitroso-Caged Rhodamine. *Chem. Commun.* **2018**, *54*, 2842–2845. [CrossRef] [PubMed]
36. Liu, Q.; Liu, C.; Jiao, X.; Cai, S.; He, S.; Zhao, L.; Zeng, X.; Wang, T. Lysosome-Targeted near-Infrared Fluorescent Dye and Its Application in Designing of Probe for Sensitive Detection of Cysteine in Living Cells. *Dyes Pigment.* **2021**, *190*, 109293. [CrossRef]
37. Gao, M.; Yu, F.; Chen, H.; Chen, L. Near-Infrared Fluorescent Probe for Imaging Mitochondrial Hydrogen Polysulfides in Living Cells and in Vivo. *Anal. Chem.* **2015**, *87*, 3631–3638. [CrossRef]

38. Liu, C.; Chen, W.; Shi, W.; Peng, B.; Zhao, Y.; Ma, H.; Xian, M. Rational Design and Bioimaging Applications of Highly Selective Fluorescence Probes for Hydrogen Polysulfides. *J. Am. Chem. Soc.* **2014**, *136*, 7257–7260. [CrossRef]
39. Han, Q.; Ru, J.; Wang, X.; Dong, Z.; Wang, L.; Jiang, H.; Liu, W. Photostable Ratiometric Two-Photon Fluorescent Probe for Visualizing Hydrogen Polysulfide in Mitochondria and Its Application. *ACS Appl. Bio Mater.* **2019**, *2*, 1987–1997. [CrossRef]
40. Dong, H.-Q.; Wei, T.-B.; Ma, X.-Q.; Yang, Q.-Y.; Zhang, Y.-F.; Sun, Y.-J.; Shi, B.-B.; Yao, H.; Zhang, Y.-M.; Lin, Q. 1,8-Naphthalimide-Based Fluorescent Chemosensors: Recent Advances and Perspectives. *J. Mater. Chem. C* **2020**, *8*, 13501–13529. [CrossRef]
41. Yao, S.; Belfield, K.D. Two-Photon Fluorescent Probes for Bioimaging. *Eur. J. Org. Chem.* **2012**, *2012*, 3199–3217. [CrossRef]
42. Han, Q.; Yang, L.; Song, Y.; Ru, J.; Zhang, H.; Jiang, H.; Wang, X. A Ratiometric Fluorescent Probe for Monitoring the Changes in the Level of Hydrogen Polysulfides in Mitochondria during Stimulus-Induced Redox Imbalance. *Dye. Pigment.* **2021**, *188*, 109190. [CrossRef]
43. Yu, F.; Gao, M.; Li, M.; Chen, L. A Dual Response Near-Infrared Fluorescent Probe for Hydrogen Polysulfides and Superoxide Anion Detection in Cells and in Vivo. *Biomaterials* **2015**, *63*, 93–101. [CrossRef] [PubMed]
44. Huang, Y.; Yu, F.; Wang, J.; Chen, L. Near-Infrared Fluorescence Probe for in Situ Detection of Superoxide Anion and Hydrogen Polysulfides in Mitochondrial Oxidative Stress. *Anal. Chem.* **2016**, *88*, 4122–4129. [CrossRef] [PubMed]
45. Meng, W.; Shi, W.; Chen, Y.; Zhang, H.; Zhao, J.; Li, Z.; Xiao, K. A Red Emitting Fluorescent Probe for Imaging Mitochondrial Hydrogen Polysulfide in Living Cells and Tissues. *Sens. Actuators B Chem.* **2019**, *281*, 871–877. [CrossRef]
46. Chen, W.; Rosser, E.W.; Matsunaga, T.; Pacheco, A.; Akaike, T.; Xian, M. The Development of Fluorescent Probes for Visualizing Intracellular Hydrogen Polysulfides. *Angew. Chem. Int. Ed.* **2015**, *54*, 13961–13965. [CrossRef]
47. Choi, H.J.; Lim, C.S.; Cho, M.K.; Kang, J.S.; Park, S.J.; Park, S.M.; Kim, H.M. A Two-Photon Ratiometric Probe for Hydrogen Polysulfide (H_2S_n): Increase in Mitochondrial H_2S_n Production in a Parkinson's Disease Model. *Sens. Actuators B Chem.* **2019**, *283*, 810–819. [CrossRef]
48. Han, L.; Shi, R.; Xin, C.; Ci, Q.; Ge, J.; Liu, J.; Wu, Q.; Zhang, C.; Li, L.; Huang, W. Mitochondrial Specific H_2S_n Fluorogenic Probe for Live Cell Imaging by Rational Utilization of a Dual-Functional-Photocage Group. *ACS Sens.* **2018**, *3*, 1622–1626. [CrossRef]
49. Liu, C.; Wu, H.; Han, B.; Zhu, B.; Zhang, X. A Highly Selective Fluorescent Chemodosimeter for Imaging Hydrogen Sulfide in Living Cells. *Dye. Pigment.* **2014**, *110*, 214–218. [CrossRef]
50. Velusamy, N.; Thirumalaivasan, N.; Bobba, K.N.; Wu, S.-P.; Bhuniya, S. A Hydrogen Sulfide Triggered Self-Immolative Fluorescent Probe for Lysosome Labeling in Live Cells. *New J. Chem.* **2018**, *42*, 1590–1594. [CrossRef]
51. Lee, K.-S.; Kim, T.-K.; Lee, J.H.; Kim, H.-J.; Hong, J.-I. Fluorescence Turn-on Probe for Homocysteine and Cysteine in Water. *Chem. Commun.* **2008**, *46*, 6173–6175. [CrossRef]
52. Cheng, X.; Xu, K.; Qu, S.; Ruan, Z. Ratiometric Fluorescent Probe for Homocysteine and CysteineBased on the Aldehyde Functionalized Coumarin and SuccessfulBioimaging Application. *Chin. J. Org. Chem.* **2019**, *39*, 2835. [CrossRef]
53. Huang, Z.; Wu, C.; Li, Y.; Zhou, Z.; Xie, R.; Pang, X.; Xu, H.; Li, H.; Zhang, Y. A Fluorescent Probe for the Specific Detection of Cysteine in Human Serum Samples. *Anal. Methods* **2019**, *11*, 3280–3285. [CrossRef]
54. Gao, M.; Wang, R.; Yu, F.; You, J.; Chen, L. Imaging and Evaluation of Sulfane Sulfur in Acute Brain Ischemia Using a Mitochondria-Targeted near-Infrared Fluorescent Probe. *J. Mater. Chem. B* **2018**, *6*, 2608–2619. [CrossRef]
55. Chen, W.; Liu, C.; Peng, B.; Zhao, Y.; Pacheco, A.; Xian, M. New Fluorescent Probes for Sulfane Sulfurs and the Application in Bioimaging. *Chem. Sci.* **2013**, *4*, 2892–2896. [CrossRef]
56. Shieh, M.; Ni, X.; Xu, S.; Lindahl, S.P.; Yang, M.; Matsunaga, T.; Flaumenhaft, R.C.; Akaike, T.; Xian, M. Shining a light on SSP4: A comprehensive analysis and biological applications for the detection of sulfane sulfurs. *Redox Biol.* **2022**, *56*, 102433. [CrossRef] [PubMed]
57. Gao, M.; Wang, R.; Yu, F.; Chen, L. Evaluation of Sulfane Sulfur Bioeffects via a Mitochondria-Targeting Selenium-Containing near-Infrared Fluorescent Probe. *Biomaterials* **2018**, *160*, 1–14. [CrossRef] [PubMed]
58. Meng, W.; Chen, Y.; Feng, Y.; Zhang, H.; Xu, Q.; Sun, M.; Shi, W.; Cen, J.; Zhao, J.; Xiao, K. An off-on Fluorescent Probe for the Detection of Mitochondria-Specific Protein Persulfidation. *Org. Biomol. Chem.* **2018**, *16*, 6350–6357. [CrossRef]
59. Casey, J.R.; Grinstein, S.; Orlowski, J. Sensors and regulators of intracellular pH. *Nat. Rev. Mol. Cell Biol.* **2010**, *11*, 50–61. [CrossRef]
60. Choi, N.E.; Lee, J.Y.; Park, E.C.; Lee, J.H.; Lee, J. Recent Advances in Organelle-Targeted Fluorescent Probes. *Molecules* **2021**, *26*, 217. [CrossRef]
61. Abeywickrama, C.S.; Bertman, K.A.; Mcdonald, L.J.; Alexander, N.; Dahal, D.; Baumann, H.J.; Salmon, C.R.; Wesdemiotis, C.; Konopka, M.; Tessier, C.A.; et al. Synthesis of highly selective lysosomal markers by coupling 2-(2′-hydroxyphenyl)benzothiazole (HBT) with benzothiazolium cyanine (Cy): The impact of substituents on selectivity and optical properties. *J. Mater. Chem. B* **2019**, *7*, 7502–7514. [CrossRef]
62. Ponsford, A.H.; Ryan, T.A.; Raimondi, A.; Cocucci, E.; Wycislo, S.A.; Frölich, F.; Swan, L.E.; Stagi, M. Live imaging of intra-lysosome pH in cell lines and primary neuronal culture using a novel genetically encoded biosensor. *Autophagy* **2021**, *17*, 1500–1518. [CrossRef] [PubMed]
63. Yang, X.-Z.; Xu, B.; Shen, L.; Sun, R.; Xu, Y.-J.; Song, Y.-L.; Ge, J.-F. Series of Mitochondria/Lysosomes Self-Targetable Near-Infrared Hemicyanine Dyes for Viscosity Detection. *Anal. Chem.* **2020**, *92*, 3517–3521. [CrossRef] [PubMed]

64. Ren, Y.; Zhang, L.; Zhou, Z.; Luo, Y.; Wang, S.; Yuan, S.; Gu, Y.; Xu, Y.; Zha, X. A new lysosome-targetable fluorescent probe with a large Stokes shift for detection of endogenous hydrogen polysulfides in living cells. *Anal. Chim. Acta* **2019**, *1056*, 117–124. [CrossRef] [PubMed]
65. Chen, S.; Li, H.; Hou, P. A novel imidazo [1,5-α]pyridine-based fluorescent probe with a large Stokes shift for imaging hydrogen sulfide. *Sens. Actuators B Chem.* **2018**, *256*, 1086–1092. [CrossRef]
66. Xiang, C.; Li, C.; Xiang, J.; Luo, Y.; Peng, J.; Deng, G.; Wang, J.; Kolemen, S.; Li, H.; Zhang, P.; et al. An easily available lysosomal-targeted ratiometric fluorescent probe with aggregation induced emission characteristics for hydrogen polysulfide visualization in acute ulcerative colitis. *Mater. Chem. Front.* **2021**, *5*, 7638–7644. [CrossRef]
67. Liang, L.; Li, W.; Zheng, J.; Li, R.; Chen, H.; Yuan, Z. A new lysosome-targetable fluorescent probe for detection of endogenous hydrogen polysulfides in living cells and inflamed mouse model. *Biomater. Sci.* **2020**, *8*, 224–231. [CrossRef]
68. Volpi, G.; Magnano, G.; Benesperi, I.; Saccone, D.; Priola, E.; Gianotti, V.; Milanesio, M.; Conterosito, E.; Barolo, C.; Viscardi, G. One pot synthesis of low cost emitters with large Stokes' shift. *Dye. Pigment.* **2017**, *137*, 152–164. [CrossRef]
69. Han, Q.; Liu, X.; Wang, X.; Yin, R.; Jiang, H.; Ru, J.; Liu, W. Rational design of a lysosomal-targeted ratiometric two-photon fluorescent probe for imaging hydrogen polysulfides in live cells. *Dye. Pigment.* **2020**, *173*, 107877. [CrossRef]
70. Han, Q.; Mou, Z.; Wang, H.; Tang, X.; Dong, Z.; Wang, L.; Dong, X.; Liu, W. Highly Selective and Sensitive One- and Two-Photon Ratiometric Fluorescent Probe for Intracellular Hydrogen Polysulfide Sensing. *Anal. Chem.* **2016**, *88*, 7206–7212. [CrossRef]
71. Tian, M.; Xu, J.; Ma, Q.; Li, L.; Yuan, H.; Sun, J.; Zhu, N.; Liu, S. A novel lysosome-located fluorescent probe for highly selective determination of hydrogen polysulfides based on a naphthalimide derivative. *Spectrochim. Acta A Mol. Biomol. Spectrosc.* **2022**, *268*, 120708. [CrossRef]
72. Zhou, H.; Tang, J.; Sun, L.; Zhang, J.; Chen, B.; Kan, J.; Zhang, W.; Zhang, J.; Zhou, J. H_2S_2-Triggered off-on Fluorescent Indicator with Endoplasmic Reticulum Targeting for Imaging in Cells and Zebrafishes. *Sens. Actuators B Chem.* **2019**, *278*, 64–72. [CrossRef]
73. Hoskere, A.A.; Sreedharan, S.; Ali, F.; Smythe, C.G.; Thomas, J.A.; Das, A. Polysulfide-Triggered Fluorescent Indicator Suitable for Super-Resolution Microscopy and Application in Imaging. *Chem. Commun.* **2018**, *54*, 3735–3738.
74. Montoya, L.A.; Pluth, M.D. Selective Turn-on Fluorescent Probes for Imaging Hydrogen Sulfide in Living Cells. *Chem. Commun.* **2012**, *48*, 4767–4769. [CrossRef] [PubMed]
75. Naha, S.; Wu, S.-P.; Velmathi, S. Naphthalimide Based Smart Sensor for $CN^−/Fe^{3+}$ and H_2S. Synthesis and Application in RAW264.7 Cells and Zebrafish Imaging. *RSC Adv.* **2020**, *10*, 8751–8759. [CrossRef] [PubMed]
76. Kim, W.Y.; Won, M.; Koo, S.; Zhang, X.; Kim, J.S. Mitochondrial H_2S_n-Mediated Anti-Inflammatory Theranostics. *Nano-Micro Lett.* **2021**, *13*, 168. [CrossRef] [PubMed]

Disclaimer/Publisher's Note: The statements, opinions and data contained in all publications are solely those of the individual author(s) and contributor(s) and not of MDPI and/or the editor(s). MDPI and/or the editor(s) disclaim responsibility for any injury to people or property resulting from any ideas, methods, instructions or products referred to in the content.

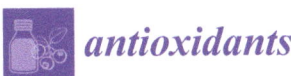

Review

Recent Development of the Molecular and Cellular Mechanisms of Hydrogen Sulfide Gasotransmitter

Jianyun Liu [1,*], Fikir M. Mesfin [1], Chelsea E. Hunter [1], Kenneth R. Olson [2], W. Christopher Shelley [1], John P. Brokaw [1], Krishna Manohar [1] and Troy A. Markel [1,*]

[1] Department of Surgery, Section of Pediatric Surgery, Indiana University School of Medicine, Riley Hospital for Children at Indiana University Health, Indianapolis, IN 46202, USA
[2] Department of Physiology, Indiana University School of Medicine—South Bend, South Bend, IN 46617, USA
* Correspondence: jealiu@iupui.edu (J.L.); tmarkel@iupui.edu (T.A.M.)

Abstract: Hydrogen sulfide has been recently identified as the third biological gasotransmitter, along with the more well studied nitric oxide (NO) and carbon monoxide (CO). Intensive studies on its potential as a therapeutic agent for cardiovascular, inflammatory, infectious and neuropathological diseases have been undertaken. Here we review the possible direct targets of H_2S in mammals. H_2S directly interacts with reactive oxygen/nitrogen species and is involved in redox signaling. H_2S also reacts with hemeproteins and modulates metal-containing complexes. Once being oxidized, H_2S can persulfidate proteins by adding -SSH to the amino acid cysteine. These direct modifications by H_2S have significant impact on cell structure and many cellular functions, such as tight junctions, autophagy, apoptosis, vesicle trafficking, cell signaling, epigenetics and inflammasomes. Therefore, we conclude that H_2S is involved in many important cellular and physiological processes. Compounds that donate H_2S to biological systems can be developed as therapeutics for different diseases.

Keywords: gasotransmitter; persulfidation; reactive sulfur species; reactive species interactome

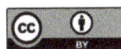

1. Introduction

Hydrogen sulfide (H_2S) was first discovered as a toxic gas and an environmental pollutant three centuries ago [1–3]. Exposure to high concentrations of H_2S for a long periods of time causes neurological, cardiovascular and pulmonary symptoms, which may eventually lead to death. However, it has also been noted that at low concentrations (<100 ppm), H_2S triggers minimal clinical impairment [2]. Recently, a plethora of work has identified H_2S as the third gasotransmitter, in addition to the two more heavily studied ones: nitric oxide (NO) and carbon monoxide (CO) [4,5]. Several enzymes, such as cystathionine-β-synthase (CBS), cystathionine-γ-lyase (CTH, also known as CSE) and 3-mercapto-sulfurtransferase (MPST, also known as 3-MST) were identified in mammals that directly or indirectly metabolize L-cysteine and produce endogenous H_2S. H_2S is mostly synthesized by these H_2S synthases in the cytosol. However, hypoxia and other stressors can trigger translocation of these H_2S synthases into mitochondria to generate H_2S, where the Cys concentration is three-fold higher than that of the cytosol [6]. The discovery of these endogenous H_2S synthases further confirms that H_2S exists inside mammals and likely plays important physiological functions, such as cell differentiation, development, cardioprotection, vasodilation and immune responses [1].

In addition to endogenous H_2S, exogenous sources from the consumption of natural H_2S-producing compounds, such as those present in vegetables, or the administration of synthetic H_2S donors can achieve similar physiological effects [7]. Currently, studies are ongoing toward the development of H_2S donors as therapeutic drugs for various diseases [8–11]. Among them, sulfide salts (Na_2S and NaHS) are considered fast H_2S donors. Once dissolved in aqueous solution, sulfide salts release large amounts of H_2S within a few seconds, which does not resemble the physiological condition [12,13]. Many slow-releasing H₂S donors have been developed [8,9]. GYY4137 (Figure 1) has become the most widely used slow-releasing H₂S donor in research, because it is commercially available and simple to handle [9]. H₂S is slowly released by hydrolysis when GYY4137 is dissolved in a neutral aqueous solution [14]. GYY4137 was originally described as an accelerant to harden natural rubber. In 2008, GYY4137 was re-discovered as a slow-releasing H₂S compound that can maintain low blood pressure by causing vasodilation and suppressing hypertension two weeks after in vivo injection in rats [12].

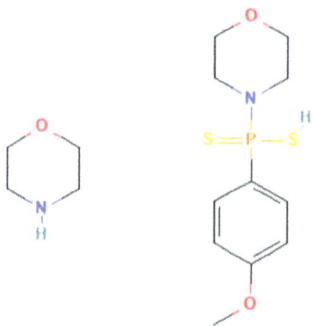

Figure 1. Chemical structure of GYY4137.

H₂S has been the topic of numerous review articles due to its promising therapeutic potential for many different diseases. H₂S donors can be divided into two major groups: (1) naturally occurring donors from food, such as diallyl disulfide (DADS) from garlic and oinons; (2) synthetic donors. Synthetic donors can be further divided into two subgroups: fast-releasing donors, such as Na₂S and NaHS, and slow-releasing donors, such as GYY4137. Based on disease scenarios, different delivery approaches can be utilized to apply H₂S donors-of-choice to patients to reach optimal results. The readers may refer to a few recent reviews on the different types of H₂S donors and their potential clinical applications [8–11,15]. To write this review, we performed a literature search on recent publications related to H₂S donors and the molecular and cellular responses after the treatment of H₂S donors in in vitro and in vivo disease models. We will first discuss the direct targets of H₂S and then examine the different cellular functions impacted by H₂S donors. Our review will help understand the possible mechanisms of how H₂S donors regulate different cellular pathways and functions to exert their therapeutical effects.

2. The Direct Target of H₂S

H₂S is a small molecule with reducing capacity. The small size makes it possible for H₂S to penetrate through cell membrane. The reducing capacity of H₂S enables it to interact with many different molecules [1]. H₂S exists in three forms (Figure 2): the disprotonated (H₂S), monoanion (HS⁻) and dianion (S²⁻) forms. All three forms are collectively referred to as hydrogen sulfide [16]. Because the pK_{a1} is ~6.8 and pK_{a2} is > 12 at 37 °C, hydrogen sulfide most likely exists as HS⁻ at physiological condition (pH ~5–7.8, 37 °C). H₂S as gas can easily diffuse across membranes, but HS⁻ may only be transported by anion channels [17].

$$\underline{H_2S} \leftrightarrow \underline{HS^-} + H^+ \leftrightarrow \underline{S^{2-}} + 2H^+$$

Figure 2. Three forms of H₂S are underlined.

2.1. Targeting ROS/RNS and Forming Reactive Species Interactome (RSI)

The concept of reactive oxygen species (ROS) and reactive nitrogen species (RNS) has been widely explored. ROS include many derivatives of oxygen produced in the normal physiological process, such as hydrogen peroxide (H_2O_2) and superoxide (O_2^-).

At a low steady-state level, ROS contributes to many normal cellular processes, including cell proliferation, differentiation and migration. However, too many ROS cause oxidative stress and result in inflammation, apoptosis and tumor growth [18]. Similarly, nitric oxide reacts with superoxide (O_2^-) and forms different derivatives called reactive nitrogen species (RNS), such as peroxynitrite ($ONOO^-$). RNS production in macrophages and neutrophils is important for their anti-microbial function in eliminating pathogens, but overproduction of RNS can be harmful and result in tissue damage [19].

H_2S, as a reducing agent, also reacts with ROS and RNS and participate in redox signaling. For example, H_2S can directly interact with peroxynitrite ($ONOO^-$) and produce ·HSO and ·NO [6,16]. It is suggested that H_2S may be oxidized either in the mitochondria or via metal-catalyzed H_2S oxidation [6,16].

Although H_2S can directly interact with ROS and act as an ROS scavenger, this is probably a very minor role of H_2S in most living cells [20,21]. The more important function of H_2S in removing ROS is to regulate the expression of ROS scavengers, such as superoxide dismutase (SOD). H_2S binds to SOD and enhances the rate of superoxide anion scavenging [22].

H_2S can also suppress ROS indirectly by preserving antioxidants. There are many antioxidants that can counterbalance ROS, such as cellular reduced glutathione (GSH), GSH/GSSG ratio and thioredoxin (Trx-1). These cellular non-enzymatic antioxidants in H_2S-treated cells can be maintained for long periods to counteract ROS, even though H_2S no longer exists in the cultured media. Furthermore, H_2S can reduce cystine to cysteine and facilitate GSH synthesis, indirectly suppressing ROS activity [21].

In fact, it is believed that H_2S forms reactive sulfur species (RSS) that played a critical role in redox signaling when the earth had more sulfur than oxygen in the atmosphere about a billion years ago [6,23]. RSS, together with ROS and RNS, form reactive species interactome (RSI), mediating complex signaling pathways in cells. The RSI is robust and flexible, allowing efficient sensing and adaptation to environmental changes to enhance fitness and resilience [23].

2.2. Binding to HEME Proteins

H_2S can directly interact with the amino acid histidine in heme-containing proteins, such as hemoglobin, and form sulfheme complexes in many invertebrates living in sulfide-rich environments [24]. In vertebrates, sulfide-ferric heme complexes may provide the storage, transport and detoxification of H_2S [25,26]. H_2S directly binds to the ferric heme structure in Cytochrome c oxidase (CcO), the last enzyme in the respiratory electron transport chain in mitochondria, and modifies its activity [27]. At low concentration (1:1 stoichiometry), H_2S acts as a substrate to CcO without inhibiting its activity. At moderate to high concentration (1:2–3 stoichiometry), H_2S inhibits CcO, resulting in the well-known toxicity of H_2S [26]. Amino acids at the distal site in hemeproteins are important in stabilizing H_2S-ferric binding. For example, in ferrous myeloperoxidase, a common distal arginine may stabilize the binding of sulfide [25]. In vertebrates, H_2S also binds to oxygenated hemoglobin and myoglobin, which forms sulfhemoglobin and sulfmyoglobin. These sulfheme protein complexes are essential to H_2S degradation in vivo [24]. Although H_2S binding to hemeproteins is expected to be essential to many biological functions, little is known regarding the sulfide-heme binding mechanisms. The physiologic functions of sulfide-hemeprotein complexes still need to be further addressed [24,25].

2.3. Persulfidation

One type of post-translational modification of proteins is persulfidation (S-sulfhydration). This occurs by adding a sulfur molecule, usually from oxidized H_2S, to an existing thiol (-SH) group of a cysteine residue [28,29]. Protein persulfidation can either stabilize and enhance its activity or inhibit its function [16]. Gao et al. developed a proteomics approach to quantitatively measure S-sulfhydrated cysteines. They found that elevated H_2S promoted the persulfidation of metabolic enzymes and stimulated glycolytic flux in pancreatic β cells experiencing endoplasmic reticulum (ER) stress [30]. NaHS treatment persulfidated the Kir6.1 subunit of the KATP channel at Cys43 and enhanced the binding of Kir6.1 to the signaling molecule PIP2, leading to KATP channel activation [31]. H_2S also persulfidated and inactivated phosphatase PTP1B, playing an important role during the response to ER stress [32]. Protein disulfide isomerase (PDI) is a key enzyme of protein folding in the ER. Jiang et al. showed that NaHS and GYY4137 treatments enhanced PDI activity, which was inhibited by mutating four cysteines in potential sulfhydrated sites of PDI [33].

Endothelial nitric oxide synthase (eNOS) is one of the three isoforms of NOS enzymes which synthesizes nitric oxide in endothelial cells. eNOS exists in either monomer or dimer formats. The dimeric eNOS is considered to be the active form [34]. NaHS treatment enhanced the persulfidation of eNOS at Cys443 and stabilized eNOS dimers, resulting in enhanced eNOS activity [35]. Nrf2 (Nuclear factor-erythroid factor 2-related factor 2) is an important transcriptional factor that regulates the expression of antioxidant proteins. Kelch-like ECH associating protein 1 (Keap1) binds to Nrf2 and acts as a negative regulator of Nrf2 [36]. NaHS treatment caused persulfidation in Keap1 at cysteine-151, resulting in Nrf2 dissociation from Keap1. Dissociated Nrf2 then translocated to the nucleus and enhanced the mRNA expression of Nrf2-targeted downstream genes [37]. P66Shc, an upstream activator of mitochondrial redox signaling, was persulfidated at Cysteine-59 when treated with NaHS. This attenuated the function of p66Shc and resulted in diminished mitochondrial ROS production [38].

2.4. NO/CO Feedback Loop

These three gasotransmitters, NO, CO and H_2S, also directly and indirectly interact with each other to regulate the signaling pathways. For example, H_2S can persulfidate eNOS and facilitate NO production, as mentioned above in 2.3 [35]. Heme oxygenase-1 (HO-1) and HO-2, endogenous CO synthases, are Nrf2 downstream targeting genes. H_2S can persulfidate Keap1 Cys151 and activate the Keap1/Nrf2 system, as mentioned in 2.3 [39]. On the other hand, both NO and CO can bind to the heme sites of H_2S synthase, CBS, and modify its function in vivo, impacting H_2S homeostasis [40]. As mentioned in 2.1, NO and H_2S can directly bind to each other, resulting in GSNO, HSNO/ONS. Therefore, adding exogenous H_2S will affect the redox states of the cells and modify NO and CO signaling.

In conclusion, H_2S can directly bind to small molecules and macromolecules to deliver its physiological function in vivo.

3. H_2S Regulates Different Cellular Processes and Functions

H_2S has the capacity to directly target many important signaling molecules and functional proteins. As a result, it plays a key role in many cellular processes and functions. Recent works have suggested that H_2S donors can modify many cellular processes and exert therapeutic effects.

3.1. Cell Signaling Pathways
3.1.1. PI3K/Akt Signaling Pathway

Many investigations have shown that H_2S can activate the PI3K/Akt signaling pathway, which is highly conserved and tightly regulated among almost all cells and tissues. Phosphoinositide 3-kinase (PI3K) is activated by extracellular stimuli through membrane-bound receptors, such as receptor tyrosine kinase (RTK), which is a G-protein-coupled receptor (GPCR). Activated PI3K phosphorylates the 3' hydroxyl of the inositol head group of phosphoinositides PIP2 and produces the lipid second messenger PIP3 [41]. Akt, also called protein kinase B (PKB), is an important serine/threonine kinase. Akt can be activated in a PI3K-dependent and independent manner. As the downstream mediator of PI3K, the lipid products (PI3, 4P2 and PIP3) of PI3K directly bind to the pleckstrin homology (PH) domain of Akt to activate this serine/threonine kinase. Akt activity can also be regulated by other proteins. For example, Akt can be activated by PIP3-dependent protein kinase 1 (PDK1) phosphorylating T308 of Akt. Phosphatases, such as PP2A and PHLPP, can dephosphorylate Akt at T308 and S473, to inactivate Akt. PTEN also suppresses Akt activity by dephosphorylating the lipid second messenger PIP3 [42]. Activated Akt can directly phosphorylate many downstream targets, including transcription factors, protein kinases, cell cycle regulators, etc. The Forkhead box O 1 (FOXO1) transcription factor is one of the well-studied targets of Akt. FOXO1 is considered a repressor of adipogenesis and insulin stimulated genes. Once phosphorylated by Akt, FOXO1 binds to 14-3-3 family of phospho-binding proteins and is transported from the nucleus to the cytosol. By removing FOXO1 from the nucleus, Akt activates adipogenesis gene expression [42] (Figure 3).

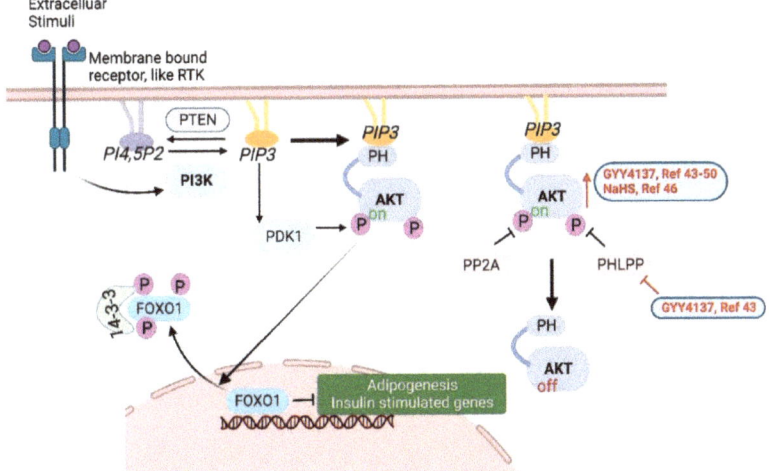

Figure 3. The PI3K/Akt signaling pathway. H_2S donors (GYY4137 and NaHS) increase Akt activation, as shown in red font, arrow and lines [43–50]. Created with BioRender.com.

High glucose in diabetic mice and cell culture is associated with increased levels of PHLPP-1 and reduced p-Akt. GYY4137 pre-treatment prevented change in the expression of PHLPP-1 and p-Akt [43]. In a myocardial ischemia/reperfusion rat model, GYY4137 treatment protected the heart and increased p-Akt. This effect was abrogated by co-treating with PI3K inhibitor LY294002. These results suggested that GYY4137 exerted cardioprotective effects by activating the PI3K/Akt signaling pathway [44]. In an ipsilateral epididymis injury rat model, GYY4137 alleviated sperm damage and epididymis injury by the activation of the PI3K/Akt pathway [45].

In a liver ischemia/reperfusion (I/R) injury rat model, GYY4137 and/or NaHS treatment elevated the plasma levels of H_2S, upregulated miR-21 and resulted in activation of the Akt pathway. Blocking miR-21 prevented the protection from NaHS by inactivating the Akt pathway, suggesting that miR-21 was important in mediating the protective effects of H_2S in I/R-induced liver injury [46].

In an aortic cross-clamping rat model that induces acute lung injury, GYY4137 increased p-Akt and the downstream factors GSK3β and S6K and attenuated the increase of Angiopoietin-2 (Ang2, promotes cell death and disrupting vascularization) in lung tissue, caused by aortic cross-clamping [47].

Homocysteine (HHcy) treatment induces apoptosis (more details in Section 3.4) and matrix remodeling in mesangial cells. HHcy inactivates Akt and therefore activates the downstream FOXO1, resulting in the induction of apoptosis and the synthesis of excessive ECM protein. However, GYY4137 prevented the dephosphorylation of Akt and increased the nuclear translocation of FOXO1 in HHcy-treated cells, indicating that H_2S regulates the Akt/FOXO1 pathway [48].

In a rat stomach culture model, GYY4137 increased phosphorylation of Akt and suppressed the secretion of the hunger hormone Ghrelin [49]. In apolipoprotein E KO mice, GYY4137 activated the PI3K/Akt pathway and reduced TLR4 expression, which was critical in preventing atherosclerotic plaque formation [50].

3.1.2. NF-κB and MAPK Signaling Pathways

Besides the PI3K/Akt signaling pathway, NF-κB and MAPK pathways are also shown to be impacted by H_2S treatment. Nuclear Factor-κB (NF-κB) is a family of inducible transcription factors that regulates a myriad of genes involved in inflammatory and immune responses. There are five main members in the NF-κB family: NF-κB1 (also named p50), NF-κB2 (also named p52), RelA (also named p65), RelB and c-Rel. In normal conditions, NF-κB are inactive and suppressed by a family of inhibitory proteins, such as IκB. Upon stimulation, a multi-subunit IκB kinase (IKK) complex is formed. IKK phosphorylates and degrades IkB proteins trigger the activation of NF-κB proteins [51,52] (Figure 4).

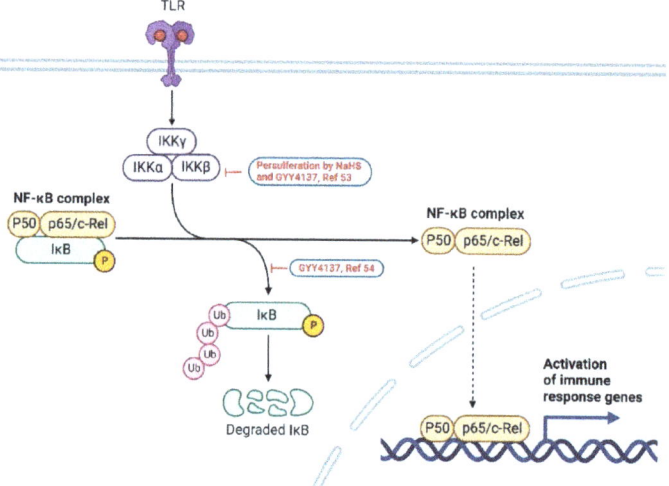

Figure 4. NF-κB signaling pathway. H_2S donors (GYY4137 and NaHS) suppress the upregulation of phospho-IκB, as shown in red, and LPS-induced inflammation [53,54]. Created with BioRender.com.

Cisplatin is a chemotherapy agent which can cause extensive nephrotoxicity. In cisplatin-treated renal tubular cells, H_2S donors (NaHS and GYY4137) persulfidated STAT3 and IKKβ, resulting in the suppression of an NF-κB-mediated inflammatory cascade, which could potentially ameliorate renal damage caused by chemotherapy [53]. In murine macrophage RAW264.7 cells, LPS treatment increased the p-IκB and nuclear translocation of p65. The addition of GYY4137 suppressed the upregulation and therefore inhibited the LPS-induced activation of RAW264.7 cells [54].

The mitogen-activated protein kinase (MAPK) cascades are a chain of conserved proteins that communicate extracellular stimuli from the cell surface all the way to the DNA in the nucleus, resulting in cell proliferation, differentiation, motility and apoptosis [55]. There are three MAPKs: ERK, JNK and p38. Upon activation, these MAPKs are activated by their upstream kinases, MAP4K, MAP3K and MAPKK. Activated MAPKs phosphorylate their downstream substrates, mostly transcription factors, such as c-Myc, c-Jun, CREB, etc. [55,56] (Figure 5). Cisplatin induces the phosphorylation of ERK, JNK and p38 MAPKs, causing cell apoptosis. H_2S donors NaHS and GYY4137 attenuated cisplatin-induced cell death by suppressing MAPK activation caused by cisplatin treatment. Cisplatin also suppressed H_2S synthase CSE and CBS. The overexpression of CSE provided resistance to cisplatin-induced cell death. H_2S donors also inhibited cisplatin-induced NADPH oxidase activation and p47phox phosphorylation, possibly by inducing the persulfidation of p47phox [57]. However, in the absence of mitogens like cisplatin, H$_2$S donors themselves may act as mitogens and activate MAPK pathways. In a cell line that secretes glucagonlike peptide-1 (GLP-1), H$_2$S donors NaHS and GYY4137 activated p38 MAPK and stimulated GLP-1 secretion [58]. In cultured mouse neurons, GYY4137 activated ERK but not p38 or JNK, resulting in the upregulation of acid-sensing ion channels (ASICs) [59].

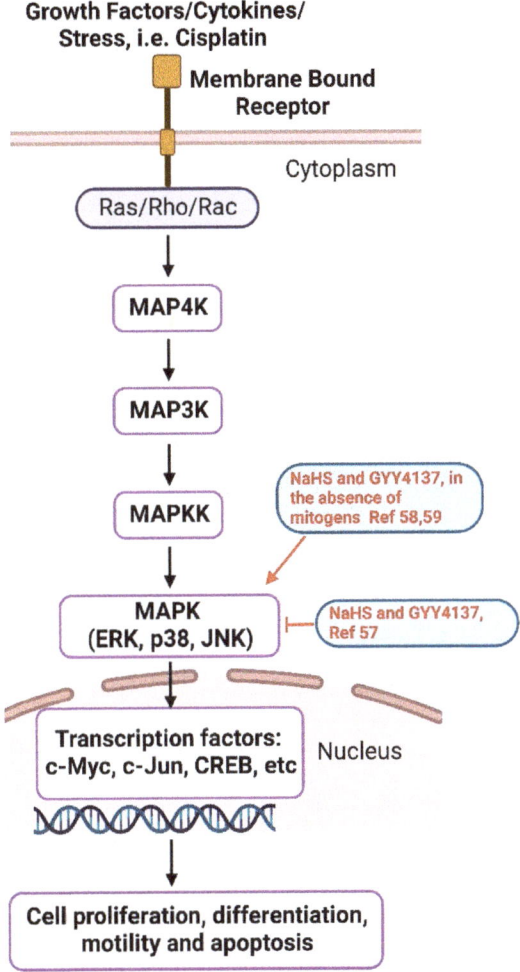

Figure 5. MAPK signaling pathway. H$_2$S donors (NaHS and GYY4137) regulate MAPK activation, as shown in red [57–59]. Created with BioRender.com.

3.2. Tight Junctions

Tight junctions are special structures in epithelia and endothelia that form barriers to separate different compartments. Tight junctions comprise transmembrane proteins (MARVEL-domain proteins, Claudins, E-cadherin, etc.) and a complex protein network in the cytosol called junctional plaque components (ZO1, ZO2, ZO3 and some other adaptor signaling proteins) that connect the transmembrane proteins to the cytoskeleton (microtubules and actin filaments). Tight junctions in epithelia and endothelia determine the body intactness. Mutations in tight junction proteins or tight junction disruption by microbial infections are linked to many diseases [60]. H$_2$S slow-releasing donor GYY4137 treatment was shown to preserve the barrier function in tight junctions in mouse models of endotoxemia and sepsis [61,62]. Sodium deoxycholate (SDC), a bile acid salt, interrupted the tight junctions and increased phosphorylation of myosin light chain kinase (MLCK) and myosin light chain (MLC) in Caco-2 cells. The addition of GYY4137 to cultured Caco-2 cells suppressed the phosphorylation of MLCK and MLC induced by SDC. Mice that received SDC by oral gavage developed colitis. The intraperitoneal injection of GYY4137 in SDC-treated mice also preserved the integrity of the intestine and alleviated the colitis [63]. Zhao et al. demonstrated that GYY4137 treatment reduced intestinal permeability and upregulated tight junctions in a Dextran sulfate sodium (DSS)-induced mouse colitis model [64]. It is so far unknown what the direct targets of H$_2$S are in enhancing tight junctions and preserving intestinal integrity.

3.3. Autophagy

When mammalian cells are under stress, such as infection, nutrient deprivation and hypoxia, they will start an adaptive process called autophagy to guarantee nutrients for vital cellular functions [65]. Autophagy is also essential in removing harmful cytosolic materials to prevent diseases such as neurodegeneration and cancer [65]. The process of autophagy typically starts with the recruitment of autophagy-related proteins (ATGs) to a specific subcellular location and the formation of a phagophore, a cup-shaped membrane structure. The phagophore keeps elongating and encircles cytosolic material to form a round double-membrane vesicle called autophagosome. Autophagosomes eventually fuse with lysosomes to form autolysosomes where the engulfed cytosolic material and autophagic body are degraded and recycled. In addition to ATGs, there are many other proteins participating in the process of autophagy, such as the serine/threonine protein kinase ULK1, ubiquitin, LC3s, etc. These autophagic proteins are highly regulated. Autophagy has been proven to be essential to cellular homeostasis by extensive research in recent years. Disorders in autophagy are linked to diseases such asneurodegeneration, immunological diseases and cancer, as well as aging [65].

In human umbilical vein endothelial cells (HUVECs), GYY4137 treatment enhanced autophagic flux by increasing LC3BII expression, exerting cytoprotective function. This process was shown to be dependent on Sirt1/FoxO1 pathway [66]. In an experimental periodontitis model, GYY4137 prevented excessive inflammation by inducing autophagy [67]. In a streptozotocin-induced diabetic model, NaHS treatment activated the AMPK/mTOR pathway and increased the levels of ATGs. Increased autophagic ultrastructures and LC3-I/LC3-II conversion were also observed in the NaHS-treated group, further confirming that H$_2$S activated autophagy [68].

3.4. Apoptosis

Apoptosis is the process of programmed cell death, which can be induced either through intrinsic or extrinsic pathways. The release of Cytochrome *c* from mitochondria often intrinsically triggers the process of apoptosis, including the formation of apoptosomes and caspase 3 activation. BCL-2 family proteins are a group of conserved proteins that share Bcl-2 homology domains and are well known as the regulators of apoptosis. Some BCL-2 family proteins, such as BIM, BID, PUMA, BAX and BAK1, are pro-apoptotic, while others, such as BCL-2, BCL-Xl, BCL-W, BCL-2-A1 and MCL1, are anti-apoptotic. The expression and function of BCL-2 family proteins can be regulated by Cyclin-dependent kinases (CDKs) and p53. Apoptosis can also be induced by cell membrane proteins called death receptors, including Fas, TNFR1, TNFR2 and TRAIL receptors. Upon binding to their ligands, death receptors are activated, triggering the recruitment of adaptor proteins FADD and the caspase cascade. The activation of caspases leads to the cleavage of BID, the activation of pro-apoptotic BCL-2 family proteins and the release of Cytochrome *c* from mitochondria [69]. Many groups have demonstrated that H$_2$S protects cells against apoptosis and/or promotes autophagy, as discussed in Section 3.3. Li et al. showed that GYY4137 treatment in cardiomyocytes attenuated high glucose-induced apoptosis by decreasing caspase-3 activity and pro-apoptotic BAX and increasing anti-apoptotic BCL-2. The effect was probably mediated via the inhibiting STAT3/HIF-1α pathway [70]. Cardiomyocyte HL-1 cells preconditioned with GYY4137 were protected from nutrient deprivation-induced apoptosis. Furthermore, GYY4137 pretreatment reduced the level of cleaved caspase-3 and preserved ATP in isolated rat heart [71]. In a pathological infertility rat model, as mentioned in Section 3.1, GYY4137 treatment increased the level of antioxidant superoxide dismutase (SOD), the phosphorylation of PI3K p85 and Akt. The treatment also suppressed the pro-apoptotic marker active caspase-3 and Bax, resulting in the alleviation of sperm damage [45]. In a neuropathic pain mouse model, pretreatment with GYY4137 and diallyl disulfide (DADS) improved the antiallodynic effects of opiate agonists morphine and UFP-512. GYY4137 and DADS treatment also suppressed the increased pro-apoptotic Bax expression in the medial septum of mice with neuropathic pain [72].

Type 2 diabetes is an independent risk factor for a failed lung transplant. Jiang et al. showed that GYY4137 treatment in a lung I/R/type 2 diabetic rat model suppressed lung cell apoptosis by using TUNEL staining. Their data suggested that GYY4137 treatment rescued SIRT1 expression, lung function, oxidative damage and inflammation. GYY4137's effectiveness was likely from the activation of SIRT1 signaling pathways, as the SIRT1 inhibitor, EX527, was shown to abolish all these effects [73].

Dexamethasone (Dex), a glucocorticoid that treats inflammation, was found to induce osteoporosis (loss of bone mass). At the same time, Dex suppressed serum H_2S and H_2S-generating enzymes in the bone marrow in vivo. In Dex-treated rats, GYY4137 alleviated osteoporosis by rescuing cell proliferation and the expression of signature proteins (i.e., Runx2, alkaline phosphatase) in osteoblasts, cells specialized in bone matrix synthesis and mineralization. GYY4137 also suppressed Dex-induced apoptosis by increasing the ratio of Bcl-2/Bax in osteoblasts [74].

The high level of plasma homocysteine is common in patients with chronic kidney diseases and the integrity of mesangial cells is essential to the function of kidney. Homocysteine induces apoptosis in cultured mouse mesangial cells. The addition of GYY4137 to the homocysteine-treated mesangial cells prevented apoptosis with reduced cleaved-Caspase 3. GYY4137 also blocked Akt/FOXO1 activation, ROS production, matrix protein induction and mitochondrial dysfunction [48]. In a diabetic cardiomyopathy rat model, GYY4137 also suppressed high-glucose-induced oxidative stress and apoptosis. However, in this model, GYY4137 induced FOXO1 phosphorylation [75], which is consistent with the previous discussion in Section 3.1.1, indicating that H_2S donors promote the PI3K/Akt/FOXO1 pathway.

GYY4137 treatment prevented mitochondria-mediated apoptosis in both cultured cells and mice deficient in H_2S-generating enzymes. Further experiments suggested that mitochondrial protein ATP synthase ATP5A1 could be persulfidated by H_2S. When Cys244 in ATP5A1 was mutated into serine (C244S), GYY4137 no longer prevented mitochondria-mediated apoptosis, suggesting that persulfidation by H_2S is a possible mechanism in regulating mitochondria function and cytoprotection [76]. Osteoarthritis is characterized by cartilage erosion. Chondrocytes, the only cell type present and essential to cartilage development, goes through apoptosis when under oxidative stress. Treatment with GYY4137 ameliorated chemical-induced ROS production and apoptosis in chondrocytes. GYY4137 also suppressed stress-induced mTOR and P70S6K activation in chondrocytes. GYY4137-treated chondrocytes showed an increased LC3II/LC3I ratio, implying GYY4137 also promoted autophagy in these cells [77].

3.5. Vesicle Trafficking: Exocytosis/Endocytosis/Pinocytosis

Vesicle trafficking is essential to the function of all live mammalian cells. Molecules are transported in between specific membrane-enclosed compartments inside the cell as well as between a cell and its environment to maintain the functional organization of cells. Vesicle trafficking can be divided into many different processes based on the direction of trafficking (endocytosis, exocytosis, transcytosis) as well as cargo specificity (pinocytosis, phagocytosis, clathrin-dependent and -independent endocytosis, COP-mediated vesicle transport, etc.) [78]. Here we will focus on three types of vesicle trafficking: exocytosis, endocytosis and pinocytosis.

Exocytosis is the process through which intracellular vesicles fuse with the plasma membrane and release their cargo to the extracellular environment. In excitable cells, such as neurons and endocrine cells, this process is highly regulated and the cells can release large amounts of neurotransmitters or hormones within milliseconds after being triggered [78]. In pancreatic β cells, glucose stimulation can trigger the influx of ions, a second messenger, and results in a signaling cascade leading to exocytosis and the release of insulin [79]. Chromaffin cells are neuroendocrine cells found mostly in the adrenal glands in mammals. Exogenous H_2S can regulate intracellular calcium in chromaffin cells, and therefore, facilitate exocytosis and the release of the neurotransmitter catecholamines [80].

Endocytosis is the process that a wide range of cargo molecules can be transported from outside to the inside of the cells. Clathrin is a protein that coats vesicles and forms complexes with other adaptor/signal proteins to transport vesicles to specific compartments [81]. Endocytosis can be divided into well-studied clathrin-dependent endocytosis and less-studied clathrin-independent endocytosis. Clathrin-independent endocytosis utilizes cholesterol-rich membrane domains called lipid rafts and contains scaffold protein caveolins [82]. Pinocytosis, "cell drinking", is a type of endocytosis that uptakes liquid content, such as lipid droplets. The size of vesicles in pinocytosis is very small and clear compared to those in other endocytosis [83]. NaHS treatment inhibited Na^+/K^+-ATPase activity by enhancing Na^+/K^+-ATPase endocytosis in rat renal tubular epithelial cells [84]. Further studies found that H_2S directly bound and activated EGFR by persulfidation at Cys797 (human) or Cys798 (rat), triggering its downstream Gab1/PI3K/Akt pathway and enhanced endocytosis. An intravenous injection of NaHS increased water and sodium excretion in the rat kidney, suggesting H_2S can be developed as therapeutics for diseases related to renal sodium homeostasis dysfunction [84]. In a different study, inhibiting H_2S synthesis enhanced and NaHS treatment inhibited CXCR2 endocytosis in mouse neutrophils in a K(ATP)(+) channel-dependent mechanism [85].

3.6. Epigenetics

Epigenetics is a process that alters gene activity but does not change the DNA sequence, including but not limited to DNA methylation, chromatin modification and noncoding RNAs. Epigenetics can be regulated by genetic, developmental and environmental factors [86]. SIRT1 is a deacetylase and can deacetylate histones and modify chromatin structures [87]. Previous work has shown that H_2S can increase SIRT1 expression. Furthermore, H_2S can persulfidate SIRT1 and stabilize it. Therefore, H_2S can enhance SIRT1 activity and promote deacetylation to regulate the expression of inflammatory proteins [88]. In HUVECs, H_2S treatment enhanced the deacetylase activity of SIRT1, which induced the deacetylation of FOXO1 and the nucleus translocation of FOXO1 [66].

MicroRNAs are small single-stranded noncoding RNAs (~22 nucleotides) that function as post-transcriptional regulators of gene expression. Hundreds of different miRNAs have been discovered in humans and many of them are conserved in other mammals [89]. As mentioned in Section 3.1, H_2S donor treatment elevated the plasma levels of H_2S, enhanced microRNA-21 (miR-21) expression and activated the Akt pathway in a rat liver I/R model. Anti-miR-21 annulled the protective effects of H_2S donor and inactivated the Akt pathway in the same model [46]. miR-129 was downregulated in a chronic kidney disease mouse model. The treatment of GYY4137 ameliorated the disease and rescued miR-129 expression in this model [90]. In a diabetic mouse model, there were decreased H_2S in plasma, reduction in miR-194, collagen deposition and fibrosis in the diabetic kidney. GYY4137 treatment rescued plasma miR-194 expression and mitigated renal disease symptoms [91]. In cardiomyocytes, Na_2S-treamtent upregulated miR-133a expression, which inhibited cardiomyocytes hypertrophy [92].

3.7. NLRP3 Inflammasome

Upon sensing pathogen-associated molecular patterns (PAMPs) or damage-associated molecular patterns (DAMPs) in the cytoplasm, proteins, such as the nucleotide-binding oligomerization domain (NOD) and leucine rich repeat (LRR)-containing receptors (NLRs), will form a multimeric protein complex with adaptor molecule ASC and the cysteine protease procaspase-1. Besides NOD and LRR domains, NLRs also contain pyrin domains which can bind to the pyrin domains of adaptor protein ASC. ASC has two domains: an N-terminal pyrin domain and a carboxy-terminal caspase recruitment domain (CARD), connecting NLRs to procaspase-1. Multiple NLRs, ASCs and procaspase-1s bind together and form a speck-like structure to induce the self-cleavage of procaspase-1, producing the active form caspase-1. Caspase-1 can cleave many precursors of proinflammatory cytokines, such as interleukin-1β, IL-18 and Gasdermin-D, triggering inflammation and pyroptosis (a form of cell death triggered by inflammatory signals) [93,94]. NLRP3 inflammasomes are the most studied PAPMs/ DAMPs sensing NLRs. Mutations in NLRP3 have been associated with autoinflammatory disorders [93,94].

Monosodium urate (MSU) crystals, the factor contributing to gout arthritis, activate the NLRP3 inflammasomes. Using mouse models and in vitro cell culture, researchers observed increased inflammation after treatment with MSU crystals, which resulted in a deficiency of CSE. The addition of GYY4137-ameliorated caspase-1 activity, ASC oligomerization, IL-1β secretion and inflammation, suggests that H_2S inhibits NLRP3 inflammasome activity [95].

GYY4137 treatment suppressed NLRP3 expression both in vivo and in vitro using a diabetes-accelerated atherosclerosis model. Furthermore, GYY4137 treatment reduced plaque formation in vivo and ICAM1/VCAM1 levels in vitro [96]. In a mouse sepsis model, GYY4137 treatment reduced NLRP3 and caspase-1, and alleviated lung injury [97]. In a sepsis mouse model, GYY4137 treatment attenuated sepsis-induced cardiac dysfunction in WT but not Nlrp3 KO mice, suggesting that GYY4137 inhibited the inflammasome pathway. In fact, GYY4137 suppressed NLRP3 inflammasome activities in macrophages and reduced the infiltration of macrophages in septic heart tissue [98].

3.8. Ion Channels

There are protein complexes on the cell surface and in the intracellular membrane that form pores to allow ions (Na, K, Ca, Cl, etc.) to be transported. These complexes are called ion channels. Some ion channels are gated by voltages while others are voltage-insensitive and gated by other mediators [56]. H_2S has been shown to regulate and modify ATP-sensitive potassium (KATP) channels and calcium channels. The KATP channel has eight subunits: four pore-forming Kir6.X subunits (either Kir6.1 or Kir6.2) and four regulatory sulfonylurea receptor (SUR) subunits. Kir6.X contains a highly conserved sequence that allows permeating K^+ ion. It also has binding sites for ATP and phosphatidylinositol 4,5-bisphosphate (PIP2), which inhibits and activates KATP channel, respectively. SUR subunits contain nucleotide-binding sites, which also regulate the opening/closure of KATP channels [99]. KATP channels are common to many cell types but mostly studied in cardiomyocytes and pancreatic β-cells regulating metabolism [99]. Calcium channels are important to the function of the brain, heart and muscle. There are many different isoforms of calcium channels which perform multiple physiological functions [100]. H_2S donors NaHS and GYY4137 persulfidated Kv2.1, a subunit in voltage-gated K (+) channels and inhibited its function in rat neurons [101]. In rat atria, treatment with NaHS or Na_2S augmented stretch-induced atrial natriuretic peptide (ANP) secretion and this effect was blocked by pretreatment with a KATP channel inhibitor, suggesting that H_2S stimulates ANP secretion via the KATP channel [102]. In a mouse paclitaxel-induced neuropathic pain model, GYY4137 treatment demonstrated anti-hyperalgesic activity and co-treatment with a KATP channel inhibitor blocked this anti-hyperalgesic activity [103]. In cultured carotid body, a cluster of chemoreceptor cells from bilateral sensory organs in the peripheral nervous system, NaHS treatment triggered transient calcium influx, which depended on the calcium in the culture media, suggesting that H$_2$S regulates calcium channels in carotid bodies [104].

4. Conclusions

Our current knowledge suggests that H$_2$S can directly persulfidate proteins and metabolites, and likely influence the NO/CO feedback loop. H$_2$S modifies the metal-binding complex in hemeproteins to regulate their functions. It can also directly modulate ROS/RNS and affect redox signaling. These direct effects may impact cellular functions, such as regulating tight junctions, autophagy/apoptosis, signaling pathways, epigenetics and ion channels, resulting in physiological changes, such as vasodilation, cardioprotection, cell differentiation, etc. (Figure 6). However, more work is needed to precisely identify the working mechanisms of H$_2$S as a gasotransmitter in mammals. For instance, methods for the precise measurement of H$_2$S concentration in different tissues are still lacking [1,105]. Although a useful tool in studying H$_2$S function, GYY4137 has a few drawbacks. For example, GYY4137 releases byproducts other than H$_2$S after hydrolysis, which may contribute to the observed physiological function in vivo and in vitro [9]. So far, no H$_2$S donor has been approved in clinical trials. This is partly due to the lack of a reliable method measuring free H$_2$S in human samples, resulting in difficulties in studying the pharmacokinetics of H$_2$S donors [106]. Nonetheless, H$_2$S functioning as a neuromodulator was only first reported in the 1990s [5] and as a gasotransmitter in 2001 [107]. With promising data from animal disease models and more research emerges, H$_2$S donors have great potential as future therapeutic agents for many cardiovascular, neurological and inflammatory diseases.

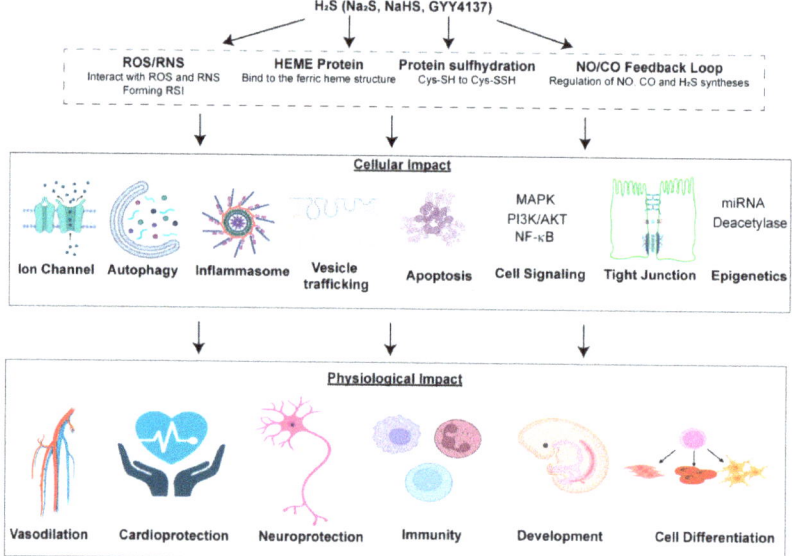

Figure 6. Illustration of the direct targets of H$_2$S and the downstream cellular/physiological impacts.

Author Contributions: J.L. and T.A.M. drafted the manuscript. F.M.M., C.E.H., W.C.S., J.P.B., K.M. and K.R.O. made critical revisions. All authors have read and agreed to the published version of the manuscript.

Funding: This work was supported by the following: National Institute of Health R01HD105301 (TAM); American College of Surgeons Clowe's Memorial Research Fund (TAM); Gerber Foundation (TAM); Riley Children's Foundation (TAM); National Science Foundation IOS2012106 (KRO); and funds from Indiana University Department of Surgery.

Conflicts of Interest: TAM serves as a consultant for Noveome Biotherapeutics. All other authors declare no conflict of interest.

Abbreviations

Akt—serine/threonine protein kinase, aka. protein kinase B (PKB); AMPK—AMP-activated protein kinase; Ang2—Angiopoietin-2; ANP—atrial natriuretic peptide; ASC—adaptor protein in inflammasomes; ATG—autophagy-related protein; ATP5A1—mitochondrial ATP synthase subunit alpha; BAK1—BCL2 antagonist/killer 1; BAX—BCL-2-associated X; BCL-2—B-cell lymphoma 2; BID—a member of BCL-2 family proteins; BIM—Bcl-2-like protein 11; CARD—carboxy-terminal caspase recruitment domain; CBS—cystathionine β-synthase; CcO—cytochrome c oxidase; CDK—Cyclin-Dependent Kinase; CO—carbon monoxide; COP—coat protein; CREB—cAMP response element-binding protein; CTH—aka. CSE, cystathionine γ-lyase; CXCR2—CXC chemokine receptor 2; DADS—diallyl disulfide, a slow-releasing naturally occurring H_2S donor; DAMP—damage-associated molecular pattern; Dex—Dexamethasone; DSS—Dextran sulfate sodium; ECM—extracellular matrix; EGFR—epidermal growth factor receptor; eNOS—endothelial nitric oxide synthase; ERK—Extracellular signal-regulated kinase; FADD—Fas-associated death domain protein; FOXO1—Forkhead box O 1; Gab—Grb2-associated binder 1; GLP-1—glucagonlike peptide-1; GSH—reduced glutathione; GSK—Glycogen synthase kinase; GSSG—glutathione disulfide; GYY4137—(p-methoxyphenyl) morpholino-phosphinodithioic acid; H_2S—hydrogen sulfide; HIF-1α—hypoxia-inducible factor 1 alpha; HO-1—Heme oxygenase-1; HUVECs—human umbilical vein endothelial cells; I/R—ischemia/ reperfusion; ICAM1—intercellular adhesion molecule 1; IKK—IκB kinase; JNK—c-jun N-terminal kinase; KATP—ATP-dependent potassium channel; Keap1—kelch-like ECH associating protein 1; Kir6.1—pore-forming subunit of KATP channels; KO—knock-out; Kv—voltage-gated potassium channel; LC3—microtubule-associated protein 1A/1B-light chain 3; LPS—lipopolysaccharide; LRR—leucine rich repeat; MAPK—mitogen-activated protein kinase; MARVEL—a four transmembrane-helix architecture referred to as the MARVEL domain; MCL1—myeloid cell leukemia sequence 1; miR—microRNA; MLC—myosin light chain; MLCK—myosin light chain kinase; MPST—aka. 3-MST, 3-mercaptopyruvate sulfurtransferase; MSU—monosodium urate; mTOR—mammalian target of rapamycin; Na_2S—sodium sulfide; NADPH—reduced form of nicotinamide adenine dinucleotide phosphate ($NADP^+$); NaHS—sodium hydrogen sulfide; NLR—NOD-like receptor; NLRP3—NOD, LRR- and pyrin domain-containing protein 3; NO—nitric oxide; NOD—Nucleotide-binding and oligomerization domain; Nrf2—nuclear factor erythroid 2–related factor 2; P66Shc—a member of adaptor protein family, encoded by ShcA; PAMP—pathogen-associated molecular pattern; PDK1—PIP3-dependent protein kinase 1; PHLPP—pleckstrin homology domain leucine-rich repeat protein phosphatase; PI3K—phosphoinositide 3-kinase; PIP2—phosphatidylinositol 4,5-bisphosphate; PIP3—phosphatidylinositol (3,4,5)-trisphosphate; PP2A—protein phosphatase 2A; PTEN—phosphatase and tensin homologue; PTP1B—protein tyrosine phosphatase 1B; PUMA—p53 upregulated modulator of apoptosis; RNS—reactive nitrogen species; ROS—reactive oxygen species; RSI—reactive species interactome; RSS—reactive sulfur species; S6K—ribosomal protein S6 kinase beta-1; SDC—sodium deoxycholate; SIRT1—sirtuin 1; SOD—superoxide dismutase; STAT3—signal transducer and activator of transcription 3; SUR—sulfonylurea receptor; TNFR—tumor necrosis factor receptor; TRAIL—TNF-related apoptosis-inducing ligand; Trx-1—thioredoxin; TUNEL—terminal deoxynucleotidyl transferase dUTP nick end labeling; ULK—Unc-51 like autophagy activating kinase; VACM1—vascular cell adhesion molecule 1; ZO—zonula occludens.

References

1. Wang, R. Physiological implications of hydrogen sulfide: A whiff exploration that blossomed. *Physiol. Rev.* **2012**, *92*, 791–896. [CrossRef]
2. Reiffenstein, R.J.; Hulbert, W.C.; Roth, S.H. Toxicology of hydrogen sulfide. *Annu. Rev. Pharmacol. Toxicol.* **1992**, *32*, 109–134. [CrossRef]
3. Cirino, G.; Szabo, C.; Papapetropoulos, A. Physiological roles of hydrogen sulfide in mammalian cells, tissues and organs. *Physiol. Rev.* 2022, in press. [CrossRef]
4. Wang, R. Two's company, three's a crowd: Can H_2S be the third endogenous gaseous transmitter? *FASEB J.* **2002**, *16*, 1792–1798. [CrossRef]

5. Abe, K.; Kimura, H. The possible role of hydrogen sulfide as an endogenous neuromodulator. *J. Neurosci.* **1996**, *16*, 1066–1071. [CrossRef] [PubMed]
6. Olson, K.R. Are Reactive Sulfur Species the New Reactive Oxygen Species? *Antioxid. Redox Signal.* **2020**, *33*, 1125–1142. [CrossRef] [PubMed]
7. Zhang, H.; Bai, Z.; Zhu, L.; Liang, Y.; Fan, X.; Li, J.; Wen, H.; Shi, T.; Zhao, Q.; Wang, Z. Hydrogen sulfide donors: Therapeutic potential in anti-atherosclerosis. *Eur. J. Med. Chem.* **2020**, *205*, 112665. [CrossRef] [PubMed]
8. Zhao, Y.; Biggs, T.D.; Xian, M. Hydrogen sulfide (H_2S) releasing agents: Chemistry and biological applications. *Chem. Commun.* **2014**, *50*, 11788–11805. [CrossRef] [PubMed]
9. Powell, C.R.; Dillon, K.M.; Matson, J.B. A review of hydrogen sulfide (H_2S) donors: Chemistry and potential therapeutic applications. *Biochem. Pharmacol.* **2018**, *149*, 110–123. [CrossRef]
10. Song, Z.L.; Zhao, L.; Ma, T.; Osama, A.; Shen, T.; He, Y.; Fang, J. Progress and perspective on hydrogen sulfide donors and their biomedical applications. *Med. Res. Rev.* **2022**, *42*, 1930–1977. [CrossRef]
11. Corvino, A.; Frecentese, F.; Magli, E.; Perissutti, E.; Santagada, V.; Scognamiglio, A.; Caliendo, G.; Fiorino, F.; Severino, B. Trends in H_2S-Donors Chemistry and Their Effects in Cardiovascular Diseases. *Antioxidants* **2021**, *10*, 429. [CrossRef] [PubMed]
12. Li, L.; Whiteman, M.; Guan, Y.Y.; Neo, K.L.; Cheng, Y.; Lee, S.W.; Zhao, Y.; Baskar, R.; Tan, C.H.; Moore, P.K. Characterization of a novel, water-soluble hydrogen sulfide-releasing molecule (GYY4137): New insights into the biology of hydrogen sulfide. *Circulation* **2008**, *117*, 2351–2360. [CrossRef] [PubMed]
13. Lee, Z.W.; Zhou, J.; Chen, C.S.; Zhao, Y.; Tan, C.H.; Li, L.; Moore, P.K.; Deng, L.W. The slow-releasing hydrogen sulfide donor, GYY4137, exhibits novel anti-cancer effects in vitro and in vivo. *PLoS ONE* **2011**, *6*, e21077. [CrossRef] [PubMed]
14. Alexander, B.E.; Coles, S.J.; Fox, B.C.; Khan, T.F.; Maliszewski, J.; Perry, A.; Pitak, M.B.; Whiteman, M.; Wood, M.E. Investigating the generation of hydrogen sulfide from the phosphonamidodithioate slow-release donor GYY4137. *Medchemcomm* **2015**, *6*, 1649–1655. [CrossRef]
15. Ascenção, K.; Szabo, C. Emerging roles of cystathionine β-synthase in various forms of cancer. *Redox Biol.* **2022**, *53*, 102331. [CrossRef]
16. Mishanina, T.V.; Libiad, M.; Banerjee, R. Biogenesis of reactive sulfur species for signaling by hydrogen sulfide oxidation pathways. *Nat. Chem. Biol.* **2015**, *11*, 457–464. [CrossRef]
17. Olson, K.R. H_2S and polysulfide metabolism: Conventional and unconventional pathways. *Biochem. Pharmacol.* **2018**, *149*, 77–90. [CrossRef]
18. Sies, H.; Jones, D.P. Reactive oxygen species (ROS) as pleiotropic physiological signalling agents. *Nat. Rev. Mol. Cell Biol.* **2020**, *21*, 363–383. [CrossRef]
19. Adams, L.; Franco, M.C.; Estevez, A.G. Reactive nitrogen species in cellular signaling. *Exp. Biol. Med.* **2015**, *240*, 711–717. [CrossRef]
20. Chen, T.; Tian, M.; Han, Y. Hydrogen sulfide: A multi-tasking signal molecule in the regulation of oxidative stress responses. *J. Exp. Bot.* **2020**, *71*, 2862–2869. [CrossRef]
21. Xie, Z.Z.; Liu, Y.; Bian, J.S. Hydrogen Sulfide and Cellular Redox Homeostasis. *Oxidative Med. Cell. Longev.* **2016**, *2016*, 6043038. [CrossRef] [PubMed]
22. Searcy, D.G.; Whitehead, J.P.; Maroney, M.J. Interaction of Cu, Zn superoxide dismutase with hydrogen sulfide. *Arch. Biochem. Biophys.* **1995**, *318*, 251–263. [CrossRef] [PubMed]
23. Cortese-Krott, M.M.; Koning, A.; Kuhnle, G.G.C.; Nagy, P.; Bianco, C.L.; Pasch, A.; Wink, D.A.; Fukuto, J.M.; Jackson, A.A.; van Goor, H.; et al. The Reactive Species Interactome: Evolutionary Emergence, Biological Significance, and Opportunities for Redox Metabolomics and Personalized Medicine. *Antioxid. Redox Signal.* **2017**, *27*, 684–712. [CrossRef] [PubMed]
24. Ríos-González, B.B.; Román-Morales, E.M.; Pietri, R.; López-Garriga, J. Hydrogen sulfide activation in hemeproteins: The sulfheme scenario. *J. Inorg. Biochem.* **2014**, *133*, 78–86. [CrossRef] [PubMed]
25. Boubeta, F.M.; Bieza, S.A.; Bringas, M.; Palermo, J.C.; Boechi, L.; Estrin, D.A.; Bari, S.E. Hemeproteins as Targets for Sulfide Species. *Antioxid. Redox Signal.* **2020**, *32*, 247–257. [CrossRef] [PubMed]
26. Pietri, R.; Román-Morales, E.; López-Garriga, J. Hydrogen sulfide and hemeproteins: Knowledge and mysteries. *Antioxid. Redox Signal.* **2011**, *15*, 393–404. [CrossRef] [PubMed]
27. Collman, J.P.; Ghosh, S.; Dey, A.; Decréau, R.A. Using a functional enzyme model to understand the chemistry behind hydrogen sulfide induced hibernation. *Proc. Natl. Acad. Sci. USA* **2009**, *106*, 22090–22095. [CrossRef]
28. Filipovic, M.R. Persulfidation (S-sulfhydration) and H_2S. *Handb. Exp. Pharmacol.* **2015**, *230*, 29–59. [CrossRef]
29. Filipovic, M.R.; Zivanovic, J.; Alvarez, B.; Banerjee, R. Chemical Biology of H_2S Signaling through Persulfidation. *Chem. Rev.* **2018**, *118*, 1253–1337. [CrossRef]
30. Gao, X.H.; Krokowski, D.; Guan, B.J.; Bederman, I.; Majumder, M.; Parisien, M.; Diatchenko, L.; Kabil, O.; Willard, B.; Banerjee, R.; et al. Quantitative H_2S-mediated protein sulfhydration reveals metabolic reprogramming during the integrated stress response. *eLife* **2015**, *4*, e10067. [CrossRef]
31. Mustafa, A.K.; Sikka, G.; Gazi, S.K.; Steppan, J.; Jung, S.M.; Bhunia, A.K.; Barodka, V.M.; Gazi, F.K.; Barrow, R.K.; Wang, R.; et al. Hydrogen sulfide as endothelium-derived hyperpolarizing factor sulfhydrates potassium channels. *Circ. Res.* **2011**, *109*, 1259–1268. [CrossRef] [PubMed]

32. Krishnan, N.; Fu, C.; Pappin, D.J.; Tonks, N.K. H$_2$S-Induced sulfhydration of the phosphatase PTP1B and its role in the endoplasmic reticulum stress response. *Sci. Signal.* **2011**, *4*, ra86. [CrossRef] [PubMed]
33. Jiang, S.; Xu, W.; Chen, Z.; Cui, C.; Fan, X.; Cai, J.; Gong, Y.; Geng, B. Hydrogen sulphide reduces hyperhomocysteinaemia-induced endothelial ER stress by sulfhydrating protein disulphide isomerase to attenuate atherosclerosis. *J. Cell. Mol. Med.* **2021**, *25*, 3437–3448. [CrossRef] [PubMed]
34. Andrew, P.J.; Mayer, B. Enzymatic function of nitric oxide synthases. *Cardiovasc. Res.* **1999**, *43*, 521–531. [CrossRef]
35. Altaany, Z.; Ju, Y.; Yang, G.; Wang, R. The coordination of S-sulfhydration, S-nitrosylation, and phosphorylation of endothelial nitric oxide synthase by hydrogen sulfide. *Sci. Signal.* **2014**, *7*, ra87. [CrossRef]
36. Zang, H.; Mathew, R.O.; Cui, T. The Dark Side of Nrf2 in the Heart. *Front. Physiol.* **2020**, *11*, 722. [CrossRef]
37. Yang, G.; Zhao, K.; Ju, Y.; Mani, S.; Cao, Q.; Puukila, S.; Khaper, N.; Wu, L.; Wang, R. Hydrogen sulfide protects against cellular senescence via S-sulfhydration of Keap1 and activation of Nrf2. *Antioxid. Redox Signal.* **2013**, *18*, 1906–1919. [CrossRef]
38. Xie, Z.Z.; Shi, M.M.; Xie, L.; Wu, Z.Y.; Li, G.; Hua, F.; Bian, J.S. Sulfhydration of p66Shc at cysteine59 mediates the antioxidant effect of hydrogen sulfide. *Antioxid. Redox Signal.* **2014**, *21*, 2531–2542. [CrossRef]
39. Xie, L.; Gu, Y.; Wen, M.; Zhao, S.; Wang, W.; Ma, Y.; Meng, G.; Han, Y.; Wang, Y.; Liu, G.; et al. Hydrogen Sulfide Induces Keap1 S-sulfhydration and Suppresses Diabetes-Accelerated Atherosclerosis via Nrf2 Activation. *Diabetes* **2016**, *65*, 3171–3184. [CrossRef]
40. Giuffrè, A.; Vicente, J.B. Hydrogen Sulfide Biochemistry and Interplay with Other Gaseous Mediators in Mammalian Physiology. *Oxidative Med. Cell. Longev.* **2018**, *2018*, 6290931. [CrossRef]
41. Hennessy, B.T.; Smith, D.L.; Ram, P.T.; Lu, Y.; Mills, G.B. Exploiting the PI3K/AKT pathway for cancer drug discovery. *Nat. Rev. Drug. Discov.* **2005**, *4*, 988–1004. [CrossRef] [PubMed]
42. Manning, B.D.; Toker, A. AKT/PKB Signaling: Navigating the Network. *Cell* **2017**, *169*, 381–405. [CrossRef] [PubMed]
43. Qiu, Y.; Wu, Y.; Meng, M.; Luo, M.; Zhao, H.; Sun, H.; Gao, S. GYY4137 protects against myocardial ischemia/reperfusion injury via activation of the PHLPP-1/Akt/Nrf2 signaling pathway in diabetic mice. *J. Surg. Res.* **2018**, *225*, 29–39. [CrossRef] [PubMed]
44. Karwi, Q.G.; Whiteman, M.; Wood, M.E.; Torregrossa, R.; Baxter, G.F. Pharmacological postconditioning against myocardial infarction with a slow-releasing hydrogen sulfide donor, GYY4137. *Pharmacol. Res.* **2016**, *111*, 442–451. [CrossRef]
45. Xia, Y.Q.; Ning, J.Z.; Cheng, F.; Yu, W.M.; Rao, T.; Ruan, Y.; Yuan, R.; Du, Y. GYY4137 a H$_2$S donor, attenuates ipsilateral epididymis injury in experimentally varicocele-induced rats via activation of the PI3K/Akt pathway. *Iran J. Basic Med. Sci.* **2019**, *22*, 729–735. [CrossRef]
46. Lu, M.; Jiang, X.; Tong, L.; Zhang, F.; Ma, L.; Dong, X.; Sun, X. MicroRNA-21-Regulated Activation of the Akt Pathway Participates in the Protective Effects of H$_2$S against Liver Ischemia-Reperfusion Injury. *Biol. Pharm. Bull.* **2018**, *41*, 229–238. [CrossRef]
47. Tang, B.; Ma, L.; Yao, X.; Tan, G.; Han, P.; Yu, T.; Liu, B.; Sun, X. Hydrogen sulfide ameliorates acute lung injury induced by infrarenal aortic cross-clamping by inhibiting inflammation and angiopoietin 2 release. *J. Vasc. Surg.* **2017**, *65*, 501–508.e501. [CrossRef]
48. Majumder, S.; Ren, L.; Pushpakumar, S.; Sen, U. Hydrogen sulphide mitigates homocysteine-induced apoptosis and matrix remodelling in mesangial cells through Akt/FOXO1 signalling cascade. *Cell. Signal.* **2019**, *61*, 66–77. [CrossRef]
49. Slade, E.; Williams, L.; Gagnon, J. Hydrogen sulfide suppresses ghrelin secretion in vitro and delays postprandial ghrelin secretion while reducing appetite in mice. *Physiol. Rep.* **2018**, *6*, e13870. [CrossRef]
50. Zheng, Y.; Lv, P.; Huang, J.; Ke, J.; Yan, J. GYY4137 exhibits anti-atherosclerosis effect in apolipoprotein E (-/-) mice via PI3K/Akt and TLR4 signalling. *Clin. Exp. Pharmacol. Physiol.* **2020**, *47*, 1231–1239. [CrossRef]
51. Liu, T.; Zhang, L.; Joo, D.; Sun, S.-C. NF-κB signaling in inflammation. *Signal Transduct. Target. Ther.* **2017**, *2*, 17023. [CrossRef] [PubMed]
52. Taniguchi, K.; Karin, M. NF-κB, inflammation, immunity and cancer: Coming of age. *Nat. Rev. Immunol.* **2018**, *18*, 309–324. [CrossRef] [PubMed]
53. Sun, H.J.; Leng, B.; Wu, Z.Y.; Bian, J.S. Polysulfide and Hydrogen Sulfide Ameliorate Cisplatin-Induced Nephrotoxicity and Renal Inflammation through Persulfidating STAT3 and IKKβ. *Int. J. Mol. Sci.* **2020**, *21*, 7805. [CrossRef] [PubMed]
54. Zhuang, R.; Guo, L.; Du, J.; Wang, S.; Li, J.; Liu, Y. Exogenous hydrogen sulfide inhibits oral mucosal wound-induced macrophage activation via the NF-κB pathway. *Oral Dis.* **2018**, *24*, 793–801. [CrossRef]
55. Plotnikov, A.; Zehorai, E.; Procaccia, S.; Seger, R. The MAPK cascades: Signaling components, nuclear roles and mechanisms of nuclear translocation. *Biochim. Biophys. Acta* **2011**, *1813*, 1619–1633. [CrossRef]
56. Alexander, S.P.H.; Mathie, A.; Peters, J.A. Ion Channels. *Br. J. Pharmacol.* **2011**, *164* (Suppl. S1), S137–S174. [CrossRef]
57. Cao, X.; Xiong, S.; Zhou, Y.; Wu, Z.; Ding, L.; Zhu, Y.; Wood, M.E.; Whiteman, M.; Moore, P.K.; Bian, J.S. Renal Protective Effect of Hydrogen Sulfide in Cisplatin-Induced Nephrotoxicity. *Antioxid. Redox Signal.* **2018**, *29*, 455–470. [CrossRef]
58. Pichette, J.; Fynn-Sackey, N.; Gagnon, J. Hydrogen Sulfide and Sulfate Prebiotic Stimulates the Secretion of GLP-1 and Improves Glycemia in Male Mice. *Endocrinology* **2017**, *158*, 3416–3425. [CrossRef]
59. Peng, Z.; Kellenberger, S. Hydrogen Sulfide Upregulates Acid-sensing Ion Channels via the MAPK-Erk1/2 Signaling Pathway. *Function* **2021**, *2*, zqab007. [CrossRef]
60. Zihni, C.; Mills, C.; Matter, K.; Balda, M.S. Tight junctions: From simple barriers to multifunctional molecular gates. *Nat. Rev. Mol. Cell Biol.* **2016**, *17*, 564–580. [CrossRef]

61. Chen, S.; Bu, D.; Ma, Y.; Zhu, J.; Sun, L.; Zuo, S.; Ma, J.; Li, T.; Chen, Z.; Zheng, Y.; et al. GYY4137 ameliorates intestinal barrier injury in a mouse model of endotoxemia. *Biochem. Pharmacol.* **2016**, *118*, 59–67. [CrossRef] [PubMed]
62. Cui, W.; Chen, J.; Yu, F.; Liu, W.; He, M. GYY4137 protected the integrity of the blood-brain barrier via activation of the Nrf2/ARE pathway in mice with sepsis. *FASEB J.* **2021**, *35*, e21710. [CrossRef] [PubMed]
63. Chen, Z.; Tang, J.; Wang, P.; Zhu, J.; Liu, Y. GYY4137 Attenuates Sodium Deoxycholate-Induced Intestinal Barrier Injury Both In Vitro and In Vivo. *Biomed. Res. Int.* **2019**, *2019*, 5752323. [CrossRef] [PubMed]
64. Zhao, H.; Yan, R.; Zhou, X.; Ji, F.; Zhang, B. Hydrogen sulfide improves colonic barrier integrity in DSS-induced inflammation in Caco-2 cells and mice. *Int. Immunopharmacol.* **2016**, *39*, 121–127. [CrossRef] [PubMed]
65. Dikic, I.; Elazar, Z. Mechanism and medical implications of mammalian autophagy. *Nat. Rev. Mol. Cell Biol.* **2018**, *19*, 349–364. [CrossRef]
66. Zhu, L.; Duan, W.; Wu, G.; Zhang, D.; Wang, L.; Chen, D.; Chen, Z.; Yang, B. Protective effect of hydrogen sulfide on endothelial cells through Sirt1-FoxO1-mediated autophagy. *Ann. Transl. Med.* **2020**, *8*, 1586. [CrossRef]
67. Ni, K.; Hua, Y. Hydrogen sulfide exacerbated periodontal inflammation and induced autophagy in experimental periodontitis. *Int. Immunopharmacol.* **2021**, *93*, 107399. [CrossRef]
68. Yang, F.; Zhang, L.; Gao, Z.; Sun, X.; Yu, M.; Dong, S.; Wu, J.; Zhao, Y.; Xu, C.; Zhang, W.; et al. Exogenous H_2S Protects Against Diabetic Cardiomyopathy by Activating Autophagy via the AMPK/mTOR Pathway. *Cell. Physiol. Biochem.* **2017**, *43*, 1168–1187. [CrossRef]
69. Carneiro, B.A.; El-Deiry, W.S. Targeting apoptosis in cancer therapy. *Nat. Rev. Clin. Oncol.* **2020**, *17*, 395–417. [CrossRef]
70. Li, J.; Yuan, Y.Q.; Zhang, L.; Zhang, H.; Zhang, S.W.; Zhang, Y.; Xuan, X.X.; Wang, M.J.; Zhang, J.Y. Exogenous hydrogen sulfide protects against high glucose-induced apoptosis and oxidative stress by inhibiting the STAT3/HIF-1α pathway in H9c2 cardiomyocytes. *Exp. Ther. Med.* **2019**, *18*, 3948–3958. [CrossRef]
71. Garcia, N.A.; Moncayo-Arlandi, J.; Vazquez, A.; Genovés, P.; Calvo, C.J.; Millet, J.; Martí, N.; Aguado, C.; Knecht, E.; Valiente-Alandi, I.; et al. Hydrogen Sulfide Improves Cardiomyocyte Function in a Cardiac Arrest Model. *Ann. Transpl.* **2017**, *22*, 285–295. [CrossRef] [PubMed]
72. Bai, X.; Batallé, G.; Balboni, G.; Pol, O. Hydrogen Sulfide Increases the Analgesic Effects of μ- and δ-Opioid Receptors during Neuropathic Pain: Pathways Implicated. *Antioxidants* **2022**, *11*, 1321. [CrossRef] [PubMed]
73. Jiang, T.; Yang, W.; Zhang, H.; Song, Z.; Liu, T.; Lv, X. Hydrogen Sulfide Ameliorates Lung Ischemia-Reperfusion Injury Through SIRT1 Signaling Pathway in Type 2 Diabetic Rats. *Front. Physiol.* **2020**, *11*, 596. [CrossRef] [PubMed]
74. Ma, J.; Shi, C.; Liu, Z.; Han, B.; Guo, L.; Zhu, L.; Ye, T. Hydrogen sulfide is a novel regulator implicated in glucocorticoids-inhibited bone formation. *Aging* **2019**, *11*, 7537–7552. [CrossRef] [PubMed]
75. Ye, P.; Gu, Y.; Zhu, Y.R.; Chao, Y.L.; Kong, X.Q.; Luo, J.; Ren, X.M.; Zuo, G.F.; Zhang, D.M.; Chen, S.L. Exogenous hydrogen sulfide attenuates the development of diabetic cardiomyopathy via the FoxO1 pathway. *J. Cell Physiol.* **2018**, *233*, 9786–9798. [CrossRef]
76. Wang, C.; Du, J.; Du, S.; Liu, Y.; Li, D.; Zhu, X.; Ni, X. Endogenous H_2S resists mitochondria-mediated apoptosis in the adrenal glands via ATP5A1 S-sulfhydration in male mice. *Mol. Cell Endocrinol.* **2018**, *474*, 65–73. [CrossRef]
77. Wu, J.; Yang, F.; Zhang, X.; Chen, G.; Zou, J.; Yin, L.; Yang, D. Hydrogen sulfide inhibits endoplasmic reticulum stress through the GRP78/mTOR pathway in rat chondrocytes subjected to oxidative stress. *Int. J. Mol. Med.* **2021**, *47*, 4867. [CrossRef]
78. Liang, K.; Wei, L.; Chen, L. Exocytosis, Endocytosis, and Their Coupling in Excitable Cells. *Front. Mol. Neurosci.* **2017**, *10*, 109. [CrossRef]
79. Trexler, A.J.; Taraska, J.W. Regulation of insulin exocytosis by calcium-dependent protein kinase C in beta cells. *Cell Calcium* **2017**, *67*, 1–10. [CrossRef]
80. de Pascual, R.; Baraibar, A.M.; Méndez-López, I.; Pérez-Ciria, M.; Polo-Vaquero, I.; Gandía, L.; Ohia, S.E.; García, A.G.; de Diego, A.M.G. Hydrogen sulphide facilitates exocytosis by regulating the handling of intracellular calcium by chromaffin cells. *Pflug. Arch.* **2018**, *470*, 1255–1270. [CrossRef]
81. Pearse, B.M. Clathrin: A unique protein associated with intracellular transfer of membrane by coated vesicles. *Proc. Natl. Acad. Sci. USA* **1976**, *73*, 1255–1259. [CrossRef] [PubMed]
82. Allen, J.A.; Halverson-Tamboli, R.A.; Rasenick, M.M. Lipid raft microdomains and neurotransmitter signalling. *Nat. Rev. Neurosci.* **2007**, *8*, 128–140. [CrossRef] [PubMed]
83. Canton, J. Macropinocytosis: New Insights Into Its Underappreciated Role in Innate Immune Cell Surveillance. *Front. Immunol.* **2018**, *9*, 2286. [CrossRef] [PubMed]
84. Ge, S.N.; Zhao, M.M.; Wu, D.D.; Chen, Y.; Wang, Y.; Zhu, J.H.; Cai, W.J.; Zhu, Y.Z.; Zhu, Y.C. Hydrogen sulfide targets EGFR Cys797/Cys798 residues to induce Na(+)/K(+)-ATPase endocytosis and inhibition in renal tubular epithelial cells and increase sodium excretion in chronic salt-loaded rats. *Antioxid. Redox Signal.* **2014**, *21*, 2061–2082. [CrossRef] [PubMed]
85. Dal-Secco, D.; Cunha, T.M.; Freitas, A.; Alves-Filho, J.C.; Souto, F.O.; Fukada, S.Y.; Grespan, R.; Alencar, N.M.; Neto, A.F.; Rossi, M.A.; et al. Hydrogen sulfide augments neutrophil migration through enhancement of adhesion molecule expression and prevention of CXCR2 internalization: Role of ATP-sensitive potassium channels. *J. Immunol.* **2008**, *181*, 4287–4298. [CrossRef] [PubMed]
86. Cavalli, G.; Heard, E. Advances in epigenetics link genetics to the environment and disease. *Nature* **2019**, *571*, 489–499. [CrossRef]
87. Zhang, T.; Kraus, W.L. SIRT1-dependent regulation of chromatin and transcription: Linking NAD(+) metabolism and signaling to the control of cellular functions. *Biochim. Biophys. Acta* **2010**, *1804*, 1666–1675. [CrossRef]

88. Du, C.; Lin, X.; Xu, W.; Zheng, F.; Cai, J.; Yang, J.; Cui, Q.; Tang, C.; Cai, J.; Xu, G.; et al. Sulfhydrated Sirtuin-1 Increasing Its Deacetylation Activity Is an Essential Epigenetics Mechanism of Anti-Atherogenesis by Hydrogen Sulfide. *Antioxid. Redox Signal.* **2019**, *30*, 184–197. [CrossRef]
89. Bartel, D.P. Metazoan MicroRNAs. *Cell* **2018**, *173*, 20–51. [CrossRef]
90. Weber, G.J.; Pushpakumar, S.B.; Sen, U. Hydrogen sulfide alleviates hypertensive kidney dysfunction through an epigenetic mechanism. *Am. J. Physiol. Heart Circ. Physiol.* **2017**, *312*, H874–H885. [CrossRef]
91. John, A.; Kundu, S.; Pushpakumar, S.; Fordham, M.; Weber, G.; Mukhopadhyay, M.; Sen, U. GYY4137, a Hydrogen Sulfide Donor Modulates miR194-Dependent Collagen Realignment in Diabetic Kidney. *Sci. Rep.* **2017**, *7*, 10924. [CrossRef]
92. Nandi, S.S.; Mishra, P.K. H2S and homocysteine control a novel feedback regulation of cystathionine beta synthase and cystathionine gamma lyase in cardiomyocytes. *Sci. Rep.* **2017**, *7*, 3639. [CrossRef] [PubMed]
93. Malik, A.; Kanneganti, T.D. Inflammasome activation and assembly at a glance. *J. Cell Sci.* **2017**, *130*, 3955–3963. [CrossRef]
94. Swanson, K.V.; Deng, M.; Ting, J.P. The NLRP3 inflammasome: Molecular activation and regulation to therapeutics. *Nat. Rev. Immunol.* **2019**, *19*, 477–489. [CrossRef] [PubMed]
95. Castelblanco, M.; Lugrin, J.; Ehirchiou, D.; Nasi, S.; Ishii, I.; So, A.; Martinon, F.; Busso, N. Hydrogen sulfide inhibits NLRP3 inflammasome activation and reduces cytokine production both in vitro and in a mouse model of inflammation. *J. Biol. Chem.* **2018**, *293*, 2546–2557. [CrossRef] [PubMed]
96. Zheng, Q.; Pan, L.; Ji, Y. H2S protects against diabetes-accelerated atherosclerosis by preventing the activation of NLRP3 inflammasome. *J. Biomed. Res.* **2019**, *34*, 94–102. [CrossRef]
97. Li, J.; Ma, J.; Li, M.; Tao, J.; Chen, J.; Yao, C.; Yao, S. GYY4137 alleviates sepsis-induced acute lung injury in mice by inhibiting the PDGFRβ/Akt/NF-κB/NLRP3 pathway. *Life Sci.* **2021**, *271*, 119192. [CrossRef]
98. Zhou, T.; Qian, H.; Zheng, N.; Lu, Q.; Han, Y. GYY4137 ameliorates sepsis-induced cardiomyopathy via NLRP3 pathway. *Biochim. Biophys. Acta Mol. Basis Dis.* **2022**, *1868*, 166497. [CrossRef]
99. Pipatpolkai, T.; Usher, S.; Stansfeld, P.J.; Ashcroft, F.M. New insights into KATP channel gene mutations and neonatal diabetes mellitus. *Nat. Rev. Endocrinol.* **2020**, *16*, 378–393. [CrossRef]
100. Zamponi, G.W. Targeting voltage-gated calcium channels in neurological and psychiatric diseases. *Nat. Rev. Drug Discov.* **2016**, *15*, 19–34. [CrossRef]
101. Dallas, M.L.; Al-Owais, M.M.; Hettiarachchi, N.T.; Vandiver, M.S.; Jarosz-Griffiths, H.H.; Scragg, J.L.; Boyle, J.P.; Steele, D.; Peers, C. Hydrogen sulfide regulates hippocampal neuron excitability via S-sulfhydration of Kv2.1. *Sci. Rep.* **2021**, *11*, 8194. [CrossRef] [PubMed]
102. Yu, L.; Park, B.M.; Ahn, Y.J.; Lee, G.J.; Kim, S.H. Hydrogen sulfide donor, NaHS, stimulates ANP secretion via the K(ATP) channel and the NOS/sGC pathway in rat atria. *Peptides* **2019**, *111*, 89–97. [CrossRef] [PubMed]
103. Qabazard, B.; Masocha, W.; Khajah, M.; Phillips, O.A. H2S donor GYY4137 ameliorates paclitaxel-induced neuropathic pain in mice. *Biomed. Pharmacother.* **2020**, *127*, 110210. [CrossRef] [PubMed]
104. Gallego-Martin, T.; Prieto-Lloret, J.; Aaronson, P.I.; Rocher, A.; Obeso, A. Hydroxycobalamin Reveals the Involvement of Hydrogen Sulfide in the Hypoxic Responses of Rat Carotid Body Chemoreceptor Cells. *Antioxidants* **2019**, *8*, 62. [CrossRef]
105. Paul, B.D.; Snyder, S.H. Modes of physiologic H2S signaling in the brain and peripheral tissues. *Antioxid. Redox Signal.* **2015**, *22*, 411–423. [CrossRef]
106. Sulfagenix Australia Pty Ltd. Assessing the Safety and Ability of SG1002 to Overcome Deficits in Hydrogen Sulfide in Heart Failure Patients. ClinicalTrials.gov Identifier: NCT01989208. Available online: https://clinicaltrials.gov/ct2/show/study/NCT01989208 (accessed on 5 May 2020).
107. Zhao, W.; Zhang, J.; Lu, Y.; Wang, R. The vasorelaxant effect of H2S as a novel endogenous gaseous K(ATP) channel opener. *EMBO J.* **2001**, *20*, 6008–6016. [CrossRef]

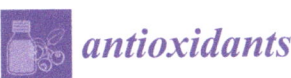

Perspective

The Reactive Species Interactome in Red Blood Cells: Oxidants, Antioxidants, and Molecular Targets

Miriam M. Cortese-Krott [1,2,3]

1. Myocardial Infarction Research Laboratory, Department of Cardiology, Pulmonology and Angiology, Medical Faculty, Heinrich-Heine-University, Universitätstrasse 1, 40225 Düsseldorf, Germany; miriam.cortese@hhu.de
2. Department of Physiology and Pharmacology, Karolinska Institutet, 17177 Stockholm, Sweden
3. CARID, Cardiovascular Research Institute, Heinrich-Heine University, 40225 Düsseldorf, Germany

Abstract: Beyond their established role as oxygen carriers, red blood cells have recently been found to contribute to systemic NO and sulfide metabolism and act as potent circulating antioxidant cells. Emerging evidence indicates that reactive species derived from the metabolism of O_2, NO, and H_2S can interact with each other, potentially influencing common biological targets. These interactions have been encompassed in the concept of the *reactive species interactome*. This review explores the potential application of the concept of *reactive species interactome* to understand the redox physiology of RBCs. It specifically examines how *reactive species* are generated and detoxified, their interactions with each other, and their targets. Hemoglobin is a key player in the *reactive species interactome* within RBCs, given its abundance and fundamental role in O_2/CO_2 exchange, NO transport/metabolism, and sulfur species binding/production. Future research should focus on understanding how modulation of the *reactive species interactome* may regulate RBC biology, physiology, and their systemic effects.

Keywords: red blood cells; reactive species interactome; nitric oxide; sulfide; antioxidant enzymes; oxidative stress; hemoglobin

1. Introduction

Oxidative stress was originally defined by Helmut Sies as *"an imbalance between antioxidants and oxidants in favor of the oxidant, which can potentially lead to molecular damage"* [1]. Excessive production of oxidants and/or consumption of antioxidant systems disrupt cellular redox control and signaling [2,3]. He also introduced the term "reactive oxygen species" (ROS) to describe oxidants derived from the metabolic utilization of oxygen, including free oxygen radicals (•OH), superoxide radical anion (•O_2^-), and hydrogen peroxide (H_2O_2).

Intracellular antioxidant systems responsible for scavenging and removal of ROS comprise molecules that act as redox couples and/or cofactors of enzymes (including the "*inevitable*" glutathione [4], as well as antioxidant enzymes, like glutathione peroxidase, catalase, and superoxide dismutase. The concept of cellular redox balance/disbalance was described by using the image of a traditional scale consisting of two plates suspended at equal distances from a fulcrum. Antioxidants were depicted on one plate, and oxidants (or ROS) were depicted on the other plate. In a weighing balance, the weighing plates level off only when a static equilibrium between the two plates is achieved, i.e., only when the masses on the two plates are equal.

According to this conceptual model, under resting conditions, the cellular redox state is maintained when the oxidant production is balanced by the intracellular antioxidant response. If the levels of oxidants exceed those of antioxidants, as a result of higher ROS levels or lower antioxidant production [1], there will be damage to the cell. ROS have been shown to react with other endogenously produced free radicals and reactive species containing nitrogen (reactive nitrogen species, RNS) and sulfur (reactive sulfur species, RSN), which have also been proven to be potent oxidants and disturb normal

Citation: Cortese-Krott, M.M. The Reactive Species Interactome in Red Blood Cells: Oxidants, Antioxidants, and Molecular Targets. *Antioxidants* 2023, *12*, 1736. https://doi.org/10.3390/antiox12091736

Academic Editors: John Toscano and Vinayak Khodade

Received: 2 July 2023
Revised: 27 August 2023
Accepted: 4 September 2023
Published: 7 September 2023

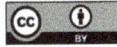

Copyright: © 2023 by the author. Licensee MDPI, Basel, Switzerland. This article is an open access article distributed under the terms and conditions of the Creative Commons Attribution (CC BY) license (https://creativecommons.org/licenses/by/4.0/).

redox homeostasis [5]. In earlier studies, the presence of enhanced oxidative stress or ROS/RNS/RSS levels was associated with diseases such as diabetes, inflammation, and mitochondrial dysfunction [1].

The study of redox biology and its conceptualization has evolved considerably since then. It was proven that ROS are not the only reactive species responsible for oxidative damage. The free radical nitric oxide (NO) was demonstrated to be produced endogenously in cells by a nitric oxide synthase (NOS) and act as a signaling molecule and a neurotransmitter. Also, H_2O_2 was found to have important signaling functions under physiological conditions and be produced under highly controlled conditions by NADPH oxidases. In recent years, sulfide has been shown to be produced endogenously in mammalian cells and tissues and shows fundamental biological and physiological effects, resembling the effects of NO in some cases. Here, the term "sulfide" is used for simplicity to indicate the mixture of all sulfide species found in equilibrium among themselves at biological pH., i.e., H_2S (g), H_2S (aq), HS^-, and S^{2-}. In water at pH 7.4, H_2S (aq) is rapidly equilibrated into HS^- (>70%) and S^{2-}. Therefore, the main biologically relevant sulfide species in cells are H_2S (aq) and HS^- (>70%). The IUPAC nomenclature of these species is as follows: H_2S, sulfane or hydrogen sulfide; HS^-, sulfanide or hydrogen(sulfide)(-1); S^{2-}, sulfide(-2) or sulfanediide.

It is also clear that these radicals and oxidants are highly compartmentalized, undergo chemical reactions and complex interactions among them, and may affect common biological targets. In other words, in a biological environment, molecules derived from the metabolism of O_2, NO, and H_2S may interact with each other and should be considered components of the same system. Therefore, we introduced the term *reactive species interactome* [5]. The *reactive species interactome* is defined as an "oxidation-reduction system consisting of chemical interactions between reactive sulfur species (RSS), reactive nitrogen species (RNS), and ROS with their thiol targets".

Red blood cells (RBCs) are simple, short-lived, anucleated cells present in almost all vertebrates, whose main function is the transport of oxygen (O_2) and carbon dioxide (CO_2) along the vascular system of vertebrates. For many years, scientists have thought that the sole function of RBCs was to deliver O_2 to body tissues. However, there is growing evidence that these cells may be involved in complex systemic redox regulation [6]. RBCs have a very complex and poorly understood *reactive species interactome*.

The presence of high concentrations of hemoglobin and its oxidized form, methemoglobin, is one of the main sources of ROS in RBCs. RBCs are particularly rich in antioxidants and detoxifying enzymes and transport high millimolar concentrations of glutathione [6,7] and glutathione persulfide $(GS(S)_nSG)$ [8].

In addition, RBCs are exposed to endothelial-derived nitric oxide (NO) and its metabolites, such as nitrite (NO_2^-), nitrate (NO_3^-), and nitrosospecies (RXNO) [9]. (RXNO indicates low-molecular-weight molecules where a "nitroso group" is bound to a cysteine (nitrosothiols) or an amino group (nitrosamine) [9].) RBCs have been shown to transport NO metabolites and NO bound to hemoglobin as nitrosylhemoglobin and s-nitrosohemoglobin. RBCs also produce NO under hypoxic conditions and release "NO bioactivity", i.e., they are able to induce vasodilatation in ex vivo bioassays. In addition, RBCs express an endothelial nitric oxide synthase (eNOS) [10]. Therefore, RBCs play a central role in the systemic regulation of NO [6].

Additionally, RBCs participate in sulfide metabolism. RBCs were shown to scavenge sulfide, transport RSS, and express a 3-mercapto sulfotransferase (3-MST) and thus potentially contribute to the endogenous enzymatic production of sulfide and its metabolites as well [11]. The potential chemical, biochemical, and pharmacological interactions of sulfide with NO in RBCs (or "cross-talk", as defined in the literature) and their reactions with hemoglobin have also been proposed [5,11–15].

Erythroid cells and reticulocytes (and therefore probably also RBCs) contain high levels of heme oxygenase 1, which catalyzes the degradation of oxidized hemoglobin and thereby also produces carbon monoxide (CO) [16]. The interaction of CO with other reactive species in RBCs (or in other compartments) has not yet been investigated in detail. In general, the role of the *reactive species interactome* in the regulation of RBC physiology and pathophysiology remains unclear. This review summarizes recent evidence on the *reactive species interactome* in RBCs and how it may affect the cardiovascular system. Specifically, we will introduce the concept of the *reactive species interactome* as it applies to RBCs, how oxidants are produced in RBCs and how they are detoxified, the role of RBCs in systemic NO and sulfide metabolism, and their cross-talk.

2. Role of RBCs in Systemic Redox Regulation—Oxidant Generation and Antioxidant Systems

RBCs contain complex redox systems that are indispensable for the preservation of cellular integrity, the control of cellular metabolism, and the modulation of cellular shape and flexibility [6]. Predominantly, the generation of ROS in RBCs arises from the autoxidation of oxyhemoglobin. This process transitions the iron from its typical ferrous state (Fe^{2+}) to a ferric state (Fe^{3+}), resulting in the formation of methemoglobin (metHb) and superoxide anion radical ($O_2^{\bullet-}$). This shift greatly diminishes the oxygen affinity of the prosthetic group of hemoglobin and is followed by protein degradation. Given the substantial concentration of hemoglobin within RBCs (32 to 36 g/dL), this reaction significantly contributes to ROS formation. However, Hb-Fe^{3+} can be reverted back to Hb-Fe^{2+} via cytochrome b5 reductase, using NADH as an electron donor [6]. Iron can also be released from metHb during its degradation, and—if not scavenged by ferritin [17]—it is a potent generator of ROS, mainly by reactions involving $O_2^{\bullet-}$ radicals or H_2O_2, culminating in the production of highly reactive hydroxyl radicals and hydroxyl anions. Interestingly, both Hb-Fe^{2+} (oxy/deoxyHb) and Hb-Fe^{3+} can react with hydrogen peroxide (H_2O_2). This reaction forms ferryl hemoglobin (Hb-Fe^{4+}=O), which is a highly oxidizing species that generates secondary radicals and ultimately liberates *free* iron. For a detailed discussion of these reactions, please refer to older but excellent reviews [18,19]. RBCs are also recognized for their ability to produce NO under both normoxic and hypoxic conditions [20]. NO may also react with $O_2^{\bullet-}$ to produce peroxynitrite, but its formation in RBCs has not been studied.

Hence, it is essential for RBCs to possess robust antioxidant systems, both enzymatic and nonenzymatic, which can neutralize these reactive species and sustain their intracellular levels to a minimum. These systems can be divided into three categories. The first category consists of antioxidant molecules and redox pairs, including reduced/oxidized glutathione (GSH), ascorbate/dehydroascorbate, and α-tocopherol [6]. GSH, a linear tripeptide, can occur in the reduced form (GSH) or in the oxidized form (GSSG, a dimer of two GSH molecules). The ratio of GSH/GSSG in RBCs is utilized to estimate the redox state of an organism; typically, reduced GSH constitutes 90–95% of the total GSH [4,5,21,22]. Ascorbate, also referred to as vitamin C, serves as a crucial antioxidant in RBCs. The redox pair ascorbate/dehydroascorbate plays a vital role in sustaining redox homeostasis within RBCs by reducing metHb and oxidants that diffuse into the cell membrane [23]. Vitamin E, or α-tocopherol, is another significant antioxidant within RBCs. It is found within the membranes of RBCs due to its lipophilic properties [24]. The second category consists of redox equivalents, such as NADH and NADPH, which play a crucial role by providing reducing equivalents for enzymes catalyzing redox reactions. They are reduced during glycolysis and the pentose phosphate pathway. The deficiency of glucose or malfunction of pentose phosphate pathways can severely impact the membrane integrity and redox homeostasis of RBCs [25–28].

The third category involves enzymatic antioxidant systems that are crucial for the survival and proper functioning of RBCs [29]. A series of detoxifying enzymes is found in RBCs, including catalase, peroxiredoxin 2, glutathione peroxidase, and glutaredoxin. For instance, catalase and glutathione peroxidase catalyze the conversion of H_2O_2 into water [30]. Peroxiredoxin and thioredoxin (which is needed to recycle peroxiredoxin) detoxify mainly lipid peroxides in the membrane [31], and play a fundamental role in

RBC redox homeostasis in vivo [32]. Glutaredoxins are responsible for keeping thiols in a reduced state; they were isolated from RBCs almost 30 years ago, but their role is still elusive [33,34].

The key function of the enzymatic and nonenzymatic redox antioxidant systems found in RBCs is to keep hemoglobin in a reduced form, thereby preserving its ability to bind oxygen. By limiting the generation of metHb, these systems reduce ROS generation and protect the cellular membrane lipids, proteins, channels, and metabolic enzymes from oxidative stress.

Furthermore, an additional fourth category of multifunctional or "moonlighting" enzymes participate in the overall redox homeostasis by coordinating and fine-tuning antioxidant response, iron homeostasis, and energy metabolism. In RBCs, these include the glyceraldehyde 3-phosphate dehydrogenase (GAPDH), which forms a membrane "metabolome" complex at the N-terminus of Band3/anion exchange 1 (AE-1) together with glycolytic enzymes and cytoskeletal proteins, and can migrate into the cytoplasmic compartment in dependency of the pO_2 [35,36]. Under oxidative stress conditions and during RBC storage (for example, in transfusion units), the oxidation of Cys152 and His179 in the catalytic pocket of GAPDH alters its metabolic function and leads to a metabolic switching from glycolysis towards the pentose phosphate pathway [37].

Deficiencies in these antioxidant systems can lead to cellular damage and dysfunction derived from the oxidation of redox switches found in cytoskeletal proteins (like spectrin, ankyrin, protein 4.2, and actin), leading to a loss of membrane integrity, altered RBC deformability, and hemolysis [38]. Genetic mutations of these proteins are linked with severe conditions like hemolytic anemia [6]. Moreover, these modifications also occur during RBC storage and are defined as a "storage lesion" [26]. Very elegant proteomics and metabolomics studies carried out in recent years have revealed how pO_2, protein–protein interactions, redox state, and metabolic control are intimately intertwined and modulate the redox physiology of RBC [37,39]. In addition, these studies may also provide new ways to prevent the "storage lesion" and prolong the therapeutic applicability of transfusion units, which is of fundamental importance in the therapy of different forms of severe anemia and blood loss in the clinic.

3. Role of RBCs in Systemic NO Metabolism

RBCs play a pivotal role in regulating the systemic availability and bioactivity of NO by scavenging, binding, and metabolizing NO and its metabolites [20]. In this way, RBCs are an important contributor to the concentrations of other NO metabolites in plasma, including nitrate, nitrite, nitrosothiols (RSNO), and nitrosamines (RNNO). The NO metabolites also show bioactivity as they can release NO (via enzymatic and nonenzymatic reactions) and cause vasodilation, and thereby can affect the cardiovascular system [40–44]. There is also evidence that nitrite may have signaling effects on its own by modulating the activity of downstream targets, including protein kinase A [45,46].

RBCs may regulate the pool of circulating NO metabolites via various mechanisms, mainly involving reactions with hemoglobin or eNOS-derived NO formation [20,47]. Oxyhemoglobin (oxyHb) captures eNOS-derived NO from the vascular endothelium under normoxic conditions in a rapid reaction that leads to the formation of nitrate, thus limiting and fine-tuning the bioactivity of endothelial NO. Under hypoxic conditions, deoxyhemoglobin can also react with NO, forming nitrosyl hemoglobin (HbNO), which is more stable under these conditions. HbNO has been proposed as an indicator of NO bioavailability in RBCs [48]. HbNO was also indicated as being an intermediate for the formation of S-nitroso hemoglobin, which, in turn, initiates a cascade of transnitrosation reactions transferring the nitroso group from one cysteine to the next and mediates hypoxic vasodilation [49–51]. In ex vivo experiments, the nitrosation of the membrane protein spectrin aids in preserving RBC deformability under oxidative stress [52]. Deoxyhemoglobin reduces nitrite to NO under hypoxic conditions [53–55]. This nitrite reductase activity of deoxyhemoglobin was shown to induce NO-dependent vasodilation under hypoxic conditions, thus offering more evidence that RBCs indeed partake in the vasodilation of vessels and do not merely serve as NO sinks.

RBCs also express an active eNOS, which is, therefore, another source of NO production and is active under normoxic conditions [10]. There is compelling in vivo evidence that endogenous NO production by eNOS in RBCs affects both circulating NO metabolites and blood pressure [56,57]. Chimera mice obtained from the transplantation of bone marrow from eNOS KO into irradiated WT mice showed decreased circulating NO metabolites and elevated systolic blood pressure and mean arterial pressure [56]. Recently, we generated a mouse model lacking eNOS in RBCs obtained by crossing eNOS$^{flox/flox}$ mice with mice expressing a Cre recombinase under the control of the hemoglobin beta chain promoter (HbbCre^{pos} mice) [57]. These mice showed hypertension and increased systemic vascular resistance, accompanied by decreased HbNO levels in RBCs, decreased nitrite/nitrate, and hypertension.

We also generated mice carrying eNOS in RBCs only and lacking eNOS in all other tissues (RBC eNOS KI mice), which we obtained by crossing mice carrying a duplicated and inverted exon 2 (conditional eNOS KO mice) and two pairs of loxP sequences with the HbbCre mice; in the presence of the Cre recombinase, the exon 2 is "flipped", and eNOS expression is restored. The reactivation of eNOS expression in RBCs rescued the hypertension phenotype and the levels of HbNO in RBCs. These data demonstrate that RBCs play a fundamental role in blood pressure regulation and NO metabolism.

4. Role of RBCs in Systemic Sulfide and Persulfide Metabolism

The role of sulfide metabolism in the canonical and noncanonical functions of RBC and/or their dysfunction has never been investigated specifically. However, independent studies have shown that RBCs can scavenge, transport, metabolize, and release sulfide and its metabolites (including thiosulfate, persulfates, and polysulfides) [11]. Therefore, RBCs are likely to play a central role in overall sulfide physiology and pharmacology, similar to their role in NO metabolism.

RBCs rapidly uptake and scavenge high concentrations of sulfide both ex vivo and in vivo [11]. It is very likely that RBCs may contribute in this way to prevent its toxic accumulation in the bloodstream, as proposed already at the beginning of the last century [58–61].

At physiological pH, sulfide primarily exists as an anion HS^-, and to a lesser extent, as dissolved H_2S. In RBCs, sulfide can permeate cell membranes, entering RBCs via the anion exchange protein Band3/AE1, which catalyzes a net acid flux exchanging HCO_3^- [59]. Interestingly, HCO_3^- has a lower affinity for Band3/AE-1 as compared to HS^-. This explains why, in buffered suspensions, RBCs rapidly take up H_2S/HS^- [59,62]. As a consequence, the uptake of sulfide by RBCs may modulate the pH of the cells and their supernatants. If these effects are also present in vivo, sulfide intake in RBCs may potentially modulate the overall homeostasis of pH in the body.

Under physiological conditions, oxyhemoglobin does not undergo a reaction with sulfide. At very high concentrations, millimolar amounts of sulfide react with oxyhemoglobin to form a stable green compound sulfhemoglobin [63–67]; the reaction requires the presence of oxidative agents and is slower. Intriguingly, sulfhemoglobin is not formed under physiologically relevant conditions, and its production is solely witnessed in RBCs in vivo subsequent to the administration of oxidizing pharmaceuticals (like phenacetin) together with sulfur-containing compounds, like hydroxylamine sulfate, sulfur dioxide, and others [11].

Notably, methemoglobin forms a reversible metHb-SH$^-$ complex with sulfide at more physiologically relevant concentrations, a finding first documented by Kellin in 1933 [68] and later reproduced by others [69,70]. The metHb-SH$^-$ adduct was shown to slowly decompose to yield inorganic polysulfides, $HS_2O_3^-$, and does not react further in the presence of millimolar concentrations of low-molecular-weight thiols, like Cys and GSH [12,69,71].

Recent investigations carried out in intact RBCs have shown that sulfide reacts with metHb to form a metHb-SH⁻ intermediate and produces polysulfide and thiosulfate [12]. Interestingly, the sulfide reactivity with metHb varies in intact cells compared to cell-free solutions. In cell-free hemoglobin solutions, the metHb-SH⁻ complex is fairly stable. Instead, in intact cells, the rapid decomposition of the metHb-SH⁻ complex leads to the formation of deoxyhemoglobin and, in the presence of oxygen, oxyhemoglobin (deoxy/oxyHb). Thus, according to these experiments, treating RBCs with sulfide leads to the reduction of methemoglobin to deoxy/oxyHb. Clearly, there must be cellular mechanisms within RBCs that facilitate metHb-SH⁻ reduction since this occurs in intact cells only and not in hemoglobin solutions.

In vivo, metHb is ubiquitously present in high concentrations within healthy RBC (ranging from 100 to 300 μM), comprising 1–3% of the total hemoglobin concentration. Therefore, metHb is a highly efficacious sulfide scavenger in vivo. As mentioned in the second chapter of this review, the conversion of metHb (which has a low affinity for oxygen) into deoxy/oxyHb (which is the oxygen-binding form) is carried out by a cytochrome C reductase, and it is key for the physiological function of RBCs. The data discussed here show that the same reaction occurs when RBCs are treated with sulfide. Accordingly, sulfide has been shown to reduce heme-containing proteins of mammalian and invertebrate origin [72]. Thus, it is tempting to speculate that in this way, endogenous sulfide may help maintain hemoglobin in an oxygen-binding state. This hypothesis needs to be verified experimentally.

Interestingly, RBCs also express 3-mercaptopyruvate sulfotransferase (3-MST, EC 2.8.1.2) [73], which may catalyze the formation of sulfur species and sulfide inside the cells [69,74–79]. 3-MST metabolizes molecules containing sulfane sulfur, i.e., a sulfur atom bound to another sulfur atom (RS-$(S)_n$-R'). High 3-MST activity has been measured in RBCs, the liver, kidneys, and adrenal cortex [75–77]. Its endogenous substrate is 3-mercaptopyruvate (3-MP), which is generated from l-cysteine and α-ketoglutarate by a cysteine aminotransferase. The main function of 3-MST is to transfer the sulfur atom of 3-MP to acceptors like cyanide, sulfite, and sulfinate, producing soluble compounds for detoxification. This process involves two steps: the formation of MST-bound persulfide and H_2S. 3-MST also uses $HS_2O_3^-$ as a substrate to produce sulfite and enzyme-bound sulfane sulfur. Patients with 3-mercapto lactate-cysteine disulfiduria and iron deficiency anemia show higher activity as compared to other patient cohorts and healthy individuals [75,76]. However, the role of 3-MST in erythropoiesis, RBCs physiology, and pathophysiology is unknown.

Besides 3-MST, RBCs contain high concentrations of several other enzymatic systems, like the glutathione system and antioxidant enzymes, which are potentially involved in sulfide/polysulfide metabolism [80–82].

There is evidence that RBCs might also participate in the biochemical and biological interaction and "cross-talk" between NO and sulfide [11]. We have shown that NO-induced methemoglobin (metHb) formation can be reversed by sulfide, which reconverts metHb back to deoxy/oxyhemoglobin, effectively restoring the oxygen-carrying capacity [12]. Moreover, we found that sulfide treatment via continuous Na_2S infusion increased nitrosyl-Hb levels in RBCs in rats, indicating that sulfide boosts the formation of nitrosyl-Hb (considered by some as a vasodilator) [14]. These findings point to an in vivo cross-talk between NO and H_2S in RBCs, which may occur via the formation of hybrid S/N molecules. The role and effects of this NO/H_2S cross-talk and its interaction with hemoglobin and antioxidant enzymes on RBC physiology and function remain unknown and warrant further investigation.

5. Summary and Perspective

This article discusses how the concept of the *reactive species interactome* pertains to the complex redox biology and physiology of RBCs. At the center of the reactive species interactome in RBC is hemoglobin and its different redox forms, i.e., the reduced form (oxy/deoxyHb) and the oxidized form (metHb). The degradation of metHb (which constitutes 1–3% of all forms) is the main source of the production of superoxide and other oxidants. This is efficiently and potently neutralized by a battery of antioxidant systems. Moreover, oxy/deoxyHb are also involved in NO metabolism, as oxyHb scavenges NO, and deoxyHb reacts with NO (forming HbNO) and produces NO from nitrite. An intracellular source of NO in RBCs is eNOS, which may participate in the formation of NO adducts of hemoglobin, like HbNO. RBCs, therefore, strongly contribute to the systemic regulation of NO metabolism and bioactivity. In addition, metHb is involved in sulfide scavenging and metabolism. Sulfide forms a stable adduct with metHb, which is then reduced—in intact cells only—into deoxy/oxyHb. 3-MST is also a potential source of sulfide/persulfide in RBCs, but its role is still elusive. The exact role that the reactive species interactome plays in the regulation of RBC physiology and pathophysiology remains an open question that needs further investigation.

Funding: This research was funded by the German Research Council (DFG) grant numbers 263779315, 220652768, 521638178, and 386517575.

Institutional Review Board Statement: Not applicable.

Informed Consent Statement: Not applicable.

Data Availability Statement: No new data were created or analyzed in this study. Data sharing is not applicable to this article.

Conflicts of Interest: The author declares no conflict of interest.

References

1. Sies, H. Oxidative stress: Introductory remarks Oxidative Stress. *N. Y. Acad. J.* **1985**, *5*, 1–8.
2. Sies, H. Oxidative stress: A concept in redox biology and medicine. *Redox Biol.* **2015**, *4*, 180–183. [CrossRef] [PubMed]
3. Sies, H.; Jones, D. Oxidative Stress. In *Encyclopedia of Stress*, 2nd ed.; Fink, G., Ed.; Academic Press: New York, NY, USA, 2007; pp. 45–48.
4. Sies, H.; Wendel, A. *Functions of Glutathione in Liver and Kidney*; Springer Science & Business Media: Berlin/Heidelberg, Germany, 2012.
5. Cortese-Krott, M.M.; Koning, A.; Kuhnle, G.G.C.; Nagy, P.; Bianco, C.L.; Pasch, A.; Wink, D.A.; Fukuto, J.M.; Jackson, A.A.; van Goor, H.; et al. The Reactive Species Interactome: Evolutionary Emergence, Biological Significance, and Opportunities for Redox Metabolomics and Personalized Medicine. *Antioxid. Redox Signal.* **2017**, *27*, 684–712. [CrossRef] [PubMed]
6. Kuhn, V.; Diederich, L.; Keller, T.C.S.t.; Kramer, C.M.; Luckstadt, W.; Panknin, C.; Suvorava, T.; Isakson, B.E.; Kelm, M.; Cortese-Krott, M.M. Red Blood Cell Function and Dysfunction: Redox Regulation, Nitric Oxide Metabolism, Anemia. *Antioxid. Redox Signal.* **2017**, *26*, 718–742. [CrossRef]
7. Van't Erve, T.J.; Wagner, B.A.; Ryckman, K.K.; Raife, T.J.; Buettner, G.R. The concentration of glutathione in human erythrocytes is a heritable trait. *Free Radic. Biol. Med.* **2013**, *65*, 742–749. [CrossRef] [PubMed]
8. Ida, T.; Sawa, T.; Ihara, H.; Tsuchiya, Y.; Watanabe, Y.; Kumagai, Y.; Suematsu, M.; Motohashi, H.; Fujii, S.; Matsunaga, T.; et al. Reactive cysteine persulfides and S-polythiolation regulate oxidative stress and redox signaling. *Proc. Natl. Acad. Sci. USA* **2014**, *111*, 7606–7611. [CrossRef] [PubMed]
9. Bryan, N.S.; Rassaf, T.; Maloney, R.E.; Rodriguez, C.M.; Saijo, F.; Rodriguez, J.R.; Feelisch, M. Cellular targets and mechanisms of nitros(yl)ation: An insight into their nature and kinetics in vivo. *Proc. Natl. Acad. Sci. USA* **2004**, *101*, 4308–4313. [CrossRef]
10. Cortese-Krott, M.M.; Rodriguez-Mateos, A.; Sansone, R.; Kuhnle, G.G.; Thasian-Sivarajah, S.; Krenz, T.; Horn, P.; Krisp, C.; Wolters, D.; Heiss, C.; et al. Human red blood cells at work: Identification and visualization of erythrocytic eNOS activity in health and disease. *Blood* **2012**, *120*, 4229–4237. [CrossRef]
11. Cortese-Krott, M.M. Red Blood Cells as a "Central Hub" for Sulfide Bioactivity: Scavenging, Metabolism, Transport, and Cross-Talk with Nitric Oxide. *Antioxid. Redox Signal.* **2020**, *33*, 1332–1349. [CrossRef] [PubMed]
12. Bianco, C.L.; Savitsky, A.; Feelisch, M.; Cortese-Krott, M.M. Investigations on the role of hemoglobin in sulfide metabolism by intact human red blood cells. *Biochem. Pharmacol.* **2018**, *149*, 163–173. [CrossRef]
13. Marcolongo, J.P.; Morzan, U.N.; Zeida, A.; Scherlis, D.A.; Olabe, J.A. Nitrosodisulfide [S_2NO]− (perthionitrite) is a true intermediate during the "cross-talk" of nitrosyl and sulfide. *Phys. Chem. Chem. Phys.* **2016**, *18*, 30047–30052. [CrossRef]
14. Cortese-Krott, M.M.; Kuhnle, G.G.; Dyson, A.; Fernandez, B.O.; Grman, M.; DuMond, J.F.; Barrow, M.P.; McLeod, G.; Nakagawa, H.; Ondrias, K.; et al. Key bioactive reaction products of the NO/H_2S interaction are S/N-hybrid species, polysulfides, and nitroxyl. *Proc. Natl. Acad. Sci. USA* **2015**, *112*, E4651–E4660. [CrossRef]
15. Fukuto, J.M.; Ignarro, L.J.; Nagy, P.; Wink, D.A.; Kevil, C.G.; Feelisch, M.; Cortese-Krott, M.M.; Bianco, C.L.; Kumagai, Y.; Hobbs, A.J.; et al. Biological hydropersulfides and related polysulfides—A new concept and perspective in redox biology. *FEBS Lett.* **2018**, *592*, 2140–2152. [CrossRef]

16. Garcia-Santos, D.; Schranzhofer, M.; Horvathova, M.; Jaberi, M.M.; Bogo Chies, J.A.; Sheftel, A.D.; Ponka, P. Heme oxygenase 1 is expressed in murine erythroid cells where it controls the level of regulatory heme. *Blood* **2014**, *123*, 2269–2277. [CrossRef]
17. Cazzola, M.; Dezza, L.; Bergamaschi, G.; Barosi, G.; Bellotti, V.; Caldera, D.; Ciriello, M.M.; Quaglini, S.; Arosio, P.; Ascari, E. Biologic and Clinical Significance of Red Cell Ferritin. *Blood* **1983**, *62*, 1078–1087. [CrossRef]
18. Reeder, B.J. The redox activity of hemoglobins: From physiologic functions to pathologic mechanisms. *Antioxid. Redox Signal.* **2010**, *13*, 1087–1123. [CrossRef] [PubMed]
19. Alayash, A.I.; Patel, R.P.; Cashon, R.E. Redox reactions of hemoglobin and myoglobin: Biological and toxicological implications. *Antioxid. Redox Signal.* **2001**, *3*, 313–327. [CrossRef]
20. Cortese-Krott, M.M.; Kramer, C.M.; Kelm, M. Chapter 14—NOS, NO, and the Red Cell A2—Ignarro, Louis, J. In *Nitric Oxide*, 3rd ed.; Freeman, B.A., Ed.; Academic Press: Cambridge, MA, USA, 2017; pp. 185–194.
21. Forman, H.J.; Zhang, H.; Rinna, A. Glutathione: Overview of its protective roles, measurement, and biosynthesis. *Mol. Asp. Med.* **2009**, *30*, 1–12. [CrossRef]
22. Flohé, L. The fairytale of the GSSG/GSH redox potential. *Biochim. Biophys. Acta (BBA)-Gen. Subj.* **2013**, *1830*, 3139–3142. [CrossRef] [PubMed]
23. Einsele, H.; Clemens, M.R.; Remmer, H. Effect of ascorbate on red blood cell lipid peroxidation. *Free Radic. Res. Commun.* **1985**, *1*, 63–67. [CrossRef] [PubMed]
24. May, J.M.; Qu, Z.C.; Mendiratta, S. Protection and recycling of alpha-tocopherol in human erythrocytes by intracellular ascorbic acid. *Arch. Biochem. Biophys.* **1998**, *349*, 281–289. [CrossRef] [PubMed]
25. Möller, M.N.; Orrico, F.; Villar, S.F.; López, A.C.; Silva, N.; Donzé, M.; Thomson, L.; Denicola, A. Oxidants and antioxidants in the redox biochemistry of human red blood cells. *ACS Omega* **2022**, *8*, 147–168. [CrossRef] [PubMed]
26. D'Alessandro, A.; Reisz, J.A.; Zhang, Y.; Gehrke, S.; Alexander, K.; Kanias, T.; Triulzi, D.J.; Donadee, C.; Barge, S.; Badlam, J.; et al. Effects of aged stored autologous red blood cells on human plasma metabolome. *Blood Adv.* **2019**, *3*, 884–896. [CrossRef] [PubMed]
27. Frewin, R. CHAPTER 27—Biochemical aspects of anaemia. In *Clinical Biochemistry: Metabolic and Clinical Aspects*, 3rd ed.; Marshall, W.J., Lapsley, M., Day, A.P., Ayling, R.M., Eds.; Churchill Livingstone: London, UK, 2014; pp. 515–532.
28. Sae-Lee, W.; McCafferty, C.L.; Verbeke, E.J.; Havugimana, P.C.; Papoulas, O.; McWhite, C.D.; Houser, J.R.; Vanuytsel, K.; Murphy, G.J.; Drew, K.; et al. The protein organization of a red blood cell. *Cell Rep.* **2022**, *40*, 111103. [CrossRef] [PubMed]
29. Mohanty, J.G.; Nagababu, E.; Rifkind, J.M. Red blood cell oxidative stress impairs oxygen delivery and induces red blood cell aging. *Front. Physiol.* **2014**, *5*, 84. [CrossRef]
30. Johnson, R.M.; Goyette, G., Jr.; Ravindranath, Y.; Ho, Y.S. Hemoglobin autoxidation and regulation of endogenous H_2O_2 levels in erythrocytes. *Free Radic. Biol. Med.* **2005**, *39*, 1407–1417. [CrossRef]
31. Matte, A.; Bertoldi, M.; Mohandas, N.; An, X.; Bugatti, A.; Brunati, A.M.; Rusnati, M.; Tibaldi, E.; Siciliano, A.; Turrini, F.; et al. Membrane association of peroxiredoxin-2 in red cells is mediated by the N-terminal cytoplasmic domain of band 3. *Free Radic. Biol. Med.* **2013**, *55*, 27–35. [CrossRef]
32. Lee, T.H.; Kim, S.U.; Yu, S.L.; Kim, S.H.; Park, D.S.; Moon, H.B.; Dho, S.H.; Kwon, K.S.; Kwon, H.J.; Han, Y.H.; et al. Peroxiredoxin II is essential for sustaining life span of erythrocytes in mice. *Blood* **2003**, *101*, 5033–5038. [CrossRef]
33. Papov, V.V.; Gravina, S.A.; Mieyal, J.J.; Biemann, K. The primary structure and properties of thioltransferase (glutaredoxin) from human red blood cells. *Protein Sci. A Publ. Protein Soc.* **1994**, *3*, 428–434. [CrossRef] [PubMed]
34. Matsui, R.; Ferran, B.; Oh, A.; Croteau, D.; Shao, D.; Han, J.; Pimentel, D.R.; Bachschmid, M.M. Redox Regulation via Glutaredoxin-1 and Protein S-Glutathionylation. *Antioxid. Redox Signal.* **2020**, *32*, 677–700. [CrossRef]
35. Puchulu-Campanella, E.; Chu, H.; Anstee, D.J.; Galan, J.A.; Tao, W.A.; Low, P.S. Identification of the components of a glycolytic enzyme metabolon on the human red blood cell membrane. *J. Biol. Chem.* **2013**, *288*, 848–858. [CrossRef] [PubMed]
36. Campanella, M.E.; Chu, H.; Low, P.S. Assembly and regulation of a glycolytic enzyme complex on the human erythrocyte membrane. *Proc. Natl. Acad. Sci. USA* **2005**, *102*, 2402–2407. [CrossRef] [PubMed]
37. Reisz, J.A.; Wither, M.J.; Dzieciatkowska, M.; Nemkov, T.; Issaian, A.; Yoshida, T.; Dunham, A.J.; Hill, R.C.; Hansen, K.C.; D'Alessandro, A. Oxidative modifications of glyceraldehyde 3-phosphate dehydrogenase regulate metabolic reprogramming of stored red blood cells. *Blood* **2016**, *128*, e32–e42. [CrossRef]
38. Barbarino, F.; Wäschenbach, L.; Cavalho-Lemos, V.; Dillenberger, M.; Becker, K.; Gohlke, H.; Cortese-Krott, M.M. Targeting spectrin redox switches to regulate the mechanoproperties of red blood cells. *Biol. Chem.* **2021**, *402*, 317–331. [CrossRef]
39. Reisz, J.A.; Tzounakas, V.L.; Nemkov, T.; Voulgaridou, A.I.; Papassideri, I.S.; Kriebardis, A.G.; D'Alessandro, A.; Antonelou, M.H. Metabolic Linkage and Correlations to Storage Capacity in Erythrocytes from Glucose 6-Phosphate Dehydrogenase-Deficient Donors. *Front. Med.* **2017**, *4*, 248. [CrossRef] [PubMed]
40. Lundberg, J.O.; Gladwin, M.T.; Ahluwalia, A.; Benjamin, N.; Bryan, N.S.; Butler, A.; Cabrales, P.; Fago, A.; Feelisch, M.; Ford, P.C.; et al. Nitrate and nitrite in biology, nutrition and therapeutics. *Nat. Chem. Biol.* **2009**, *5*, 865–869. [CrossRef]
41. Lundberg, J.O.; Weitzberg, E. Nitric oxide signaling in health and disease. *Cell* **2022**, *185*, 2853–2878. [CrossRef]
42. DeMartino, A.W.; Kim-Shapiro, D.B.; Patel, R.P.; Gladwin, M.T. Nitrite and nitrate chemical biology and signalling. *Br. J. Pharm.* **2019**, *176*, 228–245. [CrossRef] [PubMed]
43. Kapil, V.; Khambata, R.S.; Jones, D.A.; Rathod, K.; Primus, C.; Massimo, G.; Fukuto, J.M.; Ahluwalia, A. The Noncanonical Pathway for In Vivo Nitric Oxide Generation: The Nitrate-Nitrite-Nitric Oxide Pathway. *Pharm. Rev.* **2020**, *72*, 692–766. [CrossRef] [PubMed]

44. Premont, R.T.; Reynolds, J.D.; Zhang, R.; Stamler, J.S. Role of Nitric Oxide Carried by Hemoglobin in Cardiovascular Physiology: Developments on a Three-Gas Respiratory Cycle. *Circ. Res.* **2020**, *126*, 129–158. [CrossRef] [PubMed]
45. Bryan, N.S.; Fernandez, B.O.; Bauer, S.M.; Garcia-Saura, M.F.; Milsom, A.B.; Rassaf, T.; Maloney, R.E.; Bharti, A.; Rodriguez, J.; Feelisch, M. Nitrite is a signaling molecule and regulator of gene expression in mammalian tissues. *Nat. Chem. Biol.* **2005**, *1*, 290–297. [CrossRef]
46. Kamga Pride, C.; Mo, L.; Quesnelle, K.; Dagda, R.K.; Murillo, D.; Geary, L.; Corey, C.; Portella, R.; Zharikov, S.; St Croix, C.; et al. Nitrite activates protein kinase A in normoxia to mediate mitochondrial fusion and tolerance to ischaemia/reperfusion. *Cardiovasc. Res.* **2014**, *101*, 57–68. [CrossRef] [PubMed]
47. Keller, T.C.S.t.; Lechauve, C.; Keller, A.S.; Brooks, S.; Weiss, M.J.; Columbus, L.; Ackerman, H.; Cortese-Krott, M.M.; Isakson, B.E. The role of globins in cardiovascular physiology. *Physiol. Rev.* **2022**, *102*, 859–892. [CrossRef]
48. Lobysheva, I.I.; Biller, P.; Gallez, B.; Beauloye, C.; Balligand, J.-L. Nitrosylated Hemoglobin Levels in Human Venous Erythrocytes Correlate with Vascular Endothelial Function Measured by Digital Reactive Hyperemia. *PLoS ONE* **2013**, *8*, e76457. [CrossRef]
49. Pawloski, J.R.; Hess, D.T.; Stamler, J.S. Export by red blood cells of nitric oxide bioactivity. *Nature* **2001**, *409*, 622–626. [CrossRef] [PubMed]
50. Jia, L.; Bonaventura, C.; Bonaventura, J.; Stamler, J.S. S-nitrosohaemoglobin: A dynamic activity of blood involved in vascular control. *Nature* **1996**, *380*, 221–226. [CrossRef] [PubMed]
51. Scharfstein, J.S.; Keaney, J.F., Jr.; Slivka, A.; Welch, G.N.; Vita, J.A.; Stamler, J.S.; Loscalzo, J. In vivo transfer of nitric oxide between a plasma protein-bound reservoir and low molecular weight thiols. *J. Clin. Investig.* **1994**, *94*, 1432–1439. [CrossRef] [PubMed]
52. Diederich, L.; Suvorava, T.; Sansone, R.; Keller, T.C.S.; Barbarino, F.; Sutton, T.R.; Kramer, C.M.; Lückstädt, W.; Isakson, B.E.; Gohlke, H.; et al. On the Effects of Reactive Oxygen Species and Nitric Oxide on Red Blood Cell Deformability. *Front. Physiol.* **2018**, *9*, 332. [CrossRef]
53. Kim-Shapiro, D.B.; Gladwin, M.T. Chapter 6—Heme Protein Metabolism of NO and Nitrite A2—Ignarro, Louis, J. In *Nitric Oxide*, 3rd ed.; Freeman, B.A., Ed.; Academic Press: Cambridge, MA, USA, 2017; pp. 85–96.
54. Cosby, K.; Partovi, K.S.; Crawford, J.H.; Patel, R.P.; Reiter, C.D.; Martyr, S.; Yang, B.K.; Waclawiw, M.A.; Zalos, G.; Xu, X.; et al. Nitrite reduction to nitric oxide by deoxyhemoglobin vasodilates the human circulation. *Nat. Med.* **2003**, *9*, 1498–1505. [CrossRef]
55. Gladwin, M.T.; Shelhamer, J.H.; Schechter, A.N.; Pease-Fye, M.E.; Waclawiw, M.A.; Panza, J.A.; Ognibene, F.P.; Cannon, R.O. Role of circulating nitrite and S-nitrosohemoglobin in the regulation of regional blood flow in humans. *Proc. Natl. Acad. Sci. USA* **2000**, *97*, 11482–11487. [CrossRef]
56. Wood, K.C.; Cortese-Krott, M.M.; Kovacic, J.C.; Noguchi, A.; Liu, V.B.; Wang, X.; Raghavachari, N.; Boehm, M.; Kato, G.J.; Kelm, M.; et al. Circulating blood endothelial nitric oxide synthase contributes to the regulation of systemic blood pressure and nitrite homeostasis. *Arter. Thromb. Vasc. Biol.* **2013**, *33*, 1861–1871. [CrossRef] [PubMed]
57. Leo, F.; Suvorava, T.; Heuser, S.K.; Li, J.; LoBue, A.; Barbarino, F.; Piragine, E.; Schneckmann, R.; Hutzler, B.; Good, M.E.; et al. Red Blood Cell and Endothelial eNOS Independently Regulate Circulating Nitric Oxide Metabolites and Blood Pressure. *Circulation* **2021**, *144*, 870–889. [CrossRef] [PubMed]
58. Cronican, A.A.; Frawley, K.L.; Ahmed, H.; Pearce, L.L.; Peterson, J. Antagonism of Acute Sulfide Poisoning in Mice by Nitrite Anion without Methemoglobinemia. *Chem. Res. Toxicol.* **2015**, *28*, 1398–1408. [CrossRef] [PubMed]
59. Jennings, M.L. Transport of H_2S and HS^- across the human red blood cell membrane: Rapid H_2S diffusion and AE1-mediated Cl^-/HS^- exchange. *Am. J. Physiol.-Cell Physiol.* **2013**, *305*, C941–C950. [CrossRef] [PubMed]
60. Haouzi, P.; Sonobe, T.; Torsell-Tubbs, N.; Prokopczyk, B.; Chenuel, B.; Klingerman, C.M. In vivo interactions between cobalt or ferric compounds and the pools of sulphide in the blood during and after H_2S poisoning. *Toxicol. Sci.* **2014**, *141*, 493–504. [CrossRef]
61. Haggard, H.W. The fate of sulfides in the blood. *J. Biol. Chem.* **1921**, *49*, 519–529. [CrossRef]
62. Jacobs, M.H.; Stewart, D.R. The role of carbonic anydrase in certain ionic exchanges involving the erythrocyte. *J. Gen. Physiol.* **1942**, *25*, 539–552. [CrossRef]
63. Hoppe-Seyler, F. Einwirkung des Schwefelwasserstoffgases auf das Blut. *Zbl. Med. Wiss* **1863**, *1*, 433.
64. Jung, F. Über das sogenannte Sulfhämoglobin. *Naunyn-Schmiedebergs Arch. Exp. Pathol. Pharmakol.* **1939**, *194*, 16–30. [CrossRef]
65. Beauchamp, R.O.; Bus, J.S.; Popp, J.A.; Boreiko, C.J.; Andjelkovich, D.A.; Leber, P. A Critical Review of the Literature on Hydrogen Sulfide Toxicity. *CRC Crit. Rev. Toxicol.* **1984**, *13*, 25–97. [CrossRef]
66. Haouzi, P.; Sonobe, T.; Judenherc-Haouzi, A. Hydrogen sulfide intoxication induced brain injury and methylene blue. *Neurobiol. Dis.* **2020**, *133*, 104474. [CrossRef]
67. Ng, P.C.; Hendry-Hofer, T.B.; Witeof, A.E.; Brenner, M.; Mahon, S.B.; Boss, G.R.; Haouzi, P.; Bebarta, V.S. Hydrogen Sulfide Toxicity: Mechanism of Action, Clinical Presentation, and Countermeasure Development. *J. Med. Toxicol.* **2019**, *15*, 287–294. [CrossRef]
68. Keilin, D. On the combination of methaemoglobin with H_2S. *Proc. R. Soc. Lond. Ser. B Contain. Pap. A Biol. Character* **1933**, *113*, 393–404.
69. Vitvitsky, V.; Yadav, P.K.; Kurthen, A.; Banerjee, R. Sulfide oxidation by a noncanonical pathway in red blood cells generates thiosulfate and polysulfides. *J. Biol. Chem.* **2015**, *290*, 8310–8320. [CrossRef] [PubMed]

70. Bianco, C.L.; Chavez, T.A.; Sosa, V.; Saund, S.S.; Nguyen, Q.N.N.; Tantillo, D.J.; Ichimura, A.S.; Toscano, J.P.; Fukuto, J.M. The chemical biology of the persulfide (RSSH)/perthiyl (RSS.) redox couple and possible role in biological redox signaling. *Free Radic. Biol. Med.* **2016**, *101*, 20–31. [CrossRef]
71. Jensen, B.; Fago, A. Reactions of ferric hemoglobin and myoglobin with hydrogen sulfide under physiological conditions. *J. Inorg. Biochem.* **2018**, *182*, 133–140. [CrossRef] [PubMed]
72. Pietri, R.; Lewis, A.; León, R.G.; Casabona, G.; Kiger, L.; Yeh, S.-R.; Fernandez-Alberti, S.; Marden, M.C.; Cadilla, C.L.; López-Garriga, J. Factors controlling the reactivity of hydrogen sulfide with hemoproteins. *Biochemistry* **2009**, *48*, 4881–4894. [CrossRef] [PubMed]
73. Van Den Hamer, C.J.A.; Morell, A.G.; Scheinberg, I.H. A Study of the Copper Content of β-Mercaptopyruvate Trans-sulfurase. *J. Biol. Chem.* **1967**, *242*, 2514–2516. [CrossRef]
74. Valentine, W.N.; Frankenfeld, J.K. 3-mercaptopyruvate sulfurtransferase (EC 2.8.1.2): A simple assay adapted to human blood cells. *Clin. Chim. Acta* **1974**, *51*, 205–210. [CrossRef]
75. Hannestad, U.; Mårtensson, J.; Sjödahl, R.; Sörbo, B. 3-Mercaptolactate cysteine disulfiduria: Biochemical studies on affected and unaffected members of a family. *Biochem. Med.* **1981**, *26*, 106–114. [CrossRef]
76. Mårtensson, J.; Sörbo, B. Human β-mercaptopyruvate sulfurtransferase: Distribution in cellular compartments of blood and activity in erythrocytes from patients with hematological disorders. *Clin. Chim. Acta* **1978**, *87*, 11–15. [CrossRef] [PubMed]
77. Sörbo, B. On the formation of thiosulfate from inorganic sulfide by liver tissue and heme compounds. *Biochim. Biophys. Acta* **1958**, *27*, 324–329. [CrossRef] [PubMed]
78. Valentine, W.N.; Toohey, J.I.; Paglia, D.E.; Nakatani, M.; Brockway, R.A. Modification of erythrocyte enzyme activities by persulfides and methanethiol: Possible regulatory role. *Proc. Natl. Acad. Sci. USA* **1987**, *84*, 1394–1398. [CrossRef] [PubMed]
79. Nawata, M.; Ogasawara, Y.; Kawanabe, K.; Tanabe, S. Enzymatic assay of 3-mercaptopyruvate sulfurtransferase activity in human red blood cells using pyruvate oxidase. *Anal. Biochem.* **1990**, *190*, 84–87. [CrossRef] [PubMed]
80. Olson, K.R.; Gao, Y.; Arif, F.; Arora, K.; Patel, S.; DeLeon, E.R.; Sutton, T.R.; Feelisch, M.; Cortese-Krott, M.M.; Straub, K.D. Metabolism of hydrogen sulfide (H_2S) and Production of Reactive Sulfur Species (RSS) by superoxide dismutase. *Redox Biol.* **2017**, *15*, 74–85. [CrossRef]
81. Olson, K.R.; Gao, Y. Effects of inhibiting antioxidant pathways on cellular hydrogen sulfide and polysulfide metabolism. *Free Radic. Biol. Med.* **2019**, *135*, 1–14. [CrossRef]
82. Dóka, É.; Pader, I.; Bíró, A.; Johansson, K.; Cheng, Q.; Ballagó, K.; Prigge, J.R.; Pastor-Flores, D.; Dick, T.P.; Schmidt, E.E.; et al. A novel persulfide detection method reveals protein persulfide- and polysulfide-reducing functions of thioredoxin and glutathione systems. *Sci. Adv.* **2016**, *2*, e1500968. [CrossRef]

Disclaimer/Publisher's Note: The statements, opinions and data contained in all publications are solely those of the individual author(s) and contributor(s) and not of MDPI and/or the editor(s). MDPI and/or the editor(s) disclaim responsibility for any injury to people or property resulting from any ideas, methods, instructions or products referred to in the content.

MDPI
St. Alban-Anlage 66
4052 Basel
Switzerland
www.mdpi.com

Antioxidants Editorial Office
E-mail: antioxidants@mdpi.com
www.mdpi.com/journal/antioxidants

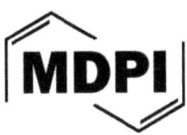

Disclaimer/Publisher's Note: The statements, opinions and data contained in all publications are solely those of the individual author(s) and contributor(s) and not of MDPI and/or the editor(s). MDPI and/or the editor(s) disclaim responsibility for any injury to people or property resulting from any ideas, methods, instructions or products referred to in the content.

www.ingramcontent.com/pod-product-compliance
Lightning Source LLC
LaVergne TN
LVHW070738100526
838202LV00013B/1265